SANTA

P9-CJC-398

Vaccine Injuries

Vaccine Injuries

Documented
Adverse Reactions
to Vaccines

2014–2015 Edition

Louis Conte and Tony Lyons

Skyhorse Publishing books may be purchased in bulk at special discounts for sales promotion, corporate gifts, fund-raising, or educational purposes. Special editions can also be created to specifications. For details, contact the Special Sales Department, Skyhorse Publishing, 307 West 36th Street, 11th Floor, New York, NY 10018 or info@skyhorsepublishing.com.

Skyhorse® and Skyhorse Publishing® are registered trademarks of Skyhorse Publishing, Inc.®, a Delaware corporation.

Visit our website at www.skyhorsepublishing.com.

10 9 8 7 6 5 4 3 2 1

Library of Congress Cataloging-in-Publication Data is available on file.

Cover design by Qualcomm
Cover photo: Thinkstock

Print ISBN: 978-1-62914-447-4
Ebook ISBN: 978-1-63220-170-6

Printed in the United States of America

"I think certainly there are dedicated groups like the National Vaccine Information Center, which used to be called Dissatisfied Parents Together, and others such as Moms Against Mercury, Safe Minds, and Generation Rescue. These are the professional anti-vaccine groups, but I think the bigger group, frankly, is made of parents who become scared. They're not sure who to trust. They're not sure what to believe. They have this vague sense that maybe pharmaceutical companies have too much influence and maybe doctors aren't to be trusted, and they're choosing to delay or withhold one or more vaccines at their children's risk."
  —Dr. Paul Offit

"As a full-time professional research scientist for 50 years, and as a researcher in the field of autism for 45 years, I have been shocked and chagrined by the medical establishment's ongoing efforts to trivialize the solid and compelling evidence that faulty vaccination policies are the root cause of the epidemic. There are many consistent lines of evidence implicating vaccines, and no even marginally plausible alternative hypotheses."
  —Bernard Rimland, PhD; Director, Autism Research Institute; Editor, Autism Research Review International; Founder, Autism Society of America

CONTENTS

PART I

HOW TO USE THIS BOOK

Vaccination has always been controversial. Proponents declare that vaccines have saved millions of lives, while critics claim that their success has been overstated and that vaccines may even be dangerous for some people. Many consider mandatory vaccinations a violation of individual rights or religious principles. Many in public health argue that vaccine mandates are justified and that anti-vaccination sentiment has reduced uptake rates in certain communities, resulting in outbreaks of preventable, and sometimes fatal, childhood illnesses. Opponents of vaccination point out that serious "vaccine preventable diseases" declined in severity and frequency before mass vaccination commenced due to better living conditions and the effectiveness of modern sanitation engineering.

The reality of vaccine injury has been horribly mishandled by the medical establishment for two hundred years, as we shall show. Denial, secrecy, and persecution of those who raise concerns about vaccine safety continue to this day. Are vaccines really safe and effective? Are the successes overstated? Are other public health initiatives more effective? Are vaccines acceptable to people with unique religious traditions? Are they contaminated? Do they sometimes spread the diseases they seek to prevent? Are they being over-used, and are severe diseases being replaced by vaccine-induced chronic diseases and conditions?

The fact is that vaccine injuries have happened in the past and continue to happen today. Even though reliance on vaccines has increased, mainstream medicine has never fully and transparently addressed the reality of vaccine injury. We must recognize that vaccines are drugs, and the more drugs one takes, the more numerous the adverse reactions to those drugs will be.

In the 1980s the United States addressed individual cases of vaccine injury by establishing the NVICP—the National Vaccine Injury Compensation Program—a controversial Department of Health and Human Resources program. The NVICP was intended to be "non-adversarial, compassionate and generous" to vaccine injury victims. However, as we write this book, Congress is considering hearings on the effectiveness of the NVICP. Many vaccine injury victims and vaccine safety advocates believe that the program is not functioning as Congress intended. The concern is that the NVICP is not an open and fair justice forum. There are also concerns that the program is keeping the reality of vaccine injury away from public inspection. While some (but perhaps not all) case decisions are posted on the United States Court of Claims website, most people don't know that the NVICP even exists.

We intend to publish *Vaccine Injuries* annually. Each year's book will feature all of the reported case decisions, by filing date, that resulted in the decision to compensate. While we have edited these cases for readability, we feel that these reported decisions, which may be referenced for legal purposes, provide an invaluable insight into the nature of vaccine injury and how the NVICP actually works. These case decisions are not easy reading. Vaccine injury can result in death and suffering. As these are public documents and petitioners have the right to file motions to redact personal information before the cases are posted, we have not removed case names. However, we ask the reader to respect the privacy of the litigants, their doctors, and expert witnesses.

We will also publish a sampling of unreported compensated cases. These cases, while public, are not reference material for legal purposes. Publishing all of the compensated cases of vaccine injury in the unreported section of the website would be excessive.

To place the current cases in context and to shed light on how the NVICP has evolved, we will also feature selected historical decisions.

The vast majority of cases filed in the NVICP do not result in compensation, as the 2013 statistical report shows.

Historically, the majority of claims have been filed for varieties of diptheria, pertussis, and tetanus and varieties of measles, mumps, and rubella vaccines. Most of these claims involved children whose alleged injuries were seizures and brain damage (encephalopathy). At the present time, the majority of cases compensated by the NVICP feature neurological injury to adults, such as Guillain-Barré syndrome (GBS), from adverse reactions to various influenza vaccines. Of the 993 NVICP cases reported for 2013, 627 were dismissed and 366 were compensated. Petitioner award amounts totaled $254,666,326.70. Since 1988, 3,540 individuals have been compensated and $2,671,223,269.97 has been paid out to victims of vaccine injury.[1]

For those who have accepted the oft-repeated claim that vaccines are safe and effective, these numbers may be shocking. However, it is critical to note that these statistics do not reflect the fact that the vast majority of vaccine injuries are not even reported to the Vaccine Adverse Event Reporting

System (VAERS) and that the vast majority of suspected injuries never result in NVICP filings.[2]

The statute of limitations for filing vaccine injury claims in the NVICP is three years. It is critical that those who claim vaccine injury have information at their fingertips so that they can act promptly.

We do not list attorney names—petitioner or respondent—in any of the cases, as we are not dispensing legal advice or providing advertising for attorneys. Be warned, however, that the burdens of acting *pro se*—on behalf of your self—in the NVICP are not to be underestimated. A list of the attorneys admitted to the bar of the program is available through the US Court of Claims website.[3] Another good resource is the National Vaccine Information Center (NVIC), which also features a listing of attorneys and other valuable information.

We recognize that many will describe this book as "anti-vaccine"—a sophistic argument. Federal aviation officials who investigate airplane accidents are not "anti-air travel." Aviation accidents result in notifications to pilots that explain the implications of these accidents. Consumers of vaccines deserve no less. Vaccines are drugs, and adverse drug reactions happen. Publicly disclosing them—as is often done on television drug commercials—allows consumers to make informed choices. Analyzing adverse drug reactions leads to safer drugs. This is our intention here.

Publication of compensated vaccine injury cases from the NVICP—something that has never been offered to the public—will allow the reader to assess vaccine injury. We hope our book serves as a jumping-off point for the reader's investigation and analysis. We hope that the information provided here will lead to family discussions about vaccines and vaccine safety. We believe in informed consent and that individuals and parents, on behalf of their children, ought to have the final decision on medical choices.

A BRIEF HISTORY OF VACCINATION

It is important to acknowledge the devastation of disease outbreaks throughout human history. Smallpox killed an estimated three hundred to five hundred million people before the last recorded case in 1979. Typhoid fever, scarlet fever, whooping cough, diptheria, tuberculosis, and even diarrhea killed untold millions. Europe lingered in the Dark Ages for hundreds of years in no small part due to the Black Death, which killed anywhere between seventy-five and two hundred million.

Disease forever altered history in the Americas as well. *Hidden Cities* author Roger Kennedy claims that North America's pre-Columbian civilization disappeared in what he termed "the Great Dying"—a plague that claimed an estimated thirty million lives due to the arrival of microbes from unknown pre-Columbian European visitors.[1] The early American historical perspective of "an open continent" was possible only because the vast majority of indigenous people had been wiped out.

It wasn't Hernando Cortez who defeated the Aztecs. It was smallpox, inadvertently transmitted by the conquistadors, that devastated the Aztec empire. Malaria has killed untold millions in Africa, Asia, and South America.

Disease has had catastrophic impacts on civilization.

The Romans suspected the importance of clean running water and personal hygiene. The Romans, like many in the ancient world, believed that "bad air"—miasma—caused disease. They designed their cities with this belief in mind. Aqueducts, sewers, and public baths were the response. It has been theorized that the fall of Rome—and the loss of Roman engineering—set the stage for the scourge of disease in the Western world.

It is not known when attempts to improve human immunity began, but it is believed that inoculation—often referred to as variolation—originated in eigth-century India. The practice involved taking exudates from a person infected with a mild case of smallpox and rubbing it into a cut on the skin of a non-infected person. The person receiving the treatment would become ill but would develop immunity to the more serious version of the disease.

Inoculation was considered by the British Royal Society in 1699 and discussed in the society's *Philosophical Transactions* in 1714 and 1716. After observing the inoculation in Turkey, Lady Mary Wortley Montagu became a champion for the technique in 1718—by publicly inoculating her children. A few years later, Edward Jenner would make the practice safer by inoculating his children with cowpox in order to protect people against smallpox.

In the new world, devastating smallpox outbreaks occurred throughout the 1600s and 1700s in New England. In Boston, the sick were often held under armed guard in "pest houses." The smallpox mortality rate for New Englanders was near 30 percent.

The Reverend Cotton Mather was inoculation's first American proponent when he learned of variolation from an African slave. Mather advocated for the practice during the smallpox outbreak of 1721. Mather publicly debated the issue with William Douglas, Boston's only trained university physician. Douglas argued that inoculation—which involved direct transfers of bodily fluids—could spread smallpox that resulted in fatalities and could also spread other diseases as well, such as syphilis. These were valid criticisms of the primitive state of the technique. Douglas also felt that Mather was undermining medical authority by carrying out inoculations in haphazard fashion.

Mather, who lost his wife and children in a measles outbreak, regarded inoculations as a gift from God. Many, however, felt that the technique was an attempt to subvert the will of God and regarded it as a heathen practice. In his 1722 sermon entitled "The Dangerous and Sinful Practice of Inoculation," English theologian Reverend Edmund Massey argued that diseases are sent by God to punish sin and that any attempt to prevent smallpox via inoculation is a "diabolical operation."

The debate was heated. Mather's house was firebombed, apparently in response to his support for inoculation. Mather ultimately convinced Dr. Zabdiel Boylston to experiment with variolation. Boylston experimented on his six-year-old son, his slave, and his slave's son. Both contracted the disease and became "gravely ill" for several days before recovering. Boylston went on to inoculate thousands in Massachusetts.[2]

Ultimately, inoculation became more accepted through the work of Edward Jenner, who noted that English milk maids didn't seem to contract smallpox and theorized that this was because they contracted non-lethal cowpox from milking cows. Jenner pioneered a new type of inoculation called "vaccination"—a word derived from the Latin word for cow—*vacca*. Jenner took cowpox virus from a cow and injected it into humans, the result being immunity from smallpox. Eventually, vaccination was embraced, and in 1840, the British government provided vaccination free of charge. Variolation was replaced by vaccination and ultimately banned. Jenner became known as the "father of immunology."

Many of America's founding fathers supported inoculation and, subsequently, vaccination. Benjamin Franklin's advocacy of inoculation was driven by the death of his son, Frankie, apparently due to smallpox. There were also rumors that Frankie died from an adverse reaction––protracted diarrhea—to inoculation.[3] Franklin denied this rumor and publicly supported inoculation.

John and Abigail Adams were also proponents. John Adams suffered a horrible two-week illness after being inoculated. Abigail also suffered an adverse reaction.

Inoculation was rough business. People in colonial America understood that the procedure often included adverse reactions, injury, and even death. The willingness to take the risks involved in early inoculation had to be weighed against the scourge of smallpox. Desperate times meant desperate measures.

Smallpox inoculation efforts triggered riots in Norfolk County, Virginia. Thomas Jefferson, then a young lawyer, defended the victims of the Norfolk riots, including a Dr. Archibald Campbell, whose house was burned down. Ultimately, it was Thomas Jefferson who became vaccination's biggest American advocate. Jefferson, who corresponded with Edward Jenner, was greatly influenced by Harvard's Benjamin Waterhouse, one of New England's only European-trained doctors. Waterhouse is largely regarded as the man who championed early vaccination in the United States.

Jefferson was, to put it mildly, distrustful of American doctors, remarking that "whenever he saw three physicians together he looked up to discover whether there was not a turkey buzzard in the neighborhood."[4] Jefferson was enamored with Waterhouse due to his European scientific training. Working with Waterhouse, Jefferson dispatched smallpox vaccines to southern cities only to find that the vaccines didn't work. Vaccine antigens were transported on pieces of cotton thread. They often failed to work because the antigen lost effectiveness. Jefferson realized that the vaccines had gone bad due to poor storage and came up with a an early form of insulated packaging—a corked bottle sealed in another corked bottle filled with water. The new packaging worked, and successful vaccination programs were established in Washington, Petersburg, Richmond, and other parts of the South. Jefferson successfully vaccinated seventy-eight family members, noting minor adverse reactions in great detail.

Despite his successes with Jefferson, Waterhouse was not without detractors. Some claimed that he was arrogant and pushed vaccination for personal profit. The primitive nature of early vaccines and the lack of sanitary procedures caused disease outbreaks because the vaccine often contained smallpox as well as cowpox. The public didn't immediately embrace vaccination, and the American medical establishment never fully embraced Waterhouse. Regardless, Waterhouse pushed his vaccine agenda and ultimately prevailed.

Mainstream medicine embraced vaccination during the late 1800s. Louis Pasteur developed the germ theory of disease in 1877, and new vaccines for other diseases soon followed. Pasteur produced the first live attenuated bacterial vaccine for chicken cholera in 1879 and a rabies vaccine in 1885. Cholera and typhoid vaccines were developed in 1896, and a vaccine for plague came in 1897.

England ultimately passed vaccination acts, which first only encouraged vaccination. In 1853, vaccination of infants became mandatory, with the highest penalty for refusal being incarceration. The 1867 law extended the requirement to fourteen-year-olds, and a backlash followed. In advance of the passage of the 1867 law, Richard Gibbs, who administered the London Free Hospital, started the first Anti-Compulsory Vaccination League in 1866. Gibbs regarded compulsory vaccination to be an infringement of individual freedom. According to Gibbs, the purpose of the League was "to overthrow this huge piece of physiological absurdity and medical tyranny . . . I believe we have hundreds of cases here, from being poisoned with vaccination, I deem incurable. One member of a family dating syphilitic symptoms from the time of vaccination, when all the other members of the family have been clear. We strongly advise parents to go to prison, rather than submit to have their helpless offspring inoculated with scrofula, syphilis, and mania."[5]

Gibbs was clearly describing what he felt were vaccine injuries. He also claimed that many family members of the vaccine-injured had presented petitions to Parliament alleging that their children had died but that these petitions had not been made public.

William Tebb, a businessman from Manchester, eventually took up the mantle from Gibbs. Tebb is described as being a radical liberal and was a member of several liberal organizations, including the Society for the Prevention of Cruelty to Children, The National Liberal Club, the New Reform Club, and the Vigilance Association for the Defence of Personal Rights. Tebb sought the repeal of the vaccination acts and was prosecuted and fined thirteen times for refusal to vaccinate his third daughter. He eventually became president of the National Anti-Vaccination League in 1896 and traveled to the United States in 1897 to campaign against smallpox vaccinations. Smallpox epidemics resumed in the United States, allegedly due to low vaccination rates. Whether this was true or not is debated, but it is certainly true that Tebb's visits spawned the establishment of American anti-vaccination leagues.

The Leicester Method

English anti-vaccination sentiment gained strength due to the popularity of an alternate disease fighting approach called the Leicester method. Advocates of the approach noted that vaccination didn't necessarily provide immunity as some vaccinated people died from smallpox—and from vaccine reactions.

The city of Leicester's "vaccination inspector" began prosecuting parents who "stupidly refused to have their children vaccinated." Arrests for defying the Vaccination Act went from two in 1869 to 1,154 in 1881. In some cases, magistrates issued fines, "but in most cases the parents deliberately allowed themselves to be sent to goal (jail)."[6]

John Thomas Biggs emerged as an opponent of compulsory vaccination and became the outspoken advocate of the Leicester method. Biggs opposed compulsory vaccination as being an infringement upon, and invasion of, personal liberty. It is said that one of his brothers suffered a vaccine injury.[7]

Biggs was a sanitary engineer, a member of the Leicester town council, and alderman, magistrate, and member of the Derwent Valley water board. He was also appointed by the Leicester Board of Guardians to develop and present its Memorial and Statistical Tables—a skill set he used to document the advantages of his Leicester method over vaccination.

Biggs kept meticulous records and studied the smallpox epidemic of 1871–1873 closely. He became convinced that vaccination wasn't efficacious and didn't prevent disease or mitigate its severity. Biggs collected data that showed that vaccination was not as effective as mainstream medicine purported. He published his findings in 1912 in *Leicester: Sanitation versus Vaccination*. The Leicester method is described by Biggs as follows:

> A new method for which great practical utility is claimed has been enforced by the sanitary committee of the Corporation for the stamping out of small-pox, and the chairman of the Committee has gone so far as to declare that small-pox is one of the least troublesome diseases with which they have to deal. The method of treatment, in a word, is this: As soon as small-pox breaks out, the

medical man and the householder are compelled under penalty to at once report the outbreak to the Corporation. The small-pox van is at once ordered by telephone to proceed to the house in question the hospital authorities are also instructed by telephone to make all arrangements, and thus, within a few hours, the sufferer is safely in the hospital. The family and inmates of the house are placed in quarantine in comfortable quarters, and the house thoroughly disinfected. The result is that in every instance the disease has been promptly and completely stamped out at a paltry expense...use plenty of water, eat good food, live in light and airy houses, and see that the Corporation kept the streets clean and the drains in order. If such details were attended to, there was no need to fear smallpox . . .

The effects of narrow, ill-conditioned streets; of imperfect drainage and improper dwellings; of circumstances of environment; and of inherited physical disability must, and will for a time, continue. These adverse elements are being gradually eliminated... the "Leicester Method" of Sanitation could bid defiance not to smallpox only, but to other infectious, if not to nearly all zymotic, diseases. Even for small-pox, not even the merest tyro among Jennerian votaries would now venture to claim that vaccination could achieve all that sanitation has accomplished. This is self-evident, because even pro-vaccinists, of the most pronounced type, now supplement the Jennerian operation with the "Leicester Method" of dealing with the disease. They dare not, as aforetime, trust solely to vaccination. To do so would, on their part, be culpable, if not in the highest degree criminal, neglect.[9]

Biggs compiled statistical data showing that his method worked just as well, if not better than, vaccination—and without vaccine injuries. Biggs took on the pro-vaccine medical establishment and produced evidence of vaccine injuries:

I presented a table (pages 417-433, Fourth Report, Royal Commission) of 109 deaths, 186 cases of injury (many of them permanent), and two of small-pox, following on vaccination, being a total of 297 cases in Leicester and neighbourhood, with the names, addresses, and details, each case being vouched for by the parents themselves. It is a harrowing, heart-rending catalogue. This gruesome testimony caused considerable questioning by the Commissioners, who, however, hesitated to accept such personal statements, unless supported by expert medical opinion! The evidence of careful, loving mothers, who had unintermittently tended their suffering little ones, was, it seems, not deemed trustworthy without being thus peculiarly confirmed! Was it likely that medical men would convict either themselves or their brethren? Manifestly, those parents (who had "accepted" vaccination) must have been in its favour, rather than against it. Otherwise their children would certainly not have been vaccinated.

The most striking points in Table 1 are:

(1) That the highest death-rates from erysipelas, both under one year, under five years, and at all ages, are concurrent with the highest years of vaccination ; and

(2) That each death-rate practically touches its lowest point coincidentally with the lowest percentage of vaccination.

By no stretch of the imagination, nor by any subterfuge, can these facts be made to tell in favour of vaccination. On the other hand, there is abundant and undeniable evidence that the practice operated most fatally.

Biggs even alleged that medical authorities were engaging in fear mongering to motivate parents to vaccinate, a claim often made by present-day vaccine safety advocates. He took on mainstream medicine's support for vaccination. British authorities attempted to prosecute Biggs on several occasions, but Biggs always prevailed. His Leicester method resonated in England and offered a viable alternative to vaccination. The 1898 vaccination law allowed for conscientious objection to compulsory vaccination. England still allows conscientious objection today.

JACOBSON V. MASSACHUSETTS

The United States in 1905 was a very different place than it is today. With the start of the Industrial Revolution, more and more people poured into cities. The streets were full of sewage and animal excrement, as modern sewage and waste disposal systems had not yet been invented. Cramped housing conditions were atrocious—cold, dark and miserable in the winter; sweltering and oppressive in the summer. Many apartments didn't have running water. The fortunate few had communal outhouses in the yard behind the building. Slaughterhouses were often located in urban centers. Many lived in sprawling shanty towns that we would compare to modern refugee camps.

These conditions–which Biggs and proponents of the Leicester method sought to mitigate–provided a breeding ground for disease.

Also driving disease was the horrendous treatment of children who were marginally educated, often forced into labor by age seven and exploited in every conceivable manner. Children were often the victims of harsh working conditions, industrial accidents, and toxic exposures.

Food was nutritionally deficient and often a source of disease. Refrigeration technology had not yet been developed, and food inspection was still years away. Clean water was often scarce, and people drank alcoholic beverages instead. People rarely bathed.

The conditions of the masses were miserable and fueled disease outbreaks that killed thousands. Proper medical care was rare. Death and misery were ubiquitous. People—and government—were desperate.

This was the reality of public health when the Jacobson case went before the US Supreme Court in 1905. Henning Jacobson, a Swedish immigrant and minister from Cambridge, Massachusetts, refused vaccination during a smallpox outbreak in 1902. Jacobson claimed that a vaccine had made him seriously ill as a child. He also claimed that a vaccine had injured his son and that he knew of others who had been injured. He refused to pay the $5.00 fine, and the Massachusetts courts rejected his arguments that the compulsory inoculation violated the state and US constitutions.

Jacobson "offered to prove that vaccination 'quite often' caused serious and permanent injury to the health of the person vaccinated; that the operation 'occasionally' resulted in death; that it was 'impossible' to tell 'in any particular case' what the results of vaccination would be, or whether it would injure the health or result in death…that vaccine matter is 'quite often' impure and dangerous to be used…that the defendant refused to submit to vaccination for the reason that he had, 'when a child,' been caused great and extreme suffering for a long period by a disease produced by vaccination; and that he had witnessed a similar result of vaccination, not only in the case of his son, but in the cases of others."[1]

The US Supreme Court didn't accept that Jacobson's fear of vaccine injury outweighed the public health authority of Massachusetts. The Supreme Court ruled that freedom of the individual must sometimes be subordinated to common welfare. The $5.00 fine was upheld—nothing more than that. The Court ruled that Massachusetts acted reasonably in fining Jacobson in the context of requiring adults to be vaccinated in an epidemic of an airborne disease.

Children were not to be subjected to the mandate, as they were believed to be too fragile

It is important to realize that mandatory vaccination today occurs in a very different context. Children are the primary targets of mandates. Vaccines today are mandatory today not because of an ongoing catastrophic epidemic of airborne disease. The seventy doses of sixteen vaccines presently recommended are mandated in the name of herd immunity. Yet refusing vaccination can have real implications for an individual's educational and even employment opportunities. Medical and religious exemptions to vaccine mandates are often subject to government review.

Jacobson is cited as the foundation of public health law but should be viewed within the realities of American culture at the turn of the twentieth century—and the diseases that affected that culture. Modern vaccines that protect against diseases that may be sexually transmitted, such as Gardasill, are qualitatively different from those designed to protect against airborne diseases, such as smallpox.

Jacobson was supported by the Massachusetts Anti-Compulsory Vaccination Association. There were a number of Anti-Vaccination Leagues emerging around the United States by the early 1900s. As it did for Henning Jacobson and J. T. Biggs, concern over vaccine injury fueled their development.

The anti-vaccine movement mobilized following the decision, and the Anti-Vaccination League of America was founded three years later in Philadelphia to promote the principle that "health is nature's greatest safeguard against disease and that therefore no State has the right to demand of anyone the impairment of his or her health." The league warned about what it believed were the dangers of vaccination and the dangers of allowing the intrusion of government and science into private life, part of the broader process identified with the progressive movement of the early twentieth century. The Anti-Vaccination League of America asked, "We have repudiated *religious* tyranny; we have rejected *political* tyranny; shall we now submit to *medical* tyranny?"[2]

CONTAMINATED "BIOLOGICS" AND A HORSE NAMED JIM

Vaccine manufacturing in the years around the time of the Jacobson decision was vastly different from today. The serum for diphtheria antitoxin was derived from horse blood.[1] There was no regulation or standardized controls over biological drugs. Like many business ventures of the time, the industry that produced vaccines and other drugs was not regulated by government.

In 1901, a retired milk wagon horse named Jim was found to be the source of contamination that caused the death of thirteen children in St. Louis, Missouri. Jim produced over seven gallons of serum over his lifetime. The tragedy was completely avoidable, as the contaminated serum could have been detected by the technology of the day, but samples from Jim, taken on different days, were mislabeled.[2]

The deaths brought the reality of vaccine injury and contaminated biologics to greater public attention. When a contaminated smallpox vaccine caused a child's death in Camden, New Jersey, enough was enough. Congress responded with the Biologics Control Act, also known as the Virus-Toxin Law, in 1902. This act is critical because for the first time, the government conducted oversight of the processes used for the production of biological products through the establishment of the Hygienic Laboratory of the US Public Health Service. The laboratory was charged with regulating the production of vaccines and antitoxins. Producers of vaccines now had to be licensed annually for the manufacture and sale of vaccines, serum, and antitoxins. Manufacturing facilities were inspected, licensed, and monitored by scientists. Products now had to be labeled by product name, expiration date, and address and license number of the manufacturer.

The deaths in St. Louis were a wake-up call that showed the danger posed by contaminated biological products. Diphtheria antitoxin was made by inoculating horses with increasingly concentrated doses of diphtheria bacteria. The horse was then bled to collect blood serum, which was bottled as antitoxin. The horse's serum was then injected into a patient suffering from diphtheria in the hopes that the antibodies in the serum would cure the patient. However, the threat of contamination loomed over every stage of the production process. The importance of the Hygienic Laboratory and the importance of its health officers became obvious. By 1907, clear standards were established to prevent contamination. The research at the laboratory led investigators into emerging sciences, such as immunology, in order to better understand why sudden deaths sometimes followed repeated injections of biologics made from foreign protein, such as horse serum.

Within a few years, Congress passed the Federal Food and Drugs Act to regulate the production of food and other products. Ultimately, the Food and Drug Administration was created. The deplorable health conditions of that time were being driven back not by vaccines–they were still an emerging technology fraught with contamination risks–but by an understanding that regulation of industry to improve medicines, foods, and other products could improve public health.

In 1914, Dr. Joseph Goldberger, an epidemiologist with the United States Public Health Service who worked at the Hygienic Laboratory, identified the cause of pellagra, a scourge of poor Southerners. Pellagra was caused by a niacin deficiency and could be cured through the use of brewer's yeast. Then Earl B. Phelps, director of the Division of Chemistry at the Hygienic Laboratory, identified how pollution affected oxygen levels in lakes and rivers.

The new public health establishment was focusing on the environmental triggers of disease, and millions of people benefited. The government was leading the way with cleaner water, healthier food, and cleaner cities through improved sanitation, as championed by J. T. Biggs and the Leicester method. Disease rates plummeted. The horrendous Industrial Revolution living conditions and abusive treatment of children were fading from American life.[3]

Few today realize that vaccine injuries ultimately opened the door to a level of federal regulation over industry that had never existed before. The result of acknowledging and focusing on vaccine injury was better vaccines and an expanded vision of the need for government regulation of industry. The result was a stunning improvement in public health and ultimately safer vaccines.

Advocates for mandatory vaccination often declare that "epidemics of diseases will return" if vaccination rates are not maintained. However, mass vaccination programs for diseases that have reportedly been eliminated by vaccines started in the 1950s after the disease rates had already plummeted. The chart on the measles vaccination on the next page clearly demonstrates this.

And when mass vaccination commenced, the specter of vaccine contamination—and vaccine injury—reared its ugly head almost immediately.

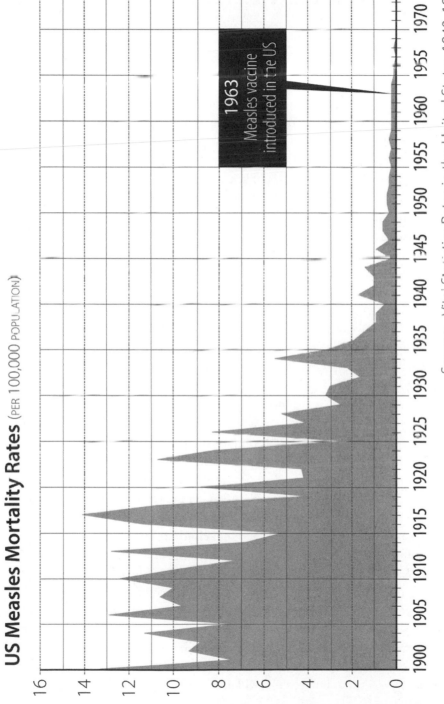

US Measles Mortality Rates (PER 100,000 POPULATION)

1963
Measles vaccine
introduced in the US

Source: Vital Statistics Rates in the United States, 1940–1960

THE CUTTER CRISIS

I n the 1950s, America was understandably gripped by fear of polio. While never causing the population-wide devastation of earlier pandemics, such as smallpox, polio was justifiably dreaded. Many people died, and many were left paralyzed. President Franklin Roosevelt was a victim. Stark images of children in iron lungs were seared into the public consciousness. The 1952 polio outbreak was the worst in the nation's history—approximately 58,000 cases were reported, causing 3,145 deaths and leaving 21,269 people with varying degrees of paralysis.[1]

Dr. Jonas Salk, a brilliant and complicated man, developed a polio vaccine that used inactivated virus. The March of Dimes heralded Salk's triumph and urged the quick development of the Salk polio vaccine. The vaccine was hailed as a huge success, and the nation justifiably celebrated Salk and his miraculous acheivment.

The Salk vaccine was competing with an oral polio vaccine created by Dr. Albert Sabin for the hearts and minds of the public health establishment. The March of Dimes supported Salk and was instrumental in getting the Salk vaccine to the market first. Given the seriousness of the polio epidemic, the public pressure to do so was enormous.

Salk believed that he had developed a technique to kill or inactivate the polio virus using a system of high-quality filters and formaldehyde. And he had. The problem was that when production of the vaccine went from a small lab to large-scale industrial production, filtration and inactivation were not as effective. At a lab run by the Cutter Company in Berkeley, California, live polio virus was getting into the final product.

Live polio virus was being injected into children.

A public health officer in Los Angeles called the National Institutes of Health (NIH) on a Friday night reporting that two children vaccinated nine days earlier now had polio. Overnight, the triumphant celebration of the conquest of polio turned into a nightmare. The polio vaccine produced at Cutter lead to eighty cases of polio in the children. These children then infected 120 other people. Approximately 75 percent of the victims were paralyzed and eleven died.

Even worse, public health officials had been made aware of problems with the Cutter vaccine but ignored the evidence.

Dr. Bernice Eddy, a microbiologist who worked at the National Institute of Health's Laboratory of Biologics Control (formerly the Hygienic Laboratory), conducted tests on the Cutter version of the polio vaccine on primates. The vaccine caused paralysis in some of the primates. Eddy turned the evidence—including photographs of the paralyzed monkeys—over to her boss, William Sebrell, the Director of the National Institutes of Health. Sebrell did nothing about Eddy's findings, and the faulty vaccines went to market.[2]

Dr. Eddy, a middle-aged woman from a mining town in West Virginia, spent her career in the "Hygienic Lab," as she still referred to it. Eddy was not a high-profile, Harvard-educated public health insider. And she was a woman working in a male-dominated profession. Eddy and her team worked around the clock to run trials that ought to have been done slowly and carefully in advance of the release of the Salk vaccine.

No one knows why Sebrell failed to act. There is no doubt that Eddy's team identified the problem and informed the hierarchy promptly. She personally delivered the results and photographs to Sebrell because "they were going to be injecting this thing into children." Sebrell accepted the photographs and responded by asking Eddy if she and her team wanted to be immunized. Eddy declined, as did the rest of her staff.[3]

As often happens with whistleblowers, Dr. Eddy was transferred. She ended up in the cancer section of the federal lab, where she discovered another vaccine contaminant: the simian virus, SV40. Eddy ran experiments showing that SV40 caused cancer in animals and grew concerned about cancer risks in humans.

As the cases of vaccine-induced polio continued to mount, the NIH was in crisis mode. Heated arguments about pulling the vaccine erupted in meetings of the NIH hierarchy. Some of the agency's leadership were reported to be in denial and refused to take the vaccines off the market. Finally, reason prevailed, and the Cutter polio vaccine was pulled. Public faith in the polio vaccine took an enormous hit.

It turned out that Cutter did follow federal standards in manufacturing the polio vaccine. Inactivating polio virus in the Salk method was a process that was difficult to accomplish in large-scale vaccine production. The Salk vaccine production ought to have received deliberate and thorough oversight. But the pressure to stop polio was enormous. The public and political leadership wanted the vaccine on the market as soon as possible. As is often the case with disasters, there was a series of mistakes by people with the best of intentions. Not acting on Dr. Eddy's research was the final mistake in a series of misjudgments.

Sebrell and other NIH administrators resigned, and public trust in vaccines was severely damaged. In court proceedings, Cutter was ultimately found not to be negligent but was still required to pay damages. In *Gottsdanker v. Cutter Laboratories* the California Court of Appeals ruled as follows:

> In returning its verdicts for plaintiffs, however, the jury drew a thoughtful and careful statement, setting forth that the jury had first considered the issue of negligence, and had "from a preponderance of the evidence concluded that the defendant, Cutter Laboratories, was not negligent either directly or by inference. . . . With regard to the law of warranty, however, we feel that we have no alternative but to conclude that Cutter Laboratories came to market . . . vaccine which when given to plaintiffs caused them to come down with poliomyelitis, thus resulting in a breach of warranty. For this cause alone we find in favor of plaintiffs.

Cutter would survive, but vaccine manufacturers bristled at having been found legally liable for vaccine injury even though they had followed federal standards. Many in the vaccine industry argued that the federal government had failed to provide proper oversight.

If vaccines are so important to public but still carry a risk of injury, should the manufacturer carry all of the liability?

The Discovery of Simian Virus 40

Dr. Maurice Hilleman picked up on Eddy's research and verified that SV40 was a contaminant in both the Salk injectable vaccine and Sabin oral vaccine. Eddy proved that SV40 caused cancer in hamsters. Hilleman found that it caused cancer in African Green Monkeys—after both vaccines had been given to over one hundred million Americans.

Hilleman came to the conclusion that SV40 induced slow-growing cancers in humans. The impact from the contaminated vaccines might not be realized for years. Hilleman presented his findings at an international polio vaccine conference in 1960. According to *Vaccine* author Arthur Allen, Hilleman was immediately attacked by the conference attendees. The Russians, who had administered the vaccine to fifty million people, quickly evacuated the room. Hilleman seems to have been stunned by the response to the information he presented.[4]

Sabin criticized Hilleman and stated that the SV40 revelation would hurt the vaccine program. Sabin confronted Hilleman and asked what he thought could happen as a result of the SV40 contamination. Hilleman answered that he obviously feared people would get cancer.

In 2004, a paper presented at the Vaccine Cell Substrate Conference noted that vaccines administered in what had been countries aligned with the former Soviet Union may have been contaminated up to 1980. Hundreds of millions may have been exposed to SV40.[5]

Even though the SV40 virus has been found in human cancer cells, mainstream medicine does not accept the view that cancer in humans is a result of the vaccine contaminant. The virus has also been described as a co-factor in the development of asbestos-related cancers—mesotheliomas. The theory in acceptance presently is that mesothelioma is caused by asbestos. However, mesothelioma-type cancers continue to increase even though asbestos exposures have been reduced. Is it possible that Bernice Eddy and Maurice Hilleman have been proven right, all these years later?

THE RISE OF "VACCINOLOGY"

The response of the vaccine establishment to Hilleman and Eddy does not leave the impression that those who are now established practitioners of what is now called "vaccinology" are open to receiving bad news about problems with vaccines. It is an impression that holds to this day. Dr. Andrew Wakefield is criticized in the media on a regular basis for a paper he published in 1998 about a case study in which parents stated that their children regressed and developed autism after receiving the MMR vaccine.

You will read cases later in this book where the National Vaccine Injury Compensation Program has compensated children for brain damage. These children also have a diagnosis of autism.[1] These are cases described as "MMR table encephalopathies." Yet the attacks on Wakefield by vaccinologists continue. The message is clear; talking about vaccine injuries is not good for your career. We have spoken to doctors who have acknowledged that a climate of fear presently exists that suppresses discourse on vaccine injuries.

Vaccinology is defined as the science of vaccine development. The National Foundation for Infectious Diseases (NFID) offers a "clinical vaccinology" course twice a year. The course is taught by highly credentialed experts in vaccinology and deals with the latest developments in the use of vaccines. The target audience is medical professionals.

The NFID receives 75 percent of its funding from pharmaceutical companies. The board of directors features public health professionals from industry, government, and academia. The pro-vaccine messages on the NFID website are crystal clear.

Those in the field of vaccinolgy now hold critical power over many of the government organs responsible for the safety of vaccines. Over the years, those involved in the development, marketing, and sale of vaccines have *become* the public health establishment. This is not just the opinion of the authors. The US House of Representatives has come to the same conclusion.

In June 2000, the House of Representatives Oversight and Government Reform Committee issued a report on *Conflicts of Interest in Vaccine Policy Making*. The introduction to the report makes the point clearly:

In August 1999, the Committee on Government Reform initiated an investigation into Federal vaccine policy. Over the last six months, this investigation has focused on possible conflicts of interest on the part of Federal policy-makers. Committee staff has conducted an extensive review of financial disclosure forms and related documents, and interviewed key officials from the Department of Health and Human Services, including the Food and Drug Administration and the Centers for Disease Control and Prevention.

This staff report focuses on two influential advisory committees utilized by Federal regulators to provide expert advice on vaccine policy:

1. The FDA's Vaccines and Related Biological Products Advisory Committee (VRBPAC);

and

2. The CDC's Advisory Committee on Immunizations Practices (ACIP).

The VRBPAC advises the FDA on the licensing of new vaccines, while the ACIP advises the CDC on guidelines to be issued to doctors and the states for the appropriate use of vaccines.

Members of the advisory committees are required to disclose any financial conflicts of interest and recuse themselves from participating in decisions in which they have an interest. The Committee's investigation has determined that conflict of interest rules employed by the FDA and the CDC have been weak, enforcement has been lax, and committee members with substantial ties to pharmaceutical companies have been given waivers to participate in committee proceedings. Among the specific problems identified in this staff report:

§ The CDC routinely grants waivers from conflict of interest rules to every member of its advisory committee.

§ CDC Advisory Committee members who are not allowed to vote on certain recommendations due to financial conflicts of interest are allowed to participate in committee deliberations and advocate specific positions.

§ The Chairman of the CDC's advisory committee until very recently owned 600 shares of stock in Merck, a pharmaceutical company with an active vaccine division.

§ Members of the CDC's advisory committee often fill out incomplete financial disclosure statements, and are not required to provide the missing information by CDC ethics officials.

§ Four out of eight CDC advisory committee members who voted to approve guidelines for the rotavirus vaccine in June 1998 had financial ties to pharmaceutical companies that were developing different versions of the vaccine.

§ 3 out of 5 FDA advisory committee members who voted to approve the rotavirus vaccine in December 1997 had financial ties to pharmaceutical companies that were developing different versions of the vaccine.

A more complete discussion of specific conflict of interest problems identified by Government Reform Committee staff can be found in Sections 4 and 5 of this report. To provide focus to the discussion, this report examines the deliberations of the two committees on one specific vaccine—the Rotavirus vaccine. Approved for use by the FDA on August 31, 1998, the Rotavirus vaccine was pulled from the market 13 months later after serious adverse reactions to the vaccine emerged.

As the House report details, investors and industry representatives involved in the development of a rotavirus vaccine voted to approve the FDA's licensing of the vaccine, as they were on the federal committee that licensed it.

Problems quickly ensued, according to the report:

A little more than one year after the Rotashield rotavirus vaccine was licensed by the Food and Drug Administration as a safe and effective vaccine, it was removed from the market due to adverse events. More than 100 cases of severe bowel obstruction, or intussusception, were reported in children who had received the vaccine.

Rotashield was licensed by FDA on August 31, 1998. Distribution began on October 1, 1998. On January 1, 1999 there were zero cases of intussusception on the Vaccine Adverse Events Reporting System (VAERS). In May 1999 there were ten cases of intussusception reported in the VAERS. Data was received from the Northern California Kaiser active surveillance system and from statewide data case control in Minnesota in early June that supported a relationship between the Rotashield vaccine and intussusception. Dr. Jeffery P. Koplan, Director of the CDC, was briefed for the first time on June 11, 1999. A subsequent meeting was held with Dr. Koplan and the CDC at which a decision was made to postpone any further use of the vaccine until further analysis was conducted. This was published in MMWR on July 16, 1999.

As of October 15, 1999, 113 cases of intussusception had been received. Nine of these reported cases were determined not to be intussusception. Of the remaining 102 cases of intussusception, 57 had received the vaccine. Of these, 29 required surgery, seven underwent bowel resection, and one five-month-old infant died after developing intussusception five days after receipt of the vaccine.[xxv] A case study was conducted that estimated that the risk of intussusception was increased by sixty percent among children who received the Rotashield.

It is alarming that it was known during clinical trials and the licensing process that there were increased incidences of intussusception in vaccinated infants. The topic was raised at a VRBPAC meeting and a reference to intussusception is listed in the ACIP recommendation, however, the committee apparently determined that the reported rate of 1 in 2010 was not to be statistically significant. The CDC continues to provide inconsistent information on their web site. One fact sheet, the Rotavirus Q & A, has not been updated since July 16, 1999 and does not provide a link to a more recent fact sheet. The fact sheet significantly plays down the seriousness of the adverse event and asserts that no association has been made. [xxvi] Another Rotavirus Vaccine Fact Sheet was updated on February 2, 2000 that indicates that the FDA and CDC confirmed the association between Rotashield and intussusception.

During the clinical trials, five children out of a total of 10,054 subjects suffered intussusception. [xxvii] If confirmed, the rate of intussusception would be 1 in 2010 children. According to the manufacturer's package insert, the adverse event was considered statistically insignificant at 0.05%. Intussusception had not previously been associated with natural rotavirus infection.

Rotashield rotavirus vaccine was removed from the U.S. market in October 1999. Development of other rotavirus vaccines continues by Merck and others.[2]

Little has changed since the publication of this report. The money made on vaccines for the pharmaceutical industry and those rewarded by it has only led to more power and influence by those invested in vaccinology. Given the way those who question vaccine safety are treated today, one wonders what kind of treatment a woman such as Bernice Eddy would receive. Would Dr. Eddy be asked to present her findings at a meeting of the Vaccine Dinner Club?

The Vaccine Dinner Club, or VDC, is an actual organization sponsored by Emory University, which many refer to as "CDC University" due to the amount of resources it receives from the Centers for Disease Control, a critical player in federal vaccine policy. The VDC offers "hot food" and "cool science." The director of the organization, in a tongue-and-cheek manner, refers to herself as "a goddess."

According to its website, the VDC exists to facilitate networking and collaboration between researchers, clinicians, policy makers, and historians/journalists who are interested in vaccination. The VDC has members from federal and state government agencies, the pharmaceutical industry, and even unnamed members of the "Fourth Estate" (print and Internet). The VDC receives funding from the Robert Woods Johnson and Gates Foundations.

The "Who We Are" section of the website is remarkable and honest because it is a listing of the powerful entities that support the field of vaccinology. As the paragraph shows, the lines between those who regulate in government and those who manufacture and distribute have become blurred.

When did this start?

In 1976 the CDC became alarmed over the possibility of a swine flu epidemic after a soldier who died at Fort Dix tested positive for the virus. A flu pandemic at the end of World War I killed thousands, and a return of the disease caused understandable alarm. The CDC urged manufacturers to quickly produce a swine flu vaccine, and Congress acted quickly to pass the Swine Flu Act. In what would ultimately become a template for the National Vaccine Injury Compensation Program, the federal government agreed to compensate flu vaccine injuries. However, unlike the NVICP, those filing vaccine injury claims would have to use the civil courts.

A swine flu epidemic never occurred. However, four thousand vaccine injury claims were filed, mostly for Guillane-Barré syndrome. The vaccine is reported to have resulted in thirty deaths, and the federal government paid an estimated $90 million in damages.

In 1979, Mike Wallace of *60 Minutes* revealed in an interview with CDC director Dr. David Sencer that the wrong strain of flu antigen had been manufactured. The vaccine produced was not based on the strain of influenza allegedly found in the soldier who had died at Fort Dix. In other words, thirty people died from having received the wrong vaccine. If there had been an actual swine flu pandemic, the vaccine that was rushed to the market would likely not have worked. Those who are now in ascendancy in vaccinology have virtually no liability for their products. The NVICP now buffers the vaccine industry from regular civil liability. Mistakes that could result in vaccine injuries don't seem to be considered on the menu of the Vaccine Dinner Club.

However, the reality of vaccine injuries is being considered critical by some in the mainstream, and controversy is sure to follow.

On May 8, 2014, evidence of a schism within vaccinology appeared in an article by journalist Lawrence Solomon of Canada's *Financial Post*. Dr. Gregory Poland of the Mayo Clinic's Vaccine Research Group made comments that many in vaccinology would regard as heresy.

"The old paradigm isn't working anymore," Poland told Solomon. The article stated that some vaccines are losing their effectiveness and that the delivery—a "one-size-fits-all" model—is outdated. Poland is promoting a new idea called "vaccinomics," in which vaccines will be tailored to an individual's genetic makeup. This theory is based on the work that the Mayo Clinic group is doing on "adversomics," which seeks to understand and analyze adverse vaccine reactions. Poland states that adverse vaccine reactions may hinge upon a person's genetic makeup.

Poland stated in Solomon's article that "a small percentage of children who get vaccine-induced fever after MMR [measles, mumps, and rubella] will develop febrile seizures. I'd like to see predictive tests or preventive therapies that could be administered with the vaccine to prevent these reactions. . . . The current science doesn't allow for an informed understanding of an individual's genetically determined risk for an adverse event due to a vaccine."

Solomon notes that Poland's notions have detractors and that he has been greeted with hostility in some quarters of the vaccinology community. However, as Solomon notes, mainstream publications such as *Scientific American* and *The Scientists* have described Poland's work as significant and innovative.

Dr. Poland opines that people ought to have risk information so that they can make informed choices. The critical issue here, however, is the matter of choice. Right now, vaccines are mandated in most parts of the United States. Many people report that they have never received information sheets about vaccine adverse reactions from doctors. Many doctors appear to be uninformed about the Vaccine Adverse Event Reporting System (VAERS), and it is generally acknowledged that approximately no more than 10 percent of all vaccine injuries are ever reported.

An important question to be answered is what data is the Mayo Clinic's Vaccine Research Group working with? Are the data kept by the pharmaceutical industry and the federal government? Is it not reasonable that this information be made available to the public so that people—as Poland suggests—can make informed medical decisions?

If a serious problem with a vaccine did arise, how would the public be aware of it if the data are unavailable? Given the hostility toward those who express concerns about vaccine safety, would those in the field of vaccinology have the courage of Dr. Bernice Eddy to stand up to those in authority? Can vaccinology be expected to police itself?

DPT: SEIZURES AND ENCEPHALOPATHY

In 1982, Lea Thompson, an investigative journalist at a Washington, DC, NBC station, produced a documentary called *DPT: Vaccine Roulette*. The documentary featured children with severe disabilities attributed to being injured by the DPT vaccine. The documentary is often blamed for generating a tremendous increase in the litigation against vaccine manufacturers.

The current narrative put forth by vaccine supporters is that Lea Thompson's journalism was flawed. She is described as having relied on parental reports and not on science. The criticism is that Thompson's documentary triggered a crisis and seemingly caused parents to believe in phenomena—DPT injury, or "DPT syndrome," as the British referred to it—that didn't exist.

The reality is that many parents in the United Kingdom and the United States had been speaking out about the effects of DPT long before Thompson's documentary. Parents were alleging that DPT had caused their children's death, often referred to as Sudden Infant Death Syndrome (SIDS). Others reported that DPT left their children with seizures and brain damage. The reports of brain damage ranged from ADHD to severe infantile spasms. Some parents claimed that DPT left their children with a disorder, rare at the time, called autism.[1] One group, led by Barbara Loe Fisher, Dissatisfied Parents Together (DPT), eventually established the National Vaccine Information Center (NVIC). Fisher became a leading vaccine safety advocate and, along with Harris Colter, wrote *A Shot in the Dark*, which documented the connection between DPT and vaccine injury.

A review of Thompson's résumé reveals a professional investigative journalist who uncovered many important stories throughout her career. The criticism of Thompson and *Vaccine Roulette* ignores the fact that DPT vaccine injuries had led to serious research on adverse reactions. The National Childhood Encephalopathy Study (NCES) was started in England in the 1970s by Dr. David Miller and others to assess whether parental reports of DPT syndrome had merit. The NCES had been underway for years, with the first phase published in 1981—a year before Thompson's documentary aired. The NCES found that, on rare occasions, DPT vaccine did result in encephalopathy.

The NCES was not a perfect study. One criticism was that there was no unvaccinated control group. At the time, the vast majority of children in the United Kingdom were vaccinated. It should be pointed out, however, that a comparative study on the health outcomes of vaccinated and unvaccinated children has never been done. Calls for such research today are often shouted down as unethical due to the belief that every child must be vaccinated.

The issue of encephalopathy as a result of vaccine injury is central in much of the modern debate around vaccine injury. *Encephalopathy* is defined by the VICP injury table as follows:

> 1. *Encephalopathy.* For purposes of paragraph (a) of this section, a vaccine recipient shall be considered to have suffered an encephalopathy only if such recipient manifests, within the applicable period, an injury meeting the description below of an acute encephalopathy, and then a chronic encephalopathy persists in such person for more than 6 months beyond the date of vaccination.
>
> (i) An acute encephalopathy is one that is sufficiently severe so as to require hospitalization (whether or not hospitalization occurred).
>
> > (A) *For children less than 18 months of age* who present without an associated seizure event, an acute encephalopathy is indicated by a significantly decreased level of consciousness lasting for at least 24 hours. Those children less than 18 months of age who present following a seizure shall be viewed as having an acute encephalopathy if their significantly decreased level of consciousness persists beyond 24 hours and cannot be attributed to a postictal state (seizure) or medication.
> >
> > (B) *For adults and children 18 months of age or older,* an acute encephalopathy is one that persists for at least 24 hours and characterized by at least two of the following:
> >
> > > (1) A significant change in mental status that is not medication related; specifically a confusional state, or a delirium, or a psychosis;
> > >
> > > (2) A significantly decreased level of consciousness, which is independent of a seizure and cannot be attributed to the effects of medication; and
> > >
> > > (3) A seizure associated with loss of consciousness.
> >
> > (C) Increased intracranial pressure may be a clinical feature of acute encephalopathy in any age group.

(D) A "significantly decreased level of consciousness" is indicated by the presence of at least one of the following clinical signs for at least 24 hours or greater (see paragraphs (b)(2)(i)(A) and (b)(2)(i)(B) of this section for applicable timeframes):

(1) Decreased or absent response to environment (responds, if at all, only to loud voice or painful stimuli);

(2) Decreased or absent eye contact (does not fix gaze upon family members or other individuals); or

(3) Inconsistent or absent responses to external stimuli (does not recognize familiar people or things).

(E) The following clinical features alone, or in combination, do not demonstrate an acute encephalopathy or a significant change in either mental status or level of consciousness as described above: Sleepiness, irritability (fussiness), high-pitched and unusual screaming, persistent inconsolable crying, and bulging fontanelle. Seizures in themselves are not sufficient to constitute a diagnosis of encephalopathy. In the absence of other evidence of an acute encephalopathy, seizures shall not be viewed as the first symptom or manifestation of the onset of an acute encephalopathy.

The NCES, the best research of the time, supported the theory that DPT vaccine was causing encephalopathy. Many vaccine advocates denied that a vaccine could ever cause brain injury. However, as the reader has likely realized, encephalopathy is exactly that. The debate around DPT-induced brain damage was heated. Many who strongly supported vaccines did concede that while it was rare, vaccines were causing serious injuries, including death, even when the vaccine was produced correctly. The legal term "unavoidably unsafe" is used to describe such a product in tort law. The reality that vaccines were just such a product ultimately led to the drafting of the National Childhood Vaccine Act.

Vaccines reportedly had a low profit margin, and DPT manufacturers had difficulty obtaining liability insurance. By 1985, only one US manufacturer of DPT remained. The pharmaceutical industry told Congress that it would get out of the vaccine production business. Plans for the rationing of DPT were actively being considered by public health authorities. In 1986, parents and industry were pressuring Congress to do something about "the vaccine crisis." The medical establishment wanted a review panel of doctors to decide vaccine injury cases, and vaccine victim advocates wanted a fair compensation program. With House Speaker Tip O'Neil's final session winding down, Representative Henry Waxman pushed the National Childhood Vaccine Injury Act, which established the Vaccine Injury Compensation Program, to a vote on the House floor. A few days later, President Ronald Regan signed the bill into law. The nation now had a no-fault administrative program under the United States Court of Claims to compensate vaccine injury victims.

And Vaccine manufacturers had an unprecedented level of liability protection.

The intent of Congress was

1. To compensate for vaccine-induced injuries
2. To make vaccines safer
3. To insulate industry and medical professionals from liability for vaccine injuries

It can reasonably be argued that the act only accomplished the third objective.

The DPT vaccine was eventually replaced by the DTaP vaccine, which appeared to be safer based on research from Japan. The DPT was a whole-cell pertussis version of the vaccine. The DTaP utilizes an attenuated-cell version. However, many vaccine advocates continue to maintain that the DPT was safe and that the children who suffered from DPT syndrome had a genetic variant—SCN1A—that triggered their seizures and developmental delays. This idea has received support in case decisions within the NVICP. However, the fact remains that the research suggesting SCN1A as the cause of DPT syndrome relied on a small population sample, only some of whom had this genetic variation. This study may well be important, as it may indicate that people with SCN1A variant may have a predisposition to develop seizure disorders. However, there has never been a population-based study of the SCN1A gene variant. We simply do not know the percentage of people in the regular population who possess this gene variation and how many do or do not have seizures or developmental delays. There is a growing consensus that genes do not determine destiny; they operate within our bodies, and our bodies are impacted by the environment.

A study recently published in *Scientific American* is reporting that the DTaP is ineffective. Many are calling for a return of the whole-cell DPT. Is it possible that those responsible for vaccine policy are willing to risk the consequences of ignoring history?

THE NATIONAL VACCINE INJURY COMPENSATION PROGRAM REFLECTION OF REALITY OR BETRAYAL OF A PROMISE?

Many feel that the NVICP has betrayed the intent of Congress and the vaccine-injured. It is not at all clear that the program has improved vaccine safety, as precious little information about vaccine injury is ever made public.

How did we get here?

It must be remembered that while many members of the medical establishment advocated for liability protection from vaccine injury, many others denied that vaccine injury ever happened.

There has always been a tension—some would say a conflict of interest—built right into the NVICP. The very existence of the program announces that vaccine injuries occur. However, the US government spends hardly any money at all publicizing the NVICP. The Department of Health and Human Services, which administers the program, is also responsible for virtually every other government organ of vaccine development, support, and promotion.

The NVICP began with a lot of promise, and many vaccine injured people were compensated justly and fairly. However, the eight special masters who presided over cases that went to hearing almost immediately faced a huge backlog of cases. A few early case decisions indicate that the Department of Justice actually resisted defending the Secretary of Health and Human Services, the respondent against whom the petitioners bring claims.

While case processing was delayed, money in the Vaccine Injury Compensation Fund continued to accrue. By 1998, the fund had amassed $1.2 billion.[1]

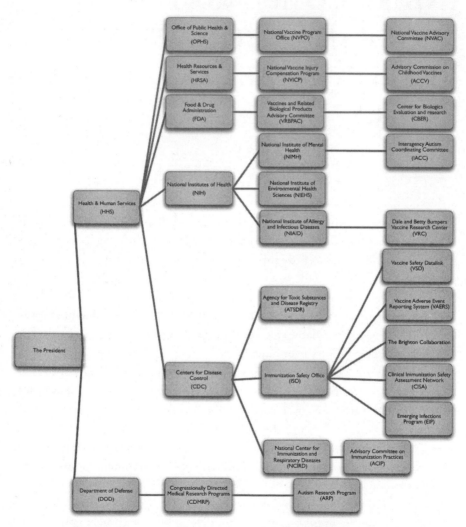

Chart courtesy of Becky Estepp

In 1995, the Secretary of Health and Human Services modified the vaccine injury table, removing residual reizure risorder (although not seizures) and tightening the criteria for encephalopathy. In a 1998 *Washington Post Magazine* article by Arthur Allen, Special Master Laura Millman questioned whether the changes had countered the will of Congress that the program be "fair, simple, and easy to administer."[2]

Had the program become unworkable?

The Secretary of Health and Human Services sided with members of the medical establishment. Dr. Gerald Fenichel of Vanderbuilt University disagreed with the findings of the NCES and disagreed with idea of accepting documented case histories of vaccine injury as sufficient proof of vaccine injury. Fenichel argued that case reports of vaccine injury—no matter how well documented—should not be accepted as "scientific proof" and published an editorial in the *Journal of the American Medical Association (JAMA)* on his perspective: "The Pertussis Vaccine Controversy: The Danger of Case Reports."

In a field bereft of research not directly funded by manufacturers, where studies on non-vaccinated groups were never done, what other kinds of proof were petitioners left with? What other kind of proof could be found? Would this bias against human observation exist in other legal arenas?

Petitioner attorneys argued that Congress didn't want petitioners to face the burdens of regular civil courts. What happened to the program Congress intended? Congress didn't intend for petitioners to prove injury with scientific certainty.

Arthur Allen's 1998 article provides important insight into what went on behind closed doors at the DVIC, the Division of Vaccine Injury Compensation:

> They don't want payments made for injuries that were not certainly caused by the vaccine. There's a larger issue, too. They want parents to immunize their children, and for that they want the record to show that vaccines are safe. "I'm not going to say that awarding too many people will undermine vaccine safety, but I look on the Internet, and I see that our statistics are taken out of context," says [Dr. Geoffrey] Evans, the medical director of the compensation program. "And so it's important that the table reflect what *we* think is really caused by the vaccines."[3]

In that same *Washington Post Magazine* article, Chief Special Master Gary Golkiewicz admitted the government had "altered the game so that it's clearly in their favor. . . . This group has a vested interest in vaccines being good. It doesn't take a mental giant to see the fundamental unfairness in this."[4]

Within ten years of the NVICP's beginning, the cases being handled by the program were quietly being held to different evidence standards than Congress had intended. Congress proscribed that the standard used in the program be preponderance of the evidence—described in law as 50 percent plus the weight of a feather. But Evans's statement indicates that a more rigorous, albeit silent standard had taken hold.

While the Division of Vaccine Injury is responsible for screening cases that enter the NVICP, it should be noted that most of the screening is now done by members of the medical and public health establishment who are under contract as experts with the DVIC.[5] The list of medical expert contractors is packed with well-credentialed members of the medical establishment, many of whom are very invested in vaccinology.

The NVICP had become a captive of the medical establishment's desire to reinforce the belief in the safety of vaccines. With the rise in autism prevalence—and a dramatic rise in petitioner's claiming autism as a vaccine injury—the problem reached a head.

THE OMNIBUS AUTISM PROCEEDINGS

In November 2013 the House of Representatives Oversight and Government Reform Committee announced plans to conduct a hearing into the the National Vaccine Injury Compensation Program. Amy Pisani, director of Every Child by Two, a pro-vaccine advocacy organization that receives significant funding from the pharmaceutical industry, called on Congress to cancel the hearing, stating that those calling for it "have a long history of claiming that vaccines cause autism, a hypothesis that has been disproved by the medical and scientific community."[1] Pisani stated further that "to dismantle the National Vaccine Injury Compensation Program in order to appease fringe groups that have had their day in court would be a great disservice to public health."[2]

The position of the public health establishment, as Ms. Pisani's letter states, is that the debate about vaccine induced autism is closed.

The NVICP agreed, and the special masters issued their rulings that vaccine injury does not result in autism. Case closed.

And this might have been the unchallenged narrative had it not been for a little girl, now known as Child Doe 77.

The Child Doe 77 case was one of the cases selected to be an Omnibus Autism Proceeding (OAP) "test case." A group of six cases was culled from the five thousand cases filed in the OAP to serve as cases that tested the prevailing theories about how vaccines may cause autism. There were MMR vaccine test cases, Thimerosal (a mercury-containing vaccine preservative) test cases, and a group under a combined theory. In 2008 the government pulled the Child Doe 77 case out of the proceedings and decided to award compensation to the child. It was decided that the nine vaccines the child received at age eleven months had aggravated an underlying mitochondrial disorder and led to seizures, encephalopathy, and "autism-like symptoms." While government representatives clung to the phrase "autism-like symptoms," it needs to be pointed out that autism is not a disease but a behavioral diagnosis that is rendered by a clinician when a child has enough of the symptoms that the *Diagnostic and Statistical Manual of Mental Disorders* delineates for autism.

Despite the twisted parlance, Child Doe 77 had autism, and the government conceded that vaccines had caused it.

The media coverage of the Child Doe 77 case was significant, and in the days and weeks that followed, other families came forward to say that they also had children who had been compensated for vaccine-induced brain injury, and these children also had autism.

However, the OAP ended with stinging dismissals. Because Child Doe 77 was pulled from the proceedings, the settlement did not establish precedent and the NVICP ruled that vaccines do not cause autism. It was as though the Child Doe 77 case had never happened.

In the Colten Snyder test case, Special Master Denise Vowel wrote, "To conclude that Colten's condition was the result of his MMR vaccine, an objective observer would have to emulate Lewis Carroll's White Queen and be able to believe six impossible (or, at least, highly improbable) things before breakfast."

What no one had yet realized was that the impossible had indeed been served for breakfast many times before in the NVICP. An investigation led by coauthor Louis Conte resulted in the publication of "Unanswered Questions from the Vaccine Injury Compensation Program: A Review of Compensated Cases of Vaccine-Induced Brain Injury" in the May 2011 *Pace Environmental Law Review*. The review's authors, Holland, Conte, Krakow, and Colin, found that the NVICP had been compensating cases for vaccine injury that featured autism for its entire history. The eighty-three cases identified, from available public records, reflected a fraction of the cases compensated by the program. Despite requests filed under the Freedom of Information Act, the government blocked investigative access to the vast majority of cases.

Those administering the NVICP never disclosed the actual history of autism within the program. Many working in the program have conceded that autism was often a sequelae—or consequence—of vaccine-induced encephalopathy. The following quote from the Health Resources and Services Administration's (HRSA's) David Bowman to investigative journalist David Kirby is telling:

From: Bowman, David (HRSA)
Sent: Friday, February 20, 2009 5:22 PM
Subject: HRSA Statement

David,

In response to your most recent inquiry, HRSA has the following statement: The government has never compensated, nor has it ever been ordered to compensate, any case based on a determination that autism was actually caused by vaccines. We have compensated cases in which children exhibited an encephalopathy, or general brain disease. Encephalopathy may be accompanied by a medical progression of an array of symptoms, including autistic behavior, autism, or seizures. Some children who have been compensated for vaccine injuries may have shown signs of autism before the decision to compensate, or may ultimately end up with autism or autistic symptoms, but we do not track cases on this basis.

Regards,
David Bowman
Office of Communications
Health Resources and Services Administration[3]

Bowman's knowledge of autism within the vaccine-injured could only have come from one source: the Division of Vaccine Injury Compensation, which screens all the cases that enter the NVICP.

After reading *Unanswered Questions*, many petitioners in the Omnibus Autism Proceedings asked why their children's autism cases were not handled the way in which previous encephalopathy cases featuring autism had been handled by the program. Eventually, those involved in the proceedings admitted that OAP was not about those cases where autism was secondary to encephalopathy. The OAP was actually about "primary" or "idiopathic" autism—not "secondary autism."

Some clinicians suggest that that primary or idiopathic autism relates to those individuals who have genetic anomalies that produce syndromes such as fragile X, Down syndrome, and tuberous sclerosis. However, *idiopathic*, defined as "arising spontaneously or from an obscure or unknown cause"—is not quite correct here. Individuals who are dealing with fragile X, Down syndrome, or tuberous sclerosis have a *known* genetic abnormality. Part of the causation of autism for these individuals is understood. However, it is also important to point out that not all individuals with these genetic issues ultimately develop autism. There are many people with these syndromes who do *not* have autism. Even in the presence of these strong genetic predispositions, autism does not always develop. It seems that something else must still occur, an injury of some sort, for autism to develop even in people with known predispositions.

In the decisions from the Omnibus Autism Proceedings, the special masters did not delineate the type of autism—primary or secondary—that they were ruling on. The terms "primary" and "secondary" autism do not appear in any of the test case decisions issued by the special masters. In the end, it was stated, in essence, that vaccines do not cause autism—all forms of autism.

Is there really a difference between primary and secondary autism? Is this really a distinction without a difference? The history of cases in the NVICP strongly indicates that brain damage induced by vaccine injury can leave the afflicted child with a diagnosis of autism, among other issues.

This understanding of autism—"secondary autism"—developing in a person who has suffered vaccine-induced brain damage is significant. A major purpose for the establishment of the NVICP was to increase the understanding of vaccine injuries. And yet this program's "understanding" about secondary autism has been acknowledged grudgingly.

Is all autism really secondary autism? If so, we are then presented with another question: How could the petitioners in the OAP ever prove that a vaccine injury could lead to primary (idiopathic) autism? How does one prove that a vaccine injury caused a disorder that arises spontaneously? If petitioners in the Omnibus Autism Proceedings were to prove primary autism, the burden was impossible, and their cases may have been doomed from the outset. Interviews with attorneys who represented petitioners in the Omnibus Autism Proceedings have reported to us that this was indeed their burden. Petitioners had to prove a different type of autism than the type that the program had quietly accepted as a sequela in the years prior to the Omnibus Autism Proceedings.

Further proof of the belief in the two types of autism is provided below. Note the footnote at the bottom of the table from a March 2012 ACCV presentation about a NVICP request to the IOM in 2009:

The footnote states,

"Secondary" autism or autistic features arising from chronic encephalopathy, mitochondrial disorders and/or other underlying disorders will be considered by the Committee. For "Primary" autism, the VICP has asked the IOM to consider the review of the medical literature post *Immunization Safety Review: Vaccines and Autism (2004)* report. In particular, VICP is interested in the Committee's review on more recent theories of "neuroinflammation" and "hyperarousal/overexcitation of the immune system via multiple antigenic stimulation."

The notion of primary and secondary autism was repeated in the March 8, 2012 report to the Advisory Commission on Childhood Vaccines, *Updating the Vaccine Injury Table Following the 2011 IOM Report on Adverse Effects of Vaccines* completed by Rosemary Johann-Liang, MD, chief medical officer, National Vaccine Injury Compensation Program

The theory of autism causation implied by the table below also explains the government's rationale for pulling the Child Doe 77 case out of the OAP, conceding the case, and awarding compensation. We now also have some understanding of why the odd phrase "resulted in autism-like symptoms" was deployed.

Attorney Robert Krakow has pointed out that one can trace the "evolution" of the Child Doe 77 case through settlement decisions to where it eventually becomes an "MMR encephalopathy table injury." MMR is emphasized even though the child received several other vaccinations that could also have been involved with her injury. As a "secondary autism" case, the MMR caused brain damage—encephalopathy. The autism was a sequela of that encephalopathy. However, the vaccine did not cause the autism; the end result just included autism.

The Mojabi case, settled in 2012, also a case from the Omnibus Autism Proceedings, seems to have gone through a similar evolution. Mojabi is another MMR table injury that resulted in encephalopathy with autism:

> No. 06-227V Chief Special Master Campbell-Smith
> Posted 12/13/12
> DECISION AWARDING DAMAGES
> Chief Special Master Campbell-Smith
> "On March 23, 2006, Saeid Mojabi and Parivash Vahabi (petitioners), as the parents and legal representatives of their minor son, Ryan, filed a petition pursuant to the National Vaccine Injury Compensation Program ("Vaccine Program"). Petitioners alleged that as a result of "all the vaccinations administered to [Ryan] from March 25, 2003, through February 22, 2005, and more specifically, measles-mumps-rubella (MMR) vaccinations administered to him on December 19, 2003 and May 10, 2004," Ryan suffered "a severe and debilitating injury to his brain, described as Autism Spectrum Disorder ('ASD')." Petition at 1. Petitioners specifically asserted that Ryan "suffered a Vaccine Table Injury, namely, an encephalopathy" as a result of his receipt of the MMR vaccination on December 19, 2003.

COMMITTEE TO REVIEW ADVERSE EFFECTS OF VACCINES
DECEMBER 2009 WORKING LIST OF ADVERSE EVENTS TO BE CONSIDERED BY THE COMMITTEE

DTaP/Tetanus Containing Vaccines	Hepatitis A Vaccine	Meningococcal Vaccine	MMR Vaccine

• Anaphylaxis or Anaphylactic Shock
• Arthropathy (Arthritis, Arthralgia)
• Autism*
• Autism Spectrum Disorders (ASD)/Pervasive Developmental Disorders (PDD)*
• Ataxia
• Bell's Palsy
• Chronic, Remitting Demyelinating Diseases:
  ▪ Chronic Inflammatory Disseminated Polyneuropathy
  ▪ Multiple Sclerosis
• Chronic Urticaria
• Complex Regional Pain Syndrome
• Convulsions:
  ▪ Febrile, Afebrile
  ▪ Infantile Spasms
  ▪ Myoclonic Epilepsy
• Encephalopathy/Encephalitis
• Fibromyalgia
• Immune Thrombocytopenic Purpura
• Insulin-dependent Diabetes Mellitus
• Monophasic Demyelinating Diseases:
  ▪ Acute Disseminating Encephalomyelitis
  ▪ Guillain-Barré Syndrome
  ▪ Transverse Myelitis
• Myocarditis
• Opsoclonus Myoclonus Syndrome
• Optic Neuritis
• Serum Sickness
• Sudden Infant Death Syndrome (SIDS)
	• Anaphylaxis or Anaphylactic Shock
	• Bell's Palsy
	• Chronic, Remitting Demyelinating Diseases:
	  ▪ Chronic Inflammatory Disseminated Polyneuropathy
	  ▪ Multiple Sclerosis
	• Hepatitis (autoimmune)
	• Monophasic Demyelinating Diseases:
	  ▪ Acute Disseminating Encephalomyelitis
	  ▪ Guillain-Barré Syndrome
	  ▪ Transverse Myelitis
		• Anaphylaxis or Anaphylactic Shock
		• Chronic Headaches
		• Chronic, Remitting Demyelinating Diseases:
		  ▪ Chronic Inflammatory Disseminated Polyneuropathy
		  ▪ Multiple Sclerosis
		• Encephalopathy/Encephalitis
		• Monophasic Demyelinating Diseases:
		  ▪ Acute Disseminating Encephalomyelitis
		  ▪ Guillain-Barré Syndrome
		  ▪ Transverse Myelitis
			• Anaphylaxis or Anaphylactic Shock
			• Arthropathy (Arthritis, Arthralgia)
			• Autism*
			• Autism Spectrum Disorders (ASD)/Pervasive Developmental Disorders (PDD)*
			• Ataxia
			• Brachial Neuritis
			• Chronic Fatigue Syndrome
			• Chronic, Remitting Demyelinating Diseases:
			  ▪ Chronic Inflammatory Disseminated Polyneuropathy
			  ▪ Multiple Sclerosis
			• Complex Regional Pain Syndrome
			• Convulsions:
			  ▪ Febrile, Afebrile
			  ▪ Infantile Spasms
			  ▪ Myoclonic Epilepsy
			• Encephalopathy/Encephalitis
			• Fibromyalgia
			• Hearing Loss
			• Hepatitis
			• Insulin-dependent Diabetes Mellitus
			• Monophasic Demyelinating Diseases:
			  ▪ Acute Disseminating Encephalomyelitis
			  ▪ Guillain-Barré Syndrome
			  ▪ Transverse Myelitis
			• Opsoclonus Myoclonus Syndrome

* "Secondary" autism or autistic features arising from chronic encephalopathy, mitochondrial disorders and/or other underlying disorders will be considered by the Committee. For "Primary" autism, VICP has asked the IOM to consider the review of the medical literature post *Immunization Safety Review: Vaccines and Autism (2004)* report. In particular, VICP is interested in the Committee's review on more recent theories of "neuroinflammation" and "hyperarousal/overexcitation of the immune system via multiple simultaneous antigenic stimulation."

In the alternative, petitioners asserted that "as a cumulative result of his receipt of each and every vaccination between March 25, 2003 and February 22, 2005, Ryan has suffered . . . neuroimmunologically mediated dysfunctions in the form of asthma and ASD."

Ryan Mojabi was compensated—$969,474.91.

The authors recently contacted individuals who retired from the NVICP and the Division of Vaccine Injury Compensation. It is now clear that many in the program had an understanding about autism that was never publicly stated. Retired employees have acknowledged that autism had always been understood to be a common occurrence in severe cases of vaccine injuries meeting requirements of the table injury for encephalopathy. One retired employee stated emphatically that the development of autism in the presence of severe encephalopathy was understood by those in the program on both sides of the bar. The disagreement in NVICP about vaccine injury leading to autism involved cases where autistic regression was gradual. Another retired employee also confirmed that autism was seen as an indication of brain damage in vaccine injury.

The understanding of autism as a result of vaccine-induced encephalopathy needs to be fully reconsidered by the public and the research community. The implications are enormous given that the increase in autism appears to coincide with the ramping up of the vaccine schedule after the passage of the 1986 law. Given the sentiment reflected in the statements of DVIC Director Dr. Geoffrey Evans in 1998—that the program reflect the beliefs of the medical community about vaccine injury—it is remarkable that so many of the cases identified as featuring autism in *Unanswered Questions* were *conceded* by the government.

The question needs to be asked; is the government withholding the truth about vaccine injury–induced autism? Here is a summary of what we know:

- The government conceded in the Child Doe 77 case that vaccine injury "resulted in autism-like symptoms," then withdrew the case from the Omnibus Autism Proceedings to avoid a case decision, which would have set precedent. Ultimately, Child Doe 77 was found to have suffered an MMR table encephalopathy.
- The government admitted to journalist David Kirby that some cases of vaccine injury featured autism but that it didn't track these cases.
- Documents from ACCV meetings refer to two types of autism—"primary" and "secondary" autism, which arises from encephalopathy and mitochondrial disorders (as in the case of Child Doe 77).

- Retired program employees have acknowledged that autism was understood to be a sequelae of vaccine injury–induced encephalopathy.
- In touching only a small percentage of compensated cases, *Unanswered Questions* found eighty-three cases of vaccine injury that also included autism. Since the publication of *Unanswered Questions*, more cases of vaccine-induced encephalopathy/autism, such as Mojabi, have emerged.

The conclusion is obvious and disturbing. The people in and around the NVICP, the Division of Vaccine Injury Compensation, and the Department of Justice "understood" that autism was associated with cases of vaccine injury but failed to disclose what they knew, even though Congress intended for the program to disclose information about the nature of vaccine injuries.

Unanswered Questions caused more than a few unanswered questions to be asked on Capitol Hill and ultimately fueled calls for a congressional hearing on what was going on in the NVICP. Representative Darrell Issa, chairman of the House of Representatives Committee on Oversight and Government Reform, announced that he would conduct hearings on the NVICP at the end of 2013. The autism issue is described as "scary" by Washington insiders. But it was once again leading to controversy about vaccine injury and how it was being addressed by the government. Pro-vaccine activists, led by Dr. Paul Offit—the same Paul Offit cited in the House Oversight and Reform Committee Report on *Conflicts of Interest in Vaccine Policy Making*—exerted enormous pressure on Congress to call the hearings off (as stated in the letter by Amy Pisani). Potential witnesses were contacted by committee staffers and nervously admitted that they faced damaging their careers if they had to testify about the "autism issue."

Congressman Issa was faced with the prospect that a hearing on the NVICP was likely to be extraordinarily contentious. Many potential witnesses contacted by the Oversight and Government Reform staff indicated that they would refuse to testify. Pro-vaccine organizations lobbied hard to shut the hearings down. Issa relented and postponed the hearing.

For the time being, vaccine advocates and the leaders of vaccinology seem to have delayed congressional questioning. But due to the lack of transparency about previous cases of vaccine-induced encephalopathy featuring autism, the decisions in the Omnibus Autism Proceedings are now regarded with suspicion. The NVICP has lost public support and is no longer seen as a true justice venue by those who claim vaccine injury.

10

VACCINE INJURY CASES

I t is worth noting that all of the cases here are actual orders issued by special masters or federal judges (on appeal or review) on compensated cases from the National Vaccine Injury Compensation Program. Some cases are compensated before reaching the hearing phase by concession or settlement between the parties.

As stated earlier, the vast majority of cases are not compensated and are dismissed. A review of the United States Court of Claims website will reveal this. One will also find interim decisions, attorney fee dismissals, and other legal actions on cases.

Some cases are compensated after settlements. HRSA now makes the curious claim on the statistics report that settlements do not necessarily mean that they agree that the case represents an actual vaccine injury. Some cases are conceded by the government, and some decisions to compensate are rendered by special masters after hearing the facts. On rare occasions, a case is decided by a US Court of Claims Judge on review or by a higher court on appeal.

We are publishing these cases with some degree of editing to reduce the length of rulings and improve readability. We welcome all to visit the Court of Claims website and review the actual cases.

These cases are publicly available on the US Court of Claims website and elsewhere on the Internet. These are cases already in the public record. Some cases are reported under "Reported Cases," meaning that they may be cited in law. Some are reported under "Unreported Cases," meaning that they may not be referenced in law. However, all of the cases in this book are publicly available, consistent with the provisions of the 1986 act. We ask the reader to respectfully consider that these injuries happened to human beings and that their suffering—and the suffering of those who love them—is real. We ask that you respect the privacy of all involved.

Immediately following are official statistics on the National Vaccine Injury Compensation. It is worthwhile to review these data to place the cases in context. The federal government has paid out over $2.6 billion to the victims of vaccine injury since 1998.

HRSA—National Vaccine Injury Compensation Program Statistics Reports

Statistics—March 5, 2014

I. Petitions Filed

Fiscal Year	Total
FY 1988	24
FY 1989	148
FY 1990	1,492
FY 1991	2,718
FY 1992	189
FY 1993	140
FY 1994	107
FY 1995	180
FY 1996	84
FY 1997	104
FY 1998	120
FY 1999	411
FY 2000	164
FY 2001	216
FY 2002	957
FY 2003	2,592
FY 2004	1,214
FY 2005	735
FY 2006	325
FY 2007	410
FY 2008	417
FY 2009	397
FY 2010	449
FY 2011	386
FY 2012	400
FY 2013	503
FY 2014	218
Total	15,100

II. Adjudications

Fiscal Year	Compensable	Dismissed	Total
FY 1989	9	12	21
FY 1990	100	33	133
FY 1991	141	447	588
FY 1992	166	487	653
FY 1993	125	588	713
FY 1994	162	446	608
FY 1995	160	575	735
FY 1996	162	408	570
FY 1997	189	198	387
FY 1998	144	181	325
FY 1999	98	139	237
FY 2000	125	104	229
FY 2001	86	87	173
FY 2002	104	103	207
FY 2003	56	99	155
FY 2004	62	233	295
FY 2005	60	121	181
FY 2006	69	191	260
FY 2007	83	120	203
FY 2008	147	134	281
FY 2009	134	231	365
FY 2010	181	292	473
FY 2011	261	1,371	1,632
FY 2012	260	2,439	2,699
FY 2013	366	627	993
FY 2014	90	68	158
Totals	3,540	9,734	13,274

III. Awards Paid

Fiscal Year	Compensated			Dismissed		Interim Fees		Total Outlays
	# of Awards	Petitioners' Award Amount	Attorneys' Fees/Costs Payments	# of Payments to Attorneys	Attorneys' Fees/Costs Payments	# of Payments to Attorneys	Attorneys' Fees/Costs Payments	
FY 1989	6	$1,317,654.78	$54,107.14	0	$0.00	0	$0.00	$1,371,761.92
FY 1990	88	$53,252,510.46	$1,379,005.79	4	$57,699.48	0	$0.00	$54,689,215.73
FY 1991	114	$95,980,493.16	$2,364,758.91	30	$496,809.21	0	$0.00	$98,842,061.28
FY 1992	130	$94,538,071.30	$3,001,927.97	118	$1,212,677.14	0	$0.00	$98,752,676.41
FY 1993	162	$119,693,267.87	$3,262,453.06	272	$2,447,273.05	0	$0.00	$125,402,993.98
FY 1994	158	$98,151,900.08	$3,571,179.67	335	$3,166,527.38	0	$0.00	$104,889,607.13
FY 1995	169	$104,085,265.72	$3,652,770.57	221	$2,276,136.32	0	$0.00	$110,014,172.61
FY 1996	163	$100,425,325.22	$3,096,231.96	216	$2,364,122.71	0	$0.00	$105,885,679.89
FY 1997	179	$113,620,171.68	$3,898,284.77	142	$1,879,418.14	0	$0.00	$119,397,874.59
FY 1998	165	$127,546,009.19	$4,002,278.55	121	$1,938,065.50	0	$0.00	$133,484,353.24
FY 1999	96	$95,917,680.51	$2,799,910.85	117	$2,306,957.40	0	$0.00	$101,024,548.76
FY 2000	136	$125,945,195.64	$4,112,369.02	80	$1,724,451.08	0	$0.00	$131,782,015.74
FY 2001	97	$105,878,632.57	$3,373,865.88	57	$2,066,224.67	0	$0.00	$111,318,723.12

Fiscal Year	Compensated			Dismissed		Interim Fees		Total Outlays
	# of Awards	Petitioners' Award Amount	Attorneys' Fees/Costs Payments	# of Payments to Attorneys	Attorneys' Fees/Costs Payments	# of Payments to Attorneys	Attorneys' Fees/Costs Payments	
FY 2002	80	$59,799,604.39	$2,653,598.89	50	$656,244.79	0	$0.00	$63,109,448.07
FY 2003	65	$82,816,240.07	$3,147,755.12	69	$1,545,654.37	0	$0.00	$87,509,650.08
FY 2004	57	$61,933,764.20	$3,079,328.55	69	$1,198,615.96	0	$0.00	$66,211,708.71
FY 2005	64	$55,065,797.01	$2,694,664.03	71	$1,790,587.29	0	$0.00	$59,551,048.33
FY 2006	68	$48,746,162.74	$2,441,199.02	54	$1,353,632.61	0	$0.00	$52,540,994.37
FY 2007	82	$91,449,433.89	$4,034,154.37	61	$1,692,020.25	0	$0.00	$97,175,608.51
FY 2008	141	$75,716,552.06	$5,270,237.04	72	$2,432,947.05	2	$117,265.31	$83,536,901.46
FY 2009	131	$74,142,490.58	$5,404,711.98	36	$1,557,139.53	28	$4,241,362.55	$85,345,704.64
FY 2010	173	$179,387,341.30	$5,961,744.40	56	$1,886,239.95	22	$1,978,803.88	$189,214,129.53
FY 2011	251	$216,319,428.47	$9,736,216.87	402	$5,425,243.19	28	$2,001,770.91	$233,482,659.44
FY 2012	250	$163,511,998.82	$9,104,488.60	1,017	$8,621,182.32	37	$5,420,257.99	$186,657,927.73
FY 2013	375	$254,666,326.70	$13,250,679.53	704	$7,052,778.84	50	$1,454,851.74	$276,424,636.81
FY 2014	135	$71,315,951.56	$3,875,092.47	388	$3,844,439.26	17	$1,275,262.25	$80,310,705.54
Total	3,535	$2,671,223,269.97	$109,305,515.01	4,761	$60,908,457.99	184	$16,489,564.69	$2,857,926,807.60

Claims Filed and Compensated or Dismissed by Vaccine, March 5, 2014

Vaccines Listed in Claims as Reported by Petitioners

Vaccine(s)	Filed			Compensated	Dismissed
	Injury	Death	Total		
DT (diphtheria-tetanus)	69	9	78	24	50
DTaP (diphtheria-tetanus-acellular pertussis)	358	76	434	170	193
DTaP-Hep B-IPV	60	24	84	27	28
DTaP-HIB	7	1	8	4	3
DTaP-IPV-HIB	16	13	29	4	7
DTP (diphtheria-tetanus-whole-cell pertussis)	3,285	696	3,981	1,269	2,704
DTP-HIB	18	8	26	4	20
Hep A-Hep B	14	0	14	8	1
Hep B-HIB	8	0	8	4	3
Hepatitis A (Hep A)	55	2	57	21	16
Hepatitis B (Hep B)	604	53	657	234	354
HIB (Haemophilus influenzae type b)	23	3	26	12	14
HPV (human papillomarvirus)	213	11	224	69	69
Influenza (Trivalent)	1,317	73	1,390	698	125
IPV (inactivated polio)	262	14	276	7	267

Vaccine(s)	Filed			Compensated	Dismissed
	Injury	Death	Total		
Measles	143	19	162	55	107
Meningococcal	34	1	35	22	3
MMR (measles–mumps–rubella)	866	57	923	357	489
MMR-varicella	28	1	29	13	6
MR	15	0	15	6	9
Mumps	10	0	10	1	9
Nonqualified	82	9	91	0	85
OPV (oral polio)	280	28	308	158	150
Pertussis	4	3	7	2	5
Pneumococcal conjugate	38	5	43	10	25
Rotavirus	57	1	58	35	16
Rubella	189	4	193	70	123
Td (tetanus-diphtheria)	180	3	183	102	64
Tdap	154	1	155	69	7
Tetanus	89	2	91	39	35
Unspecified	5,410	8	5,419	4	4,728
Varicella	75	7	82	42	20
TOTAL	13,964	1,132	15,096	3,540	9,735

National Vaccine Injury Compensation Program (VICP) Adjudication Categories by Vaccine for Claims Filed, Calendar Year 2006 to 2013

Vaccine Alleged by Petitioner	No. of Doses Distributed US CY 2006–CY 2012 (Source: CDC)	Compensable			Compensable Total	Dismissed/Non-Compensable Total	Grand Total
		Concession	Court Decision	Settlement			
DT	592,707	1	0	3	4	3	7
DTaP	68,113,573	10	16	69	95	64	159
DTaP-Hep B-IPV	38,347,667	4	6	18	28	31	59
DTaP-HIB	1,135,474	0	0	0	0	1	1
DTaP-IPV-HIB	46,633,881	0	0	5	5	8	13
DTP	0	0	1	2	3	1	4
Hep A-Hep B	10,405,325	0	0	8	8	0	8
Hep B-HIB	4,621,999	1	1	1	3	1	4
Hepaitis A (Hep A)	110,596,300	1	5	17	23	17	40
Hepatitis B (Hep B)	116,853,062	2	10	34	46	29	75
HIB	70,755,674	0	1	4	5	4	9
HPV	55,168,454	10	0	59	69	73	142
Influenza	809,000,000	18	65	616	699	134	833
IPV	52,439,162	0	0	3	3	2	5

Vaccine Alleged by Petitioner	No. of Doses Distributed US CY 2006–CY 2012 (Source: CDC)	Compensable			Compensable Total	Dismissed/Non-Compensable Total	Grand Total
		Concession	Court Decision	Settlement			
Measles	135,660	0	0	1	1	0	1
Meningococcal	51,173,032	1	1	20	22	3	25
MMR	65,864,745	16	14	48	78	64	142
MMR-varicella	8,073,618	7	0	7	14	7	21
Nonqualified	N/A	0	0	0	0	20	20
OPV	0	1	0	0	1	3	4
Pneumococcal conjugate	123,606,306	0	1	5	6	13	19
Rotavirus	61,336,583	0	2	14	16	5	21
Rubella	422,548	0	1	0	1	0	1
Td	53,009,015	4	5	47	56	15	71
Tdap	133,744,203	6	5	59	70	7	77
Tetanus	3,836,052	2	0	14	16	10	26
Unspecified	N/A	1	0	2	3	538	541
Varicella	82,534,257	3	5	17	25	10	35
GRAND TOTAL	1,968,399,297	88	139	1,073	1,300	1,063	2,363

PART II

11

SELECTED REPORTED CASES: 2013

From www.uscfc.uscourts.gov

I.D. v. Secretary of Health and Human Services, Respondent

Summary: In this decision the government has agreed to compensate the victim, identified as I.D., with $1,076,412.15 and an unspecified amount to fund an annuity after a Hepatitis B vaccination caused chronic fatigue syndrome (CFS).

Compensated Vaccine Injury: Chronic Fatigue Syndrome

Chronic fatigue syndrome, or CFS, is a debilitating and complex disorder characterized by profound fatigue that is not improved by bed rest and that may be worsened by physical or mental activity. Symptoms affect several body systems and may include weakness, muscle pain, impaired memory and/or mental concentration, and insomnia, which can result in reduced participation in daily activities.

Damages; decision based on proffer; Hepatitis B vaccine; chronic fatigue syndrome.

Case No. 04-1593V

Date Filed: April 26, 2013

I.D. v. Secretary of Health and Human Services, Respondent

DECISION AWARDING DAMAGES

The Honorable Susan G. Braden
Special Master Christian J. Moran

On October 25, 2004, I.D.'s parents filed a petition on I.D.'s behalf seeking compensation under the National Vaccine Injury Compensation Program, 42 U.S.C. §§ 300aa-1 et seq., alleging that a dose of the Hepatitis B vaccination caused I.D. to develop chronic fatigue syndrome. On April 22, 2011, the United

States Court of Federal Claims determined that I.D. is entitled to compensation under the Vaccine Act. On April 19, 2013, the undersigned issued a ruling regarding damages.

On April 26, 2013, respondent filed a Status Report on Award of Compensation, to which petitioner agrees. This status report is construed as a Proffer on Award of Compensation. Based upon the record as a whole, the special master finds the proffer reasonable and that petitioner is entitled to an award as stated in therein. Pursuant to the attached proffer, the court awards petitioner:

1. A lump sum payment of $1,076,412.15 representing compensation for life care expenses expected to be incurred during the first year after judgment ($40,357.92), lost future earnings ($838,566.45), pain and suffering ($194,580.48), and past un-reimbursable expenses ($2,907.30), in the form of a check payable to petitioner; and
2. An amount sufficient to purchase an annuity contract, subject to the conditions described in the attached Proffer (attached as Appendix A), that will provide payments for the life care items contained in the life care plan, as illustrated by the proffer's chart, paid to the life insurance company from which the annuity will be purchased. Compensation for Year Two (beginning on the first anniversary of the date of judgment) and all subsequent years shall be provided through respondent's purchase of an annuity, which annuity shall make payments directly to petitioner, only so long as petitioner is alive at the time a particular payment is due. At the Secretary's sole discretion, the periodic payments may be provided to petitioner in monthly, quarterly, annual, or other installments. The "annual amounts" set forth in the proffer's chart describe only the total yearly sum to be paid to petitioner and do not require that the payment be made in one annual installment.

IT IS SO ORDERED

Clifton Haigler and Charity Haigler, legal representatives of a minor child, Thomas Thurlow Haigler, v. Secretary of the Department of Health and Human Services

Summary: In this case decision, issued after a hearing, Special Master Dorsey rules that a varicella vaccination caused a child to suffer encephalitis, resulting in permanent brain damage.

Compensated Vaccine Injury: Encephalitis

Encephalitis is inflammation and swelling of the brain, most often due to infections.

Case No: 11-508V

Date Filed: August 9, 2011

Clifton Haigler and Charity Haigler, legal representatives of a minor child, Thomas Thurlow Haigler, v. Secretary of the Department of Health and Human Services

Dorsey, Special Master

On August 9, 2011, Clifton and Charity Haigler filed a petition for compensation under the National Vaccine Injury Compensation program, as the legal representatives of their son, Thomas Thurlow Haigler, in which they alleged that a varicella vaccination that Thomas received on October 2, 2008, caused him to suffer encephalitis. Petitioners further alleged that the vaccination "caused permanent brain damage and will continue to block [Thomas's] mental development."

FACTS

Thomas was born on September 18, 2006, in Stanly County, North Carolina. There were no observed physical abnormalities. Thomas's Apgar scores were 8 and 9, at 1 and 5 minutes, respectively. The results of the North Carolina State newborn screening blood tests were normal.

Over the next year, Thomas had a number of childhood illnesses, but was otherwise considered "normal," "alert [and] active," and "well developed." At his 10 and 12 month well-child visits, Thomas's developmental milestones were assessed by use of the "Ages & Stages Questionnaires" ("ASQ"). Thomas's communication, gross and fine motor skills, problem solving and personal social skills were noted to be normal. Thomas's hearing and vision were also noted to be normal.

On November 13, 2007, Thomas presented to his pediatrician with complaints of "tugging" his ears, nasal draining, and a cough. The assessment was bilateral otitis media, resolving. At this visit, Thomas received a number of vaccinations including the mumps-measles-rubella ("MMR") and Varivax vaccines. At his

18-month check-up, on April 24, 2008, Thomas's physical exam was normal except for slight edema of his nose. Thomas was noted to be healthy, and his 18-month ASQ reflected normal development.

On October 2, 2008, Thomas, age two, received a second full dose of the Varivax vaccine at the Stanly County Health Department. Approximately two weeks later, on October 16, 2008, Thomas was brought to his pediatrician by his mother, with complaints of fever, cough, runny nose, mouth lesions and mouth pain, decreased appetite, and an episode of shaking for approximately 10 minutes. While in the pediatrician's office, Thomas began having tonic/clonic seizures. Initially, his temperature was 100.9°F auxiliary, but it increased to 104.4°F. Thomas continued having seizures and EMS was called.

Thomas was taken from the pediatrician's office by ambulance to the Stanly Regional Emergency Department. On arrival at 1:39 P.M., Thomas was having a seizure and was unresponsive. Thomas was noted to be listless, post-ictal and unresponsive. At 3:39 P.M., he was in severe respiratory distress with rhonchi and wheezing. Thomas was intubated. Thomas was diagnosed as having status epilepticus, seizure disorder, fever, bacteremia, and pneumonitis.

At approximately 3:45 P.M., Thomas was taken by air transport from the Stanly Regional Emergency Room to the Carolinas Medical Center Pediatric Intensive Care Unit ("PICU").

On his first night in the PICU, October 16, 2008, Thomas had questionable seizure activity of symmetric, rhythmic jerking of his legs and smacking of his lips. An electroencephalogram ("EEG") was conducted on October 17, 2008, and revealed right frontal epileptiform activity. The laboratory studies were significant for elevated liver function levels, and a diagnosis of hepatitis was made.

On October 16, 2008, an initial assessment performed in the PICU revealed that Thomas had multiple ulcers on his lips with dried blood. These were also described as "several labial [mouth] ulcers." On October 18, 2008, Dr. Ahmed documented two lesions on Thomas's lips and three "crusted vesicular lesions." On October 19, 2008, the medical records state that Thomas's lip lesions and left auricle (ear) blisters had resolved. In the neurologist's progress note dated October 21, 2008, an erythematous skin rash was documented. The neurologist noted, "Question whether drug eruption or part of underlying possible infectious process."

From October 17 to 18, 2008, Thomas's neurological examinations were abnormal, and he was unresponsive. On October 18, 2008, Dr. Amina Ahmed diagnosed Thomas with meningoencephalitis and hepatitis. Tests for herpes simplex virus, enterovirus, Rocky Mountain Spotted Fever, Bartonella, cytomegalovirus, Toxoplasma, Epstein-Barr Virus, lymphocytic choriomeningitis virus and Arbovirus were negative. Additionally, bacterial and viral cultures of Thomas's blood, urine and stool were negative. There is no documentation which establishes that any of the health care providers who were treating Thomas at the time were aware that he had received the varicella vaccine two weeks prior.

On October 19, 2008, Thomas again experienced jerking of his legs and smacking of his lips. A video EEG showed suppression consistent with diffuse encephalopathy of a nonspecific nature. A repeat CT scan showed progressive loss of gray-white matter differentiation. While in the PICU, Thomas experienced episodes of teeth grinding, moaning, posturing and hypertonicity. He was intubated from October 21 to 24, 2008, due to a decline in his neurological status. An EEG performed on October 22, 2008, showed diffuse disorganization, suppression and slow brain waves, but no epileptic activity.

On October 28, 2008, Thomas was diagnosed with meningoencephalitis of unclear etiology. On October 31, 2008, the PICU attending physician diagnosed Thomas with an altered mental status secondary to a "viral meningoencephalitis." On November 2, 2008, Thomas was noted to be "neurologically devastated, likely secondary to viral meningoencephalitis."

Thomas was discharged from the Carolinas Medical Center on November 5, 2008. His discharge diagnoses included meningoencephalitis, new onset of seizures, and hepatitis. Thomas was transferred to a rehabilitation facility for physical therapy, occupational and speech therapy.

On April 17, 2009, Ms. Haigler called Thomas's pediatrician Dr. Linda Lawrence to report that Thomas had received a vaccine on October 2, 2008, and then had "an episode" on October 16, 2008, where he "broke out in blisters around his mouth and ears." Ms. Haigler asked if the varicella vaccine could have caused her son's encephalitis. She further stated that "her family physician told her that the varicella vaccine probably could have caused encephalitis." Dr. Lawrence reviewed Thomas's vaccine history, and noted that the vaccine given to him on October 2, 2008, was not his first varicella vaccine. Dr. Lawrence, or someone in her office, documented that the "medical opinion was that vaccine did not cause encephalitis."

Petitioners subsequently sought a second opinion regarding the cause of and treatment for Thomas's seizures. On April 23, 2009, Thomas was seen by Dr. Jean-Ronel Corbier, a neurologist, at his Northeast Pediatric Neurology office. Dr. Corbier diagnosed Thomas with encephalitis, encephalopathy and partial complex seizures. Dr. Corbier subsequently reviewed Thomas's medical records and ordered and reviewed his diagnostic studies.

On September 28, 2009, Dr. Corbier noted that a brain MRI performed on Thomas on August 21, 2009, showed global atrophy, and that an EEG performed on the same day showed "diffuse epileptiform discharges and slowing" compatibility with a "diffuse underlying encephalopathy." On November 9, 2009, Dr. Corbier interpreted a 24 hour video EEG performed of Thomas as showing "frequent, multifocal and generalized epileptiform discharges that at times were almost continuous." In February 2010, Thomas was diagnosed with cortical blindness.

Based on the most recent medical records from 2010, Thomas continues to have seizures, has a gastrostomy tube for nutrition, has limited motor function, and is non-verbal.

On April 1, 2013, the parties filed a joint stipulation of undisputed facts. Among other things, "[t]he parties agree that Thomas received his first varicella vaccine on November 13, 2007, and a second dose . . . on October 2, 2008." They also agree that "Thomas suffered from encephalitis and that his parents first sought medical treatment for this condition on October 16, 2008." Varicella, commonly known as chickenpox, is a member of the herpes virus family, and is caused by the varicella zoster virus ("VZV"). Potential complications of a VZV infection include neurologic complications, including encephalitis and meningitis.

To receive compensation under the Program, petitioners must prove . . . that Thomas suffered an injury that was actually caused by the varicella vaccine.

PETITIONERS' EXPERT, DR. CORBIER

Dr. Corbier became Thomas's treating pediatric neurologist in April of 2009.

Dr. Corbier opined that Thomas's October 2, 2008 varicella vaccination caused him to develop meningoencephalitis, which resulted in prolonged seizures, "global developmental delay, hypoxic ischemic encephalopathy, and very refractory epilepsy." Dr. Corbier considers all of these injuries to be part of a more generalized seizure disorder. Dr. Corbier describes Thomas's current condition as "a severe, ongoing seizure disorder . . . along with severe neurological regression . . . which persists till this day."

Dr. Corbier testified as follows:

While the research has shown that while rare, it's not a common occurrence at all, but while rare, in certain cases vaccination, including in kids with varicella, can lead to devastating neurological complications, including meningoencephalitis . . . So based on all of this information, my conclusion has been and still continues to be that the varicella vaccine much more likely than not contributed to Thomas Haigler's devastating change as far as meningoencephalitis, hypoxic ischemic encephalopathy, and the devastation that we see today.

MEDICAL LITERATURE

Dr. Corbier cites several studies which support his opinion that individuals may develop an infection after a varicella vaccination, which can lead to the development of meningoencephalitis and resulting neurological complications, including seizures.

Dr. Corbier cited the Chouliaras article, a case report of "an immunocompetent 3½ year old girl who developed encephalitis and herpes zoster opthalmieus 20 months after her immunization with varicella zoster virus vaccine." The authors concluded that the "[VZV] vaccine strain may cause encephalitis in children even in the absence of underlying immunodeficiency."

Dr. Corbier also referenced the Iyer article, where the authors described a case of "vaccine associated aseptic meningitis after herpes zoster in a previously healthy child." The authors noted that "serious adverse events have occasionally been reported with vaccine-strain varicella-zoster virus," and that the "varicella zoster virus has increasingly been implicated in central nervous system ('CNS') infections in immunocompetent individuals as well."

Dr. Corbier also referenced the Chaves article*. The authors of this article found that 5% of documented adverse events associated with the varicella vaccine were "serious." These adverse events included meningitis, fever, encephalopathy, and seizures.

Finally, Dr. Corbier referenced the Koskiniemi collaborative study, which found that the "[v]aricella-zoster virus . . . was the main agent associated with encephalitis," in a study of "3231 patients with acute central nervous system . . . symptoms of suspected viral origin." The authors found that "VZV seems to have achieved a major role in viral infections of [the central nervous system]."

RESPONDENT'S EXPERT, DR. HOLMES
Dr. Gregory Holmes, also a pediatric neurologist, testified on behalf of respondent.

Dr. Holmes estimated that he has treated five to seven patients for varicella encephalitis, and has seen "a lot of post-infectious varicella problems." None of the patients, however, had developed varicella encephalitis secondary to a vaccine.

Dr. Holmes asserted that Thomas's vaccination did not cause his injuries, although he agreed that the varicella vaccine can cause neurologic injuries, including those from which Thomas suffers. Dr. Holmes agrees with Dr. Corbier that medical reports have documented a causal relationship between the varicella vaccine and encephalitis.

He testified that the varicella vaccine contains a live virus that "could invade the central nervous system" and cause encephalitis. Although he considered it "[e]xtremely rare . . . in people that are not immunocompromised," Dr. Holmes agreed that the varicella vaccine can cause an individual to develop both encephalitis and an encephalopathy through a direct or primary varicella infection.

PETITIONERS' EXPERT, DR. CORBIER

---

* Sandra S. Chaves et al., "Safety of Varicella Vaccine after Licensure in the United States: Experience from Reports to the Vaccine Adverse Event Reporting System, 1995-2005," 197 J. Infectious Diseases S170 (2008)

Dr. Corbier opines that there is a logical sequence of cause and effect between Thomas's vaccination and his encephalitis. First, Dr. Corbier states that Thomas exhibited signs and symptoms of an infectious process shortly after his second varicella vaccination on October 2, 2008, including blisters, fever, and seizures. Dr. Corbier testified that:

Well, the logical sequence is that a young child is given a live attenuated vaccine. The vaccine is shown under—based on the information that we have in rare cases to in some patients lead to certain neurological complications. We know that Thomas was given two doses [of the varicella vaccine] that were fairly close together and . . . two weeks later he developed blisters and other changes to suggest that perhaps he developed complications from the varicella vaccine. So I believe there is a logical sequence there of events.

Dr. Corbier also based his causation opinion on the fact that Thomas had "an extensive workup which included lumbar puncture, neuroimaging, and various labs, was diagnosed with meningoencephalitis . . . and had evidence of hepatitis," and that there was no other viral explanation found for his illness." Various viruses were ruled out during Thomas's hospitalization, including HSV, EBV, LMCV, adenoviruses, Bartonella, and Arbovirus. There is no evidence to suggest that Thomas was exposed to any virus other than the VZV within a medically appropriate time frame.

Lastly, Dr. Corbier considered the time frame within which Thomas's injuries manifested after his vaccination as strong support for his opinion that they are vaccine-related. Thomas rapidly became more ill and "quickly went on to develop severe epilepsy and global devastation." Based on the timeline, Dr. Corbier opined that Thomas's clinical course provided circumstantial evidence of a "clear-cut event" of vaccine-induced harm.

EVALUATION OF THE EVIDENCE

Dr. Corbier's opinion regarding causation is straightforward. After receiving the varicella vaccine, with a live attenuated virus, Thomas developed a varicella infection, either through direct infection or reactivation, which caused encephalitis. He then developed severe epilepsy and global neurological devastation.

It is uncontested that Thomas was exposed to varicella through the vaccination, and the treating physicians and experts agree that his encephalitis is most likely due to a viral infection. As discussed, Thomas's clinical course was consistent with viral encephalitis, and there is no evidence of exposure to any other virus that would have caused it. The most likely viruses were tested for and ruled out, except that no specific testing was performed for the VZV. The only known virus to which Thomas was exposed was the VZV contained in his subject vaccination.

All of these factual findings provide sufficient circumstantial evidence for the undersigned to conclude that Thomas's subject vaccine more likely than not caused his encephalitis and resultant injuries.

CONCLUSION

For the reasons discussed above, the undersigned finds that petitioners are entitled to compensation because they have provided sufficient circumstantial evidence that preponderates in their favor.

IT IS SO ORDERED.

Katea D. Stitt, as Personal Representative of the Estate of Pamela Wanga Stitt, Petitioner v. Secretary of the Department of Health and Human Services, Respondent

Summary: In this case decision, Special Master Zane rules after a hearing that the petitioner died as a result of vaccine induced Guillain-Barré syndrome ("GBS").

Compensated Vaccine Injury: Guillain-Barré Syndrome ("GBS") Leading to Death

Guillain-Barré syndrome is a disorder in which the body's immune system attacks part of the peripheral nervous system. The first symptoms of this disorder include varying degrees of weakness or tingling sensations in the legs. In many instances, the weakness and abnormal sensations spread to the arms and upper body. These symptoms can increase in intensity until the muscles cannot be used at all and the patient is almost totally paralyzed. In these cases, the disorder is life-threatening and is considered a medical emergency. The patient is often put on a ventilator to assist with breathing. Most patients, however, recover from even the most severe cases of

Guillain-Barré syndrome (GBS), although some continue to have some degree of weakness. Guillain-Barré syndrome is rare.

Case No: 09-653V

Date Filed: May 31, 2013

Katea D. Stitt, as Personal Representative of the Estate of Pamela Wanga Stitt, Petitioner v. Secretary of the Department of Health and Human Services, Respondent

Case No: 09-653V

Date Filed: May 31, 2013

RULING ON ENTITLEMENT

Special Master Zane

This matter is before the undersigned on the issue of entitlement following a hearing. Petitioner, Katea D. Stitt ("Petitioner"), as the personal representative of the estate of her mother, Pamela Wanga Stitt ("Mrs. Stitt"), filed this petition alleging that the trivalent influenza ("flu") vaccination Mrs. Stitt received on September 25, 2008, caused Mrs. Stitt to develop Guillain-Barré Syndrome ("GBS"), which then caused her death. Petitioner seeks compensation pursuant to the National Childhood Vaccine Injury Act.

Petitioner contends that the evidence shows that it is more probable than not that the flu vaccine was a substantial factor in causing Mrs. Stitt's GBS and subsequent death. Petitioner relies on molecular mimicry as the medical theory that causally connects the flu vaccine to GBS. Petitioner argues that Mrs. Stitt's clinical picture and the results of diagnostic tests demonstrate a logical sequence of cause and effect showing the flu vaccine caused Mrs. Stitt's GBS. Finally, Petitioner maintains that the 5½ weeks between the vaccine and Mrs. Stitt's hospitalization are within the standard, medically acceptable time frame of six weeks between infection and onset of symptoms. Petitioner argues that she has satisfied her burden and shown by preponderant evidence that the flu vaccine caused her GBS, which, in turn, caused her death.

Respondent argues that Petitioner has not satisfied her burden of proof. Although Respondent acknowledges that Mrs. Stitt's GBS was one of the causes of her death, Respondent claims that Petitioner has failed to satisfy her burden of showing the flu vaccine caused Mrs. Stitt's GBS. Respondent contends that Petitioner's presentation of molecular mimicry as a theory is inadequate because Petitioner has failed to identify a specific protein in the peripheral myelin as being similar to the antigen in the flu vaccine as evidence that molecular mimicry could occur. Respondent also contends that because Petitioner could not point to any direct evidence that would specifically identify the vaccine as the cause, Petitioner did not present sufficient evidence to show a logical sequence of cause and effect. Respondent further claims that Petitioner also failed to show a logical sequence because epidemiological evidence indicates that in a majority of GBS cases, the cause is an infection. As a result, Respondent claims that the cause of Mrs. Stitt's GBS is more likely to be something other than the vaccine. Thus, according to Respondent, Petitioner fails to present sufficient evidence that the vaccine was a substantial factor in causing Mrs. Stitt's GBS and subsequent death.

For the reasons set forth below, upon review of the record as a whole, the undersigned concludes that Petitioner has satisfied her burden. She has shown by preponderant evidence that the vaccine was a substantial factor in bringing about Mrs. Stitt's GBS. And Mrs. Stitt's GBS was a substantial factor in bringing about her death. Petitioner is entitled to compensation.

FACTS
The facts as evidenced by the records and testimony are as follows:

Mrs. Stitt received an influenza ("flu") vaccination on September 25, 2008, at her local Safeway store. She was 74. At that time, Mrs. Stitt's medical condition was generally healthy, although she did have hypertension. Mrs. Stitt's medical history indicated that she had had gallbladder surgery and intermittent lower back pain over the last few years. Mrs. Stitt had also had some specific orthopedic issues, i.e., rotator cuff problems and a twisted ankle. Approximately a week after she received the flu vaccine, on October 2, 2008, Mrs. Stitt went to her orthopedist, Dr. Moskovitz, for a follow-up on her right knee and left shoulder pain (Rotator Cuff Syndrome). At that time, Mrs. Stitt mentioned a new complaint, i.e., stiffness and pain in both her hands and in her fingers, with the symptoms being greater in her right versus her left hand and fingers.

On October 30, 2008, Mrs. Stitt visited her primary care physician/internist, Dr. George Graves, for a follow-up on her hypertension. Mrs. Stitt reiterated the complaint she had made to her orthopedist of tingling in her hand up to her elbow for the past month. She denied complaints of chest pain, shortness of breath, and cough. There was no indication of any complaints of stomach problems, nausea, diarrhea or vomiting.

A few days later, on November 3, 2008, Mrs. Stitt telephoned her doctor complaining of tingling in her hands and feet. Later that same day, Mrs. Stitt was admitted to Sibley Hospital due to leg weakness. At the time of her admission, Mrs. Stitt told the admitting personnel that she had had leg weakness since the morning, that her knees buckled twice, and that she experienced shortness of breath and polyuria.

Upon admission, Dr. Mahgoub, a neurologist, provided a consult. He specifically noted that Mrs. Stitt had received a flu vaccine four weeks before admission and that the differential diagnosis, which included GBS, was well described. Having noted the receipt of the flu vaccine and possible GBS diagnosis, Dr. Mahgoub noted that the Centers for Disease Control ("CDC") and Food and Drug Administration ("FDA") had not issued an alert in connection with the flu vaccine. Nonetheless, Dr. Mahgoub made a note to contact the CDC out of concern regarding the vaccine being a possible cause. Mrs. Stitt's laboratory tests showed an elevated glucose level and elevated liver enzymes with otherwise normal results. Mrs. Stitt continued to experience leg weakness, as well as weakness in her arms.

On November 6, 2008, the results from an electrodiagnostic study confirmed that Mrs. Stitt's presentation was consistent with GBS. Mrs. Stitt was treated with a two-day course of IVIG. Because she developed shallow breathing and an increased respiratory rate on that day, Mrs. Stitt was intubated. Within a day, Mrs. Stitt developed what was diagnosed as staphylococcus pneumonia. She was treated with antibiotics. Mrs. Stitt also developed a fever and an elevated white blood cell count.

Beginning November 10, 2008, Mrs. Stitt's strength in her extremities began to return and her breathing improved. However, it was also determined that Mrs. Stitt had developed hemolytic anemia due to her IVIG treatment. As a result, her IVIG treatment was stopped after just two courses.

By November 12, 2008, Mrs. Stitt's pneumonia had resolved. Later that day, Mrs. Stitt was removed from the ventilator. Mrs. Stitt was noted to be "doing quite well" and to have a good voice. On November 13, 2008, Mrs. Stitt was again noted to be "doing well," "breathing easily," and "swallowing without difficulty," and her pneumonia had resolved. Plans were made to transfer Mrs. Stitt to the National Rehabilitation Hospital.

On November 14, 2008, Mrs. Stitt was discharged from Sibley Hospital to the National Rehabilitation Hospital. The discharge summary indicated that Mrs. Stitt was diagnosed with, *inter alia,* GBS. The doctors told Petitioner that Mrs. Stitt's GBS was caused either by the flu vaccine or some other unidentified infection.

On November 16, 2008, while at the National Rehabilitation Hospital, Mrs. Stitt experienced severe respiratory distress and was transported to Washington Hospital Center. Mrs. Stitt was intubated. A chest X-ray revealed bibasal infiltrates and an echocardiography demonstrated a nearly collapsed ventricle suggestive of hypovolemia (defined as an abnormally decreased volume of circulating blood in the body; the most common cause is hemorrhage). An evaluation for cardiac arrest revealed that Ms. Stitt had a cardiomyopathy (a general diagnostic term designating primary noninflammatory disease of the heart muscle, often of obscure or unknown etiology).

On the following day, November 17, 2008, Mrs. Stitt's EKG tests revealed changes in her ST-elevation and increased enzymes. She received cardiac catheterization, which revealed non-obstructive coronary artery disease, elevated right heart filling pressures, and takotsubo with severe liver dysfunction. Mrs. Stitt's lab results revealed no abnormalities in her stool cultures.

Mrs. Stitt was placed on a ventilator, and on November 18, 2008, she suffered hypoxic respiratory failure while on the ventilator. Mrs. Stitt was determined to have takotsubo syndrome with functional obstruction of liver outflow.

There was no change in Mrs. Stitt's status the next day, November 19, 2008. Later on November 19, 2008, Mrs. Stitt began to experience worsening hypotension due to sepsis versus takotsubo cardiomyopathy. Mrs. Stitt's mental status worsened and her family decided that she should not be resuscitated. Ms. Stitt died on November 20, 2008. Her causes of death were listed as: (A) Cardiogenic shock; (B) Cardiomyopathy; (C) GBS; and (D) Pneumonia. An autopsy was performed on January 12, 2009. The autopsy report listed the causes of death as, *inter alia,* (1) Septic shock with respiratory failure (clinical) and (2) GBS (clinical).

The parties stipulated that Mrs. Stitt had been diagnosed with GBS at the time of her discharge from Sibley Hospital to the National Rehabilitation Hospital. The parties also stipulated that the medical records listed GBS as a cause of her death. Finally, the parties stipulated that the autopsy report identified GBS as one of the causes of Mrs. Stitt's death.

DISCUSSION
A. Petitioner Has Presented Sufficient Proof of a Medical Theory Causally Connecting the Flu Vaccine to Mrs. Stitt's GBS, Satisfying *Althen*'s Prong One.

B. Petitioner Has Provided Sufficient Evidence Which Demonstrates a Logical Sequence of Cause and Effect Showing the Vaccine Was a Substantial Factor Leading to Mrs. Stitt's GBS, Satisfying *Althen*'s Prong Two.

C. Petitioner Has Shown That Mrs. Stitt's GBS Occurred Within a Medically Acceptable Time Frame, Thereby, Satisfying *Althen*'s Prong Three.

CONCLUSION
For the reasons stated above, the evidence presented demonstrates that the flu vaccine Mrs. Stitt received was a substantial factor in causing Mrs. Stitt's GBS. And, her GBS was a substantial factor in causing her death. Petitioner has established entitlement to compensation under the Vaccine Act.

IT IS SO ORDERED.

Walter Ray Graves, and Lisa Graves as Representatives of the Estate of Hayley Nicole Graves, Deceased, v. Secretary of the Department of Health and Human Services

Summary: In this case, Merow, Senior Judge Merrow rules, upon review after a hearing that the Prevnar ꞏꞏꞏꞏꞏꞏ ꞏꞏꞏꞏꞏ ꞏꞏꞏ ꞏꞏꞏꞏꞏ ꞏꞏꞏꞏꞏꞏ ꞏꞏꞏ ꞏꞏꞏꞏꞏꞏ death.

Compensated Vaccine Injury: Status Epilepticus, Leading to Death

PREVNAR

Case No: 02-0211V

Date Filed: February 25, 2013

Walter Ray Graves, and Lisa Graves as Representatives of the Estate of Hayley Nicole Graves, Deceased, v. Secretary of the Department of Health and Human Services

Merow, Senior Judge

Following the death of their infant daughter Hayley, petitioners Walter and Lisa Graves allege that a Prevnar vaccination on August 8, 2000, caused the onset of Hayley's seizures two days later. She was hospitalized immediately and continually thereafter for twenty-nine days, primarily in pediatric intensive care. Despite a battery of tests, treatment and examination by specialists, Hayley's seizures were unremitting and she died on September 24, 2000. Her death certificate documents the immediate cause of death as "[s]tatus epilepticus," and an underlying cause as "[i]ntractable seizures." Neither Hayley nor her family had a prior history of seizures.

FACTS

Hayley Graves was born on November 4, 1999 in Ft. Worth, Texas. At her well-baby check-up when she was five months old no physical abnormalities were noted. She had attained all developmental milestones.

At that August 8, 2000 appointment, at approximately 11:15 a.m., Hayley received a Hepatitis B and her second Prevnar vaccination.

According to the affidavit of Hayley's mother, Lisa Graves, filed with the Petition in this matter, the remainder of August 8, 2000, Hayley acted normally. On August 9, 2000, she was restless and stayed awake until about 10:30 or 11:00 p.m. Early on the morning of August 10, 2000, Hayley woke up about 6:45 a.m. and, according to the affidavit: "she did not appear right. The left side of her body was moving and it would not stop. We called the doctor's office and waited for a return call; however, at 7:15 a.m. when we still had not heard back from the doctor's office, we left for Cook's Children[s] Medical Center."

Hayley was admitted and transferred to the pediatric intensive care unit ("PICU") under the care of Dr. Brian Ryals, a pediatric neurologist. An EEG showed "ongoing electrical seizure activity emanating from right central brain regions." An MRI and CT scan were normal. Because barbiturate doses were prescribed, she was intubated, ventilated, and an arterial line was placed. She was continuously monitored and received regular doses of anticonvulsant medication, but her seizures did not stop.

Hayley remained in intensive care until transferred to a "regular" room for about five days until noon on August 29, 2000, when she was airlifted to the Hermann Hospital Epileptic Center in Houston, Texas for evaluation and treatment by Dr. James W. Wheless, Chief of Pediatric Neurology at the University of Tennessee College of Medicine, who later testified in these proceedings that Prevnar could and did cause her seizures and did so within a medically appropriate time.

For twenty-six days at Hermann Hospital, Hayley was evaluated by several specialists; multiple attempts were made to control her seizures without success. Tragically, her seizures which started the early morning of August 10, 2000, never stopped and Hayley died in the pediatric intensive care unit of the Hermann Hospital on September 24, 2000.

Hayley's death certificate recorded her cause of death as "[s]tatus epilepticus," caused by "[i]ntractable seizures." An autopsy performed on September 29, 2000, concluded that Hayley "died as a result of hypoxic encephalopathy which reportedly occurred following a seizure which developed following a meningitis [sic] vaccine."

PROCEDURAL BACKGROUND

Dr. Wheless was concerned that the Prevnar vaccination was the cause for Hayley's death and he referred petitioners to the office of Richard Gage. (Tr. 272- 74.) Petitioners filed a petition for vaccine injury compensation on September 16, 2002, alleging that Hayley suffered seizures and death as a result of receiving Prevnar and Hepatitis B vaccinations on August 8, 2000.

On December 26, 2007, petitioners filed a report from Hayley's treating pediatric neurologist and pediatric epilepsy specialist, Dr. James W. Wheless. Dr. Wheless opined:

Prevnar vaccine is known to cause seizures, both afebrile and febrile (without and with a fever) and these can be serious, and potentially even lead to death. It is my medical opinion that Hayley's vaccine was associated with the onset of her seizures, which proved to be intractable and her acute encephalopathy, which then progressed to chronic encephalopathy accompanied by an intractable seizure disorder, and ultimately this was fatal and responsible for her death. An extensive evaluation was performed, including obtaining her brain post-mortem, and after examining this no other cause could be found. It is established that Prevnar vaccine can contribute to this type of injury. Prevnar is established as causing this type of injury and, in this case, it is also my belief that the vaccine did cause this injury.

It is my opinion, based on a reasonable degree of medical probability, that the Prevnar vaccination, which Hayley Graves received when she was nine months old, caused her severe refractory seizure disorder that caused her death. This is a causation-in-fact opinion and is based on my role as her treating physician and as an expert in the field of pediatric epilepsy.

Giving appropriate credit to the opinion of Dr. Wheless, the treating pediatric neurologist, and given the absence of any other reason for the sudden onset of Hayley's intractable seizures which, despite her continuous specialized hospitalization, litany of tests and treatments and examination by specialists did not stop, the preponderant credible evidence bar of causation was met.

CONCLUSION

For the reasons stated herein, the court concludes that on the record as a whole, petitioners presented sufficient evidence to meet the Vaccine Act's preponderant standard for causation of the biological plausibility of the Prevnar vaccine triggering the onset of seizures, as well as increased duration and intractability of seizures, supported by reliable medical literature and expert testimony including that of Dr. Wheless, Hayley's treating physician.

The record evidence established a medical theory causally connecting the Prevnar vaccination with the instigation as well as the duration and intractability of the seizures which resulted in Hayley's death. A logical sequence of cause and effect was established that the Prevnar vaccine did cause the instigation of Hayley's seizures and the increased duration and intractability within an appropriate time frame.

Accordingly, the court determines that entitlement has been proven.

IT IS SO ORDERED.

Michael Stephen Saw, Petitioner v. Secretary of the Department of Health and Human Services, Respondent

Summary: In this decision following a hearing, Chief Special Master Patricia E. Campbell-Smith rules that the victim suffered a small nerve fiber neuropathy as a result of a hepatitis B vaccine.

Compensated Vaccine Injury: Small Nerve Fiber Neuropathy

Small Nerve Fiber Neuropathy; Finding of Entitlement to Compensation

Case No: 01-0707V

Date Filed: May 24, 2013

Michael Stephen Saw, Petitioner v. Secretary of the Department of Health and Human Services, Respondent

RULING ON ENTITLEMENT

Patricia E. Campbell-Smith
Chief Special Master

This case is before the undersigned on remand. The issue before the undersigned is whether the Hepatitis B vaccines that petitioner, Michael Shaw, received on May 5, 1999, and June 11, 1999, caused him to suffer a small nerve fiber neuropathy. The undersigned finds, by a preponderance of the evidence, that petitioner's vaccinations caused his injury.

In so finding, the undersigned notes that this ruling represents a "close call" and should accordingly be resolved in favor of petitioner.

PROCEDURAL HISTORY

On December 20, 2001, petitioner filed a petition pursuant to the National Injury Compensation Program (Vaccine Program or Program), wherein he alleged that his Hepatitis B vaccinations caused him to suffer a neuropathy. Thereafter, petitioner submitted an expert report opining that he either suffered the condition of transverse myelitis ("TM") or of chronic inflammatory demyelinating polyneuropathy ("CIDP") as a result of his vaccinations.

An evidentiary hearing was convened on March 12, 2008, to elicit the testimony of Sherri Tenpenny, D.O., an osteopathic physician, on behalf of petitioner, and Thomas Leist, M.D., a neurologist, on behalf of respondent. In a decision filed August 31, 2009, the undersigned found that petitioner failed to demonstrate entitlement to compensation. Specifically, the undersigned found that petitioner did not suffer from either of the conditions TM or CIDP as his expert, Dr. Tenpenny, had asserted in her theory of vaccine-related causation. Accordingly, the undersigned found that petitioner failed to establish a logical sequence of cause and effect as then presented, and denied compensation. Pivotal to the undersigned's finding of no entitlement in Shaw I was the finding, after a careful review, that to the extent petitioner's injury was a neurologic one, petitioner's medical records indicated that the more likely consensus diagnosis was a small fiber neuropathy. But, as Dr. Leist testified at the March 12, 2008 hearing, "small nerve fibers lack the myelin sheaths that would be harmed by the [petitioner's] proposed demyelination process." Petitioner did not rebut this testimony. Thus, relying on the unrefuted testimony of Dr. Leist, the undersigned found that petitioner's proposed theory of causation, demyelination, failed when applied to The National Vaccine Injury Compensation Program is set forth in Part 2 of the National Childhood Vaccine Injury Act of 1986.

On September 21, 2009, petitioner filed a Motion for Reconsideration of Shaw I, asserting that the undersigned's Decision was not in accordance with the law and seeking to introduce evidence, previously available but not filed, that small nerve fibers "may well" be myelinated. The undersigned denied the Motion for Reconsideration explaining that the evidence concerning small fibers was available to the petitioner two years prior to the filing of the expert report by Dr. Tenpenny and at the time of the hearing. The undersigned observed that the inability of petitioner to rebut the testimony of Dr. Leist was attributable "directly to Dr. Tenpenny's acknowledged lack of expertise in neurological matters." Moreover, the undersigned noted that the newly presented information regarding myelinated small nerve fibers was not persuasive "in the absence of any evidence presented by petitioner regarding how this evidence supports the theory of causation proposed by petitioner in this case for the specific injuries of TM and CIDP that Dr. Tenpenny's opinion contemplated."

Petitioner moved the United States Court of Federal Claims to review the undersigned's decision. Motion for Review filed September 30, 2009. On review, the court determined that the Shaw I decision—was "thorough and well reasoned"—in finding that petitioner neither suffered TM or CIDP, but rather a small fiber neuropathy. The reviewing judge upheld the undersigned's finding that the unrebutted testimony at hearing established that "Mr. Shaw's medical theory, demyelination, was incapable of causing small fiber neuropathy." However, the court concluded that "in light of the purposes and structure of the Vaccine Act, we find it in the interest of justice for the [undersigned] to consider the effect of the newly offered evidence." The court left to the discretion of the undersigned the decision whether to re-open the record beyond allowing consideration of the new evidence and permitting respondent's expert Dr. Leist an opportunity to comment on that evidence.

On remand and after consultation with the parties, the undersigned afforded petitioner an opportunity to retain an expert in neurology to explain how the newly offered evidence supported petitioner's theory of the case. Respondent's expert, Dr. Leist, also was offered an opportunity to address the newly presented evidence. Order filed March 12, 2010. Petitioner ultimately offered the opinion of Thomas Morgan, M.D., a neurologist, in support of his vaccine claim. Respondent again offered the neurologic expertise of Dr. Leist, who challenged petitioner's newly asserted theory of causation.

Another expert hearing was conducted on July 28, 2010 in Washington, D.C. The undersigned sought the testimony of Drs. Morgan and Leist on the issue of whether or not petitioner developed a small fiber neuropathy as a result of his Hepatitis B vaccine series. On remand, Mr. Shaw continued to rely on a theory of causation in fact. In support of his claim, he has filed: (1) an affidavit, (2) medical records, (3) the medical opinion of Dr. Morgan, (4) supporting medical literature, and (5) post-hearing briefs. Respondent offered: (1) the expert opinion of Dr. Leist, (2) a number of medical articles, and (3) a post-hearing memorandum to rebut petitioner's claim.

FACTS

The facts set forth below are largely derived from the undersigned's recitation of the acts in Shaw I. In general, the parties do not dispute the facts of this case, but rather the medical and legal conclusions to be drawn from them. As directed by the Vaccine Act, the undersigned has carefully considered, in addition to all other relevant medical and scientific evidence contained in the record, the diagnoses, conclusions, and medical judgments contained in the record regarding the nature, causation and aggravation of petitioner's condition as well as the results of diagnostic tests contained in the record. Declining to review here the entirety of petitioner's voluminous medical records, the undersigned focuses on the records upon which the parties have relied most heavily.

Petitioner was born on June 15, 1959. His medical history is most notable for a couple of concussive head injuries, a cracked pelvis, a chipped tailbone, a fractured nose, and broken hands and feet. Prior to receiving the vaccinations at issue in this case, petitioner traveled extensively in his professional capacity as the corporate general manager for a large, multi-national trading firm. He had responsibilities for approximately 30 offices throughout the Asian Pacific region. Recreationally, Mr. Shaw enjoyed extreme sports activities, including motor cross riding, mountain biking, roller-blading, hang gliding, parachuting, rafting and mountain climbing. He also enjoyed golf, tennis, skiing, softball and basketball.

In anticipation of scheduled business travel and as part of an employment-related immunization program, Mr. Shaw received his first Hepatitis B vaccination on May 5, 1999. He did not recall experiencing any effects after that vaccination. The next month, on June 11, 1999, he received his second Hepatitis B vaccination and a polio vaccination. The medical records indicate that on June 21, 1999, 10 days after receiving the Hepatitis B vaccination of interest, petitioner visited his primary care physician, John Roberts, M.D., of Blackhawk Medical Group, complaining of recurring numbness in his right leg below the knee. Petitioner reported that the numbness had begun on June 17, 1999, four days prior to his visit to Dr. Roberts and six days after he had received his second Hepatitis B vaccine. The numbness was "now progressing to a throbbing pain." Dr. Roberts noted a patient history of trauma associated with his motor cross riding. Dr. Roberts diagnosed petitioner with lumbar strain and nerve compression. Dr. Roberts prescribed prednisone and urged petitioner to obtain x-rays and magnetic resonance image (MRI) of his back.

Petitioner began an international business trip on June 23, 1999. In his affidavit, prepared on October 17, 2006, he recalled that: By the time I reached my first stop in England, both my feet [and] legs were affected. During business meetings in India, I began to experience tremors in my limbs, cognitive memory/speech problems, and coordination difficulties. Prior to returning home from the two-week trip, my arms were also affected. The symptoms now included not only numbness and tingling but also sharp, shooting, burning, and throbbing pain. I managed to complete the trip in defiance of significant pain. Once home, the pain continued. I experienced numbness in both of my hands and legs and had spasms in my back.

Petitioner underwent imaging of his spine on July 6, 1999. The MRI of his cervical spine produced an impression of early disc degeneration without extrusion. The MRI of his lumbar spine was normal.

On July 9, 1999, three days after his spinal MRIs, petitioner returned to his primary care provider. He complained of flu-like symptoms and of continued numbness in his right leg. Although the office notes reflect a history of numbness in petitioner left leg and hands, only a general time frame of symptom onset is specified (petitioner reporting, during a visit to his primary care physician on October 27, 1999, that his numbness had progressed to all of his extremities in late June). The diagnostic impression at the July 9, 1999 visit was sinusitis and strain in the lumbar and cervical regions of the spine. The examining physician prescribed Lorabid and Xanax and ordered physical therapy.

Treatment Sought During the First Six Months after the Hepatitis B Vaccination
Five weeks later, on August 18, 1999, petitioner visited Samuel Jorgenson,
M.D., an orthopedist. Petitioner reported a two-month history of right foot
pain and intermittent numbness and tingling in his arms, hands, and feet. Petitioner also reported that he did not continue to take the Xanax he had been
prescribed because it caused drowsiness. Dr. Jorgenson's physical examination
revealed a decreased sensation to sharp pin prick in petitioner's right foot when
compared with his left one. It was the orthopedist's assessment that petitioner
had a possible entrapment neuropathy in his lower right extremity. Lorabid is
an antibiotic indicated for the treatment of mild to moderate infections.

Dr. Jorgenson referred petitioner for an electromyogram that was conducted
on September 2, 1999. The electromyogram (or EMG) revealed no evidence
of acute or chronic lumbosacral radiculopathy, plexopathy or peripheral neuropathy. Petitioner had described symptoms of progressive burning pain and
intermittent numbness from his foot to his ankle that, at times, emanated to his
knee. The physician interpreting the EMG results noted that the patient was
most likely exhibiting very early symptoms of idiopathic peripheral neuropathy and recommended a trial of Neurontin to reduce the burning parasthesias.

Approximately two months later, on November 9, 1999, petitioner saw Janet
Lin, a neurologist, on referral from Dr. Roberts, his primary care physician.
Dr. Lin noted that petitioner's neurologic exam was normal except for some
minimal sensory abnormalities in his hands and feet. Although petitioner
reported feeling fatigued, there was no evidence of muscle weakness. Dr. Lin
believed that petitioner was suffering a post-inflammatory neuropathy related
to immunizations. During her examination nearly five months after petitioner
received the subject vaccination, Dr. Lin surmised that the culprit might be
the Hepatitis B immunization that petitioner received because petitioner had
received all the other immunizations previously.

Treatment Sought Over the Next Two Years
Petitioner sought treatment from a variety of specialists over the next two years.
An electromyogram (or EMG) is a test that is used to record the electrical activity
of muscles. When muscles are active, they produce an electrical current. This
current is usually proportional to the level of the muscle activity. . . . EMGs can
be used to detect abnormal electrical activity of muscle that can occur in many

diseases and conditions, including . . . inflammation of muscles, pinched nerves, [and] peripheral nerve damage (damage to nerves in the arms and legs).

On referral from his primary care doctor, petitioner consulted on February 28, 2000 with Benedict Villanueva, M.D., an infectious disease specialist. As reflected in the notes from the consultation, Dr. Roberts had referred petitioner to Dr. Villanueva for an evaluation of whether his symptoms of diffuse sensory neuropathy were a possible post vaccine adverse reaction. The particular vaccine under examination was the polio vaccine—not the Hepatitis B vaccine—that petitioner had received in June 1999. Dr. Villanueva noted that petitioner had a normal EMG, a basically normal MRI of his cervical and lumbar area and, with the exception of a slightly elevated protein level, a normal spinal tap. In Dr. Villanueva's assessment, among the possible etiologies for petitioner's subjective diffuse sensory polyneuropathy would be a rare/remote adverse reaction to the polio vaccine. But, Dr. Villanueva observed, such reactions occur within a few weeks after immunization and, to his knowledge, do not last for several months after the inoculation.

Approximately one month later, petitioner underwent further neurologic examination by Catherine Lomen-Hoerth, M.D., at the University of California in San Francisco. He returned to Dr. Lomen-Hoerth on May 10, 2000, for a follow-up of continuing pain and numbness. Dr. Lomen-Hoerth noted that petitioner's discomfort had progressed and was worse than when she had examined him for the first time one month earlier. It was Dr. Lomen-Hoerth's impression that petitioner had a progressive small fiber neuropathy rather than a static neuropathy related to his vaccinations last summer.

On referral from his neurologist Dr. Lomen-Hoerth, petitioner saw David Martin, M.D., a rheumatologist, on July 31, 2000. The purpose of the referral was to evaluate petitioner's severe fatigue, weight loss, intermittent burning rash on both arms and joint pain. It was Dr. Martin's impression that extensive laboratory work and physical examination failed to produce any clear evidence of connective tissue disease. In his view, petitioner suffered from an idiopathic syndrome associated with chronic fatigue and . . . possibly related to a vaccine exposure or possibly a toxin. Dr. Martin suspected that petitioner's condition had an underlying psychiatric component with possible depression.

On referral from Dr. Lomen-Hoerth, petitioner was examined by Nicholas Maragakis, M.D., a neurologist at John Hopkins Hospital on August 21, 2000, for evaluation of a possible small fiber neuropathy. Dr. Maragakis spinal tap or cerebrospinal fluid (CSF) examination that yields an elevated protein level may be indicative of an underlying infectious or inflammatory process. Noted that petitioner's "exam [was] normal, with the exception of some mild decreased pinprick sensation in the hands and feet, which is often typical for a small fiber neuropathy. Of note, quantitative sensory testing at an outside hospital was essentially normal. I think this most likely represents some form of small fiber neuropathy." In an addendum to his August 21, 2000 report, Dr. Maragakis noted that petitioner's skin biopsy "demonstrated a normal range of epidermal nerve fiber density;" however, he found the biopsy was "suggestive of early nerve fiber degeneration" and that a later biopsy "may be useful."

Over four months later, on January 3, 2001, petitioner presented to the emergency room acting strange and confused and complaining of worsening pain in his extremities. The admission notes indicate that petitioner has a neuropathic condition that has waxed and waned, but is slowly progressive. The admission notes also indicated that petitioner had experienced some changes in mental status, including poor memory, decreased alertness, and diminished concentration. The diagnosis on discharge was acute severe exacerbation of chronic neuropathy pain.

On May 8, 2001, petitioner saw Rex Chiu, M.D., an internist at Stanford Hospital and Clinics, on referral from Dr. Lomen-Hoerth. Dr. Chiu noted that petitioner experienced an onset of numbness and tingling in his left toe six days after receiving a polio vaccination and a Hepatitis B vaccination in anticipation of business travel to India. Petitioner's developing symptoms produced a concern for a post-inflammatory reaction to the immunizations, but a trial course of prednisone provided no relief. Following a series of visits to diverse medical specialists, the consensus diagnosis appears to be small fiber neuropathy. Dr. Chiu wrote that because petitioner's neurologic changes seem to have arisen after his immunization in 1999, there is question as to whether there is some type of autoimmune or other reaction to this vaccination, which may now be worsening in a progressive fashion. Dr. Chiu noted: The patient is Hepatitis B negative, referring to the lack of Hepatitis B antibodies that might be expected to appear. Dr. Chiu planned to refer petitioner for further neurologic and rheumatologic examination at Stanford.

On referral from Dr. Chiu, Yuen So, M.D., a neurologist at Stanford, examined petitioner on July 12, 2001. Dr. So noted that petitioner had seen a number of neurologists over a two-year period. Dr. So further noted that the most disabling feature of petitioner's illness was his diffuse pain. Based on a physical examination of petitioner and a review of petitioner's laboratory test results, Dr. So wrote: It is conceivable that [petitioner] had an acute, predominantly sensory polyneuropathy back in 1999. But without the records of petitioner's medical evaluation during that time period, Dr. So found it difficult to ascribe petitioner's complaint of progressive symptoms since 1999 to the received vaccinations. Disturbing to Dr. So about petitioner's condition was the a very diverse nature of petitioner's symptoms.

Also disturbing to Dr. So was the lack of objective evidence of neuropathic abnormality in a patient who has had ongoing disease for a course of two years. Contrary to normal expectations for a patient suspected of having a prior acute neuropathy, petitioner did not demonstrate a slow and steady course of improvement. Dr. So described the case as a very difficult one to diagnose and to treat.

In September 2001, petitioner and his wife moved from northern California to Delaware. Approximately two months later, on November 8, 2001, petitioner visited Gail Berkenblit, M.D., an internist at Johns Hopkins, for ongoing chronic pain. Dr. Berkenblit conducted a physical examination and reviewed the records that petitioner presented regarding his extensive laboratory work. Dr. Berkenblit took an extensive patient history and noted that petitioner's evaluations have been essentially normal, including his autonomic function testing. Petitioner's initial diagnosis was a possible post inflammatory neuropathy. Subsequently, petitioner received evaluations for a possible small fiber neuropathy. Repeated testing, however, had not disclosed any definite evidence of a small fiber neuropathy. Rather, swelling noticed in the distal leg sites during a neurologic examination at Johns Hopkins by Dr. Nicholas Maragakis was suggestive of early possible nerve fiber degeneration. During the office visit, Dr. Berkenblit addressed concerns expressed by petitioner and his wife that petitioner's symptoms resulted from his Hepatitis B vaccination. Dr. Berkenblit observed that there is no clear link between Hepatitis B vaccination and progressive neuropathic pain, but noted that if petitioner did develop symptoms of a sensory neuropathy as a consequence of the vaccine, it would most likely be as an autoimmune type mechanism and not a vaccine contamination issue as petitioner's wife speculated.

Petitioner filed his vaccine claim on December 20, 2001.

On January 15, 2002, a second skin biopsy was taken from several different places on petitioner's leg. The test result again showed a normal range of epidermal nerve fiber density, offering "no definitive evidence" of a small fiber neuropathy and "no clear progression compared to the August 2000 biopsies."

Three weeks later, on February 7, 2002, petitioner visited Lee Dresser, M.D., a neurologist, for an evaluation. Dr. Dresser noted that previous evaluations by neurologists included an assumption that petitioner had developed a sensory neuropathy as a response to his vaccination but that diagnosis was modified as extensive testing has returned negative results. It was Dr. Dresser's impression that petitioner suffers from diffuse dysesthetic pain following remote vaccinations. Of interest to Dr. Dresser was the finding of a mild elevation of petitioner's spinal fluid protein following petitioner's extensive and otherwise unremarkable testing. Dr. Dresser observed that petitioner's symptoms were essentially 100% subjective with no significant objective findings on . . . testing or examination. Dr. Dresser found petitioner's case to be a very complicated one.

Opinions of Possible Vaccine-Related Causation
To assist petitioner with his pending vaccine claim, Dr. Roberts, the primary care physician who examined petitioner when his symptoms first began in 1999, wrote a letter dated February 13, 2002. Dr. Roberts stated that petitioner had no significant neurologic symptoms prior to the petitioner's receipt of the Hepatitis B vaccination and that petitioner began to develop neurologic complaints shortly after his immunization. Id. It was Dr. Roberts' belief that the temporal relationship between the received vaccination and the onset of petitioner's symptoms strongly correlated with the hypothesis that the symptoms were caused by the vaccination. Thereafter, other treating doctors offered views about what may have caused petitioner's symptoms.

On January 21, 2003, Robert Allen, M.D., an evaluator retained by the defense in connection with the worker's compensation claim filed by petitioner, examined petitioner.

Dr. Allen observed that petitioner's neurologic evaluations (including biopsies) have not documented any progressive neurologic disease. In Dr. Allen's opinion, petitioner's clinical history and physical examination, together with the extensive objective work-up, suggested a diagnosis of fibromyalgia. He explained that the diagnosis of fibromyalgia involves the presence of widespread musculoskeletal pain, as well as multiple tender points . . . that occur both above and below the waist. He stated that the etiology of his fibromyalgia remains unclear and may have developed as a result of the June 1999 vaccinations. But, Dr. Allen acknowledged, such causation is impossible to confirm or deny. Dr. Allen was one of two evaluators to diagnose petitioner with fibromyalgia, a diagnosis that is disputed by petitioner's treating physicians. The diagnosis of fibromyalgia was first considered by the defense evaluator, Dr. Robert Allen. Another defense evaluator, Dr. Charles Skomer, diagnosed a chronic pain condition but allowed that petitioner's symptoms were possibly consistent with a finding of fibromyalgia. But, there is no evidence in either the multiple neurologic or rheumatologic evaluations contained in petitioner's medical records.

On April 29, 2003, Harold Buttram, M.D., an internist with Woodlands Healing Research Center, examined petitioner. Dr. Buttram noted that petitioner had become ill following chelation efforts to eliminate mercury, and subsequent testing indicated that mercury toxicity was not an issue for petitioner. Dr. Buttram further noted that Dr. Tenpenny, the treating physician who testified at the first hearing on petitioner's behalf, had directed petitioner's mercury detoxicification process. Aware that petitioner's vaccine claim was pending, Dr. Buttram wrote: "For the records, it is my opinion that the patient's peripheral neuropathy is directly related to (was caused by) a series of two Hepatitis B vaccines." Noting that petitioner Aha[d] been diagnosed by neurologists as having chronic neuropathic pain, Dr. Buttram prepared an opinion letter dated June 6, 2003, stating that he agreed with the diagnosis of the neurologists and reiterating that petitioner's condition was caused by a series of Hepatitis B vaccines.

On November 4, 2004, petitioner was given a diagnosis of "vaccine-induced neuroimmune dysfunction" by Vincent Natali, M.D., a general practitioner. Thereafter, on December 23, 2004, David Waldman, M.D., another physician, issued an extensive report concerning petitioner's disability status. Dr. Waldman's report was informed by his review of petitioner's medical records, his review of medical literature, and a physical examination of petitioner.

Contained in Dr. Waldman's report was a detailed, chronological summary of petitioner's medical evaluations and laboratory results. Also contained in Dr. Waldman's report was a summary of medical articles that he had reviewed, in connection with his evaluation of petitioner, concerning complications from the Hepatitis B vaccination. Dr. Waldman concluded there is no evidence within the records submitted that, prior to 6/11/99, Mr. Shaw had any neurological injury and was not able to function . . . . After the vaccinations of 6/11/99, Mr. Shaw began a very complex medical history, resulting in a chronic pain disorder syndrome. . . . Mr. Shaw has a problem with pain medicine addiction, which he did not have prior to his industrial injury. As stated within his multiple medical records, as a consequence of his work related chronic pain disorder, he has developed a drug dependence. . . . There is no evidence in review of the medical records that Mr. Shaw has a fibromyalgia syndrome. . . Rather, Mr. Shaw has developed a chronic neuropathic pain syndrome. Although the exact etiology has not been determined, based on the review of the medical records and medical literature, it is with medical probability that this syndrome was a consequence of the vaccinations received on 6/11/99. This opinion that this syndrome occurred post vaccination has also been supported by multiple clinical evaluators . . . including Dr. Janet Lin and Dr. [Catherine] Lomen-Hoerth [two neurologists] at UCSF Medical Center. This has also been supported by recent evaluations which Mr. Shaw has sought to obtain relief from his pain syndrome . . . with multiple sequelae, including drug dependence, and these conditions are industrial in nature.

Pamela P. Palmer, M.D., an anesthesiologist at the UCSF Medical Center's Pain Management Center, examined petitioner nearly nine months later on September 20, 2005. Dr. Palmer assessed petitioner as "a 46 year-old gentleman with six years of diffuse pain after vaccination, consistent with a diffuse small fiber neuropathy."

Four months later, on January 30, 2006, petitioner was evaluated by Phyllis A. Cullen, M.D., an anesthesiologist and pain specialist with the Chico Pain Clinic in Chico, California. Dr. Cullen reported petitioner's history as that of "a 46 year old man who suffered an intense reaction to a Hepatitis B vaccine in 1999, developing a small fiber neuropathy." Dr. Cullen's impression after examining petitioner was that he had a "small fiber neuropathy."

Thereafter, Robert E. Sullivan, M.D., who prescribed petitioner's medicinal cannabis, found on February 13, 2007, that petitioner's "chronic polyneuropathy persists, secondary to a Hepatitis B adverse reaction."

Petitioner testified at the 2008 hearing for his vaccine claim that he continued to experience fluctuating levels of pain. His pain is best managed by the opiate therapy he has been prescribed. A neuropsychologic evaluation was subsequently conducted by Alfred L. Scopp, Ph.D., at the request of petitioner's disability attorney. In a lengthy report dated June 25, 2008, Dr. Scopp concluded that petitioner suffered from a "progressive peripheral neuropathy subsequent to Hepatitis B inoculation."

On August 7, 2008, petitioner was seen by Oscar N. Abeliuk, M.D., a neurologist for a comprehensive neurologic consultation in connection with his disability claim. Dr. Abeliuk prepared a lengthy report, in which he determined that petitioner suffered from a "decreased perception of pinprick and light touch in a symmetrical distribution in the upper and lower extremities distally, suggestive of long-term polyneuropathy (in this case, small fiber type)." Dr. Abeliuk offered as a diagnosis, "chronic debilitating polyneuropathy, well documented by multiple tests. Doctor Lomen-Hoerth has determined the presence of small fiber polyneuropathy affecting the upper and lower extremities, as documented by a skin biopsy at Johns Hopkins, with disturbing skin sensations."

On May 18, 2009, petitioner was seen by Joel M. Rothfeld, Ph.D, M.D., for a neurologic consultation. In Dr. Rothfeld's assessment, petitioner has a "history of distal small fiber neuropathy with chronic pain refractory to multiple medication therapies." Dr. Rothfeld found that petitioner's "neurolgical exam revealed alodynic response to sensory testing distal lower extremities consistent with small fiber neuropathy neuropathic pain."

Petitioner appears to have remained under the care of his primary treating neurologist, Dr. Catherine Lomen-Hoerth. Dr. Lomen-Hoerth found after her examination of petitioner on August 26, 2009, that clinically [petitioner] appears to have a progressive small fiber neuropathy, with documentation on skin biopsy suggestive of an early small fiber neuropathy. These type of neuropathies typically have normal nerve conduction studies and normal neuroimaging, as was the case with Mr. Shaw. . . . He is unable to work due to an inability to stand or sit for any period of time and has an inability to type well due to numbness and pain.

In a letter dated November 14, 2009 to Cigna Disability Claims department, Dr. Pamela P. Palmer, the anesthesiologist who continued to treat petitioner for pain, noted that he suffers from "a clearly diagnosed small-fiber neuropathy" and urged that his disability benefits be reinstated. Likewise, his primary care physician, Katherine Julian, M.D., wrote a letter requesting reinstatement of petitioner's disability benefits. Dr. Julian explained that "it is unclear as to the . . . etiology of his neuropathy, though specialists believe the cause is likely due to a vaccine he received in the late 1990's. . . . However, he has been evaluated by neurology, and standard office-based nerve testing does reveal neuropathy."

APPLICABLE LEGAL STANDARDS

The Vaccine Act provides two separate methods by which to obtain Program compensation: (1) Vaccine Injury Table (Table) claims; and (2) causation in fact (off-Table) claims. When asserting a Table claim, a claimant is afforded a presumption of causation if he shows that he received a vaccine listed on the Table and suffered an injury listed on the Table within the prescribed time period. If unable to establish a Table claim, the claimant must show that his injury was caused in fact by the vaccine he received.

The Vaccine Act provides for the compensation of any illness, disability, injury, or condition not set forth in the Vaccine Injury Table but which was caused by a vaccine covered under the Program. The Act does not require a petitioner bringing a non-Table claim to categorize the suffered injury. Rather, a petitioner is required only to show that the vaccine in question caused injury regardless of the ultimate diagnosis. When, as in this case, the conditions at issue present with many of the same symptoms—but the underlying causes and required treatments are different—and when, as in this case, the evidence for causation depends on the particular diagnosis of petitioner's condition, a special master may consider whether the record supports the diagnosis proposed by petitioner. A petitioner may prove entitlement to Program compensation of an off-Table case by satisfying the three-part test set forth by the Federal Circuit in *Althen v. Secretary of Health & Human Services*. Concisely stated, a claimant's burden is to show by preponderant evidence that the vaccination brought about [his] injury by providing: (1) a medical theory causally connecting the vaccination and the injury; (2) a logical sequence of cause and effect showing that the vaccination was the reason for the injury; and (3) a showing of a proximate temporal relationship between vaccination and injury.

If a claimant satisfies this burden, he is entitled to recover unless the government shows, also by a preponderance of evidence, that the injury was in fact caused by factors unrelated to the vaccine. To prevail, a claimant's theory of causation must be supported by a reputable medical or scientific explanation. A claimant need not produce medical literature or epidemiologic evidence in support of his theory causation, but if such evidence is submitted, a special master may consider the scientific soundness of that evidence in reaching an informed judgment as to whether a particular vaccination more likely than not caused a particular injury.

While *Althen* contemplates that the provided support for a claimant's theory of causation is based on a reputable medical or scientific explanation, that support need not rise to the level of medical or scientific certainty for a petitioner to prevail on a vaccine claim. In *Andreu*, the Federal Circuit made clear that submitted medical literature and epidemiologic evidence must be viewed, however, not through the lens of the laboratorian, but instead from the vantage point of the Vaccine Act's preponderant evidence standard: "The standard of proof required by the [Vaccine] Act is simple preponderance of evidence; not scientific certainty. . . . [I]t is not plaintiff's burden to disprove every possible ground of causation suggested by defendant nor must the findings of the court meet the standards of the laboratorian."

When reviewing offered scientific evidence, a special master must take into account that a finding of causation in the medical community may require a much higher level of certainty than that required by the Vaccine Act to establish a prima facie case. Also reiterated in *Andreu* is the importance in vaccine cases of considering medical opinions contained in the records or presented at hearing testimony. Such opinions, explained the Circuit Court, can be quite probative since treating physicians are likely to be in the best position to determine whether a logical sequence of cause and effect show[s] that the vaccination was the reason for the injury. However, consistent with the Vaccine Act, a special master is not bound by any diagnosis, conclusion, judgment, test result, report, or summary contained in the record. A special master must consider the entire record and the course of the subject injury when evaluating the weight to be afforded to any offered diagnosis, conclusion, judgment, test result, report, or summary contained in the record.

ANALYSIS
Opinion of Petitioner's Expert Witness, Dr. Morgan

In support of his vaccine claim, on remand, Mr. Shaw relies on the opinions of the treating physicians contained in his filed medical records, as well as the offered expert report and remand hearing testimony of Dr. Morgan. Having obtained a medical degree from Meharry Medical College in 1970, Dr. Morgan is board-certified by the American Board of Psychiatry and Neurology, as well as by the American Board of Independent Medical Examiners. Dr. Morgan is a practicing neurologist, whose focus is neurologic injury and disability. Dr. Morgan is also an Assistant Professor at Brown University, School of Medicine in the Department of Clinical Neuroscience.

It is Dr. Morgan's opinion, based on the evaluations of petitioner's treating physicians, the medical records, the medical literature, as well as his own expertise, that Mr. Shaw suffers from a small fiber neuropathy. It is the further position of Dr. Morgan that petitioner's injury resulted from a demyelination of his peripheral nerves through the biological mechanism of molecular mimicry caused by the Hepatitis B vaccines he received. This theory of causation contemplates that the administered "vaccine stimulates the host's immune system to react to the Hepatitis B antigen and cross react with the myelinated nerve fibers of the host. This mistaken attack by the body's own immune system is secondary to the similarity between the foreign Hepatitis B antigen and the myelin component in the host." In sum, Dr. Morgan posits that the Hepatitis B vaccine can cause demyelination of the peripheral nerves, id., and a finding that petitioner suffers from "a small fiber neuropathy causally related to a post-vaccinal immune mediated peripheral nerve disorder," is supported by the "time of symptom onset."

Opinion of Respondent's Expert Witness, Dr. Leist
To address the opinion offered by Dr. Morgan, respondent offered the opinion and testimony of Dr. Leist, who serves as Chief of the Division of Neuroimmunology and Director of the Comprehensive Multiple Sclerosis (MS) Center at Thomas Jefferson University in Philadelphia, Pennsylvania. Possessing a doctorate in biochemistry from the University of Zurich in 1985 and a medical degree from the University of Miami in 1993, Dr. Leist augmented his studies by pursuing postgraduate training in the areas of pathology, microbiology, immunology and neurology. Board-certified by the American Board of

Psychiatry and Neurology and describing himself as a bench-trained immunologist with strong interests in general immunology and viral immunology, he has focused, through his training, on diseases that are immunologic in nature and affect the nervous system.

Dr. Leist takes issue with Dr. Morgan's opinion. Dr. Leist notes as an initial matter, that Mr. Shaw has had two skin biopsies performed to evaluate whether he has a small fiber neuropathy. In both instances, the biopsies exhibited "normal epidermal nerve fiber density"—a result that did not support a finding that petitioner suffer from a small fiber neuropathy. Leist further notes that neither the MRIs or the electrophysiologic studies that were performed for Mr.Shaw, after the vaccinations at issue, showed evidence of a demyelinating or inflammatory process in the peripheral or central nervous system. Additional evidence that in Dr. Leist's view diminishes the likelihood that petitioner's injury is vaccine-related is the negative result of the test conducted for antibodies against the Hepatitis B vaccine on September 26, 2001.That negative finding, according to Dr. Leist, indicates that petitioner's Hepatitis B vaccination did not result in the type of T-cell response necessary to precipitate demyelination.

Evaluating Whether Petitioner Suffers a Small Fiber Neuropathy
Among the issues to be resolved is whether petitioner suffers from a small fiber neuropathy. For the reasons discussed below the undersigned is persuaded that petitioner more likely than not suffers from a small fiber neuropathy. At hearing, petitioner's expert, Dr. Morgan, provided the following background information concerning small fiber neuropathy. He explained that a small fiber neuropathy is a syndrome that "primarily involves the sensory nerves." He elaborated that a "hallmark" of this condition are both "positive" and "negative" symptoms. Id. Positive symptoms are sharp pains and involve the myelinated Alpha Delta fibers; in contrast, negative symptoms are numbness and involve the unmyelinated C fibers. He testified that "small nerve fibers are nerves that are made up of both unmyelinated fibers, called C fibers; and . . . myelinated fibers called Alpha Delta fibers" which are "thinly myelinated." The medical records indicate that Mr. Shaw began to experience both the positive symptom of "pins and needles" and the negative symptom of "some numbness," approximately six days after his June 11, 1999 Hepatitis B immunization—as reported to his treating physician (noting that his numbness began on June 17, 1999, four days prior to his visit to Dr. Roberts and six days after he received his second Hepatitis B vaccine, and that numbness was "progressing to a throbbing pain").

Petitioner experienced the symptoms in his hands and feet ("glove and stocking"). According to Dr. Morgan, the numbness in all four limbs reported to petitioner's orthopedic surgeon was a negative symptom involving the unmyelinated C fibers. Contrastingly, the reported "shooting pain in the limbs with throbbing" was a positive symptom implicating the myelinated fibers. Dr. Morgan's testimony explaining the symptoms of small nerve fiber dysfunction was consistent with petitioner's filed medical literature.

Petitioner's Laboratory Tests: Dr. Morgan addressed petitioner's various medical tests and the test results, asserting that they supported or, at least, did not contradict a diagnosis of small fiber neuropathy. Referring to petitioner's skin biopsies, Dr. Morgan explained that petitioner's early test results showed a "normal range of epidermal nerve fiber density," but when considered with his other skin biopsy results, revealed abnormality. Dr. Morgan testified that petitioner's treater, Dr. Maragakis, determined from petitioner's first skin biopsy that the "nerve swellings . . . could be the beginning of a nerve degeneration" (addendum to August 21, 2000 report of Dr. Maragakis discussing the results of petitioner's first skin biopsy). Because petitioner's symptoms did not improve, but progressively worsened after that biopsy, Dr. Lomen-Hoerth, petitioner's treating neurologist, recommended repeating the skin biopsy. The second skin biopsy was taken from several different places on petitioner's leg, including she proximal thigh, his distal thigh, and his distal leg. The test result again showed a normal range of epidermal nerve fiber density offering "no definitive skin biopsy is considered the best method for diagnosing a small fiber neuropathy." A skin biopsy will report an abnormal result in 67% of small fiber neuropathy cases. Dr. Morgan testified, however, that the result was "not normal" at the proximal thigh location because petitioner's "nerve fiber distribution was borderline" normal with a patchy distribution and that some of the examined fibers were "fragmented and contained small swellings." Similarly at the distal leg the nerve fiber "distribution again is patchy." In Dr. Morgan's opinion, this "patchy" distribution of nerve fiber cells is consistent with a small fiber neuropathy. Dr. Morgan also addressed the findings of petitioner's EMG and nerve conduction exams which were documented as normal. Dr. Morgan explained that an abnormal EMG requires "some involvement of the . . . ventral nerve root," but because small fiber neuropathy "doesn't involve the ventral nerve root that supplies motor fibers," an EMG would not show abnormality.

Dr. Morgan also discussed petitioner's conduction study. Dr. Morgan offered that: Sensory nerve conduction, which is a little more sensitive than motor nerve . . . measures more . . . heavily myelinated fibers. And if that process is spared, you won't see abnormalities on the nerve conduction and the nerve conduction velocities will be normal, particularly the sensory nerve conductions. And so . . . the nerve conduction study just further supports that this petitioner's injury involves . . . small fibers, both myelinated and unmyelinated. Dr. Morgan further offered that small fiber sensory neuropathy does not involve sufficient heavily myelinated fibers to "create abnormalities in the nerve conduction testing." He added that "if there is too much involvement of the heavily myelinated fibers," the condition no longer falls within small fiber neuropathy category." Petitioner's treating neurologist, Dr. Lomen-Hoerth, commented, in her notes that petitioner's "normal nerve conduction" studies "do not exclude a small fiber neuropathy." The electromyographer, Dr. James Wei, who reviewed the nerve conduction studies agreed with Dr. Lomen-Hoerth.

The filed medical literature confirms the difficulty described by Dr. Morgan in diagnosing a small fiber neuropathy. As observed in the 2002 Lacomis article, small-fiber neuropathy is a "commonly encountered disorder" that is "frustrating to clinicians because of difficulties in proving the diagnosis and in treatment." Consistent with Dr. Morgan's testimony, Lacomis observed that to the extent routine nerve conduction studies assess large-fiber function, they are generally normal." Lacomis also states that although "heart variability can be assessed on some EMG equipment . . . it is likely that the subtle abnormalities associated with most small-fiber neuropathies will not be detected."

Respondent's expert Dr. Leist is not persuaded that petitioner suffers from a small fiber neuropathy. In his view, petitioner's test results—particularly the skin biopsies—provide evidence that "weighs against" a small fiber neuropathy diagnosis. Dr. Leist opines, "I would expect that if somebody has progressive symptoms over a period of time, that there would be evidence of a progressive underlying dysfunction. . . . would I expect . . . an objectifiable finding of, for example, nerve loss over the one and a half or two years between the two skin biopsies? Yes, I would expect this. The fact that it's not there, I would consider as less usual. . . .The fact that it doesn't show abnormality clearly doesn't support a finding of small fiber neuropathy."

The Opinions of Petitioner's Treating Doctors: Dr. Morgan also relied on the opinions of petitioner's treating physicians who variously considered a small fiber neuropathy diagnosis. Petitioner's doctors recorded different impressions about the precise nature of his injury. What is consistently reported, however, is a condition involving a progressive and chronic pain syndrome. After a careful review of petitioner's records and the expert testimony, the undersigned is persuaded that it is more likely than not that petitioner suffers from a small fiber neuropathy. Interpretation of the EMG results in September of 1999: The patient is most likely exhibiting very early symptoms of idiopathic peripheral neuropathy. Dr. Lin indicating that petitioner was suffering a post-inflammatory neuropathy related to immunizations. Dr. Villanueva discussing petitioner's subjective diffuse sensory polyneuropathy. Dr. Lomen-Hoerth's impression in May of 2000 that petitioner had a progressive small fiber neuropathy. Dr. Maragakis's view that "this most likely represents some form of small fiber neuropathy." Dr. So opining in July 2001: It is conceivable that petitioner had an acute, predominantly sensory polyneuropathy back in 1999. Dr. Waldman finding in December 2004 that "Mr. Shaw has developed a chronic neuropathic pain syndrome." Dr. Cullen's reported patient's history as that of "a 46 year old man who suffered an intense reaction to a Hepatitis B vaccine in 1999, developing a small fiber neuropathy." Dr. Palmer describing petitioner as "a 46 year-old gentleman with six years of diffuse pain after vaccination, consistent with a diffuse small fiber neuropathy." Dr. Robert Sullivan finding in February 2007 that petitioner's "chronic polyneuropathy persists." Dr. Alfred Scopp indicating that petitioner has an Axis III diagnosis of peripheral neuropathy." Dr. Oscar Abeliuk found petitioner's condition to be "suggestive of long-term polyneuropathy (in this case, small fiber type)." Dr. Rothfeld's assessment that petitioner has a "history of and current neurologic responses consistent with small fiber neuropathy with chronic pain." Petitioner's primary treating neurologist, Dr. Lomen-Hoerth, finding again in August 2009 that "clinically petitioner appears to have a progressive small fiber neuropathy, with documentation on skin biopsy suggestive of an early small fiber neuropathy." In November of 2009, Dr. Palmer, who treated petitioner for pain, noting that he suffers from "a clearly diagnosed small-fiber neuropathy."

It is true—as respondent points out, see Respondent's Post-Hearing Brief on Remand filed November 17, 2010, that many of petitioner's treating physicians did not make a definitive diagnosis of small fiber neuropathy. But, it is this diagnosis that his various treaters and evaluations most frequently considered based chiefly on petitioner's neurologic responses. Recognizing that the "objective" tests and studies do not clearly demonstrate or negate a diagnosis of small fiber neuropathy, the undersigned is persuaded that petitioner's clinical presentation (as reflected in the medical records), the opinions of petitioner's treating physicians, the expert opinion of Dr. Morgan and the cited medical literature adequately support such a finding. While the undersigned cannot find with medical certainty that petitioner suffers from a small fiber neuropathy, the undersigned does find that more likely than not petitioner is afflicted with this condition, and the undersigned is mindful that "the standard of proof required by the Vaccine Act is simple preponderance of evidence; not scientific certainty." The undersigned notes that Dr. Maragakis later indicated that he could not "make a diagnosis of peripheral neuropathy based on any of the based on any of the studies" performed.

Evaluating Petitioner's Claim under the *Althen* Prongs

As stated earlier, petitioner must prove causation by showing: (1) a medical theory causally connecting the vaccination and the injury; (2) a logical sequence of cause and effect showing the vaccination was the reason for the injury; and (3) a proximate temporal relationship between the vaccination and the injury. The undersigned addresses each of the prongs of the *Althen* standard in turn. For ease of discussion, the undersigned addresses the first and the third prongs of the *Althen* before turning to the second prong.

Petitioner's Offered Medical Theory: Petitioner must offer a medical theory causally connecting the vaccination and the injury. As discussed above, Dr. Morgan opined in his written report that petitioner's small fiber neuropathy resulted from his Hepatitis B vaccine causing a demyelination of his peripheral nerves through a biological mechanism of molecular mimicry. This theory contemplates that the "vaccine stimulates the host['s] immune system to react to the Hepatitis B antigen and cross react with the myelinated nerve fibers of the host. . . . This mistaken attack by the body's own immune system is secondary to the similarity between the foreign Hepatitis B antigen and the myelin component in the host."

At hearing, Dr. Morgan explained his theory of molecular mimicry as follows: It starts at the dorsal root ganglion and that ganglion has unmyelinated, myelinated, heavily myelinated fibers. There is an antigen antibody reaction that occurs there, disrupts the myelin and is reflected in the peripheral nerve and small fibers, specifically involving both the alpha thinly myelinated fibers and the unmyelinated C fibers. And that is caused by an immune mechanism which is the antigen from the vaccine that looks at the normal self myelin, cross reacts with it, and causes this initial inflammatory reaction. And which then leads to the gradual demyelination affecting the nerve roots, which then account for the person's—for Mr. Shaw's—symptoms. Dr. Morgan pointed to Petitioner's Trial Exhibit Number 5 to further describe this mechanism: And so you could see where if someone got an inflammatory demyelinative reaction, how the secondary effects would affect both . . . the unmyelinated fiber, which is the C fiber, which is what we see with small fiber neuropathy; but it also affects the thinly myelinated fiber, which also is part of small fiber neuropathy. And there's some suggestion that it actually affects some of even the heavier myelinated fibers but not much. If it does, then it becomes no longer a small fiber neuropathy. . . . So it's a complex understanding of it, but I think it explains why these things aren't just black and white . . . it's not one root, one root and everything is nicely fit. That's why these syndromes are called syndromes. And they overlap.

Dr. Morgan testified that inflammatory cells have likewise been observed, from autopsy slides, in the dorsal root ganglion of patients with Guillain-Barré syndrome. Dr. Morgan offered evidence supporting petitioner's theory, that molecular mimicry can cause "a post-vaccinal type of neuropathy," in the form of medical literature. Specifically, the Lacomis article notes that "in some patients with idiopathic small-fiber neuropathy, an inflammatory autoimmune basis has been hypothesized, and circumstantial evidence is available." Lacomis goes on to discuss this evidence, concluding: "Thus, there is evidence that suggests, but does not prove, that infections or autoimmune processes may cause small-fiber neuropathy. Unfortunately, there are no good laboratory markers of this autoimmune process."

But, Dr. Leist took issue with the lack of evidence that the Hepatitis B vaccination can harm unmyelinated C fibers, and was not persuaded by Dr. Morgan's explanation that the unmyelinated C fibers experience secondary effects or bystander effects from the post vaccinal inflammatory demyelinative reaction. At the first hearing in this case, Dr. Leist conceded that it is "potentially possible" that the Hepatitis B vaccine can cause auto-immune reactions. In making this statement, Dr. Leist indicated that he was relying upon "the opinion of the Institute of Medicine (IOM), which says it's possible to put a mechanism together by which Hepatitis B could cause an immune mediated injury." Notwithstanding this statement by the IOM, Dr. Leist found in this case there is not "a reputable theory by which one could explain a small fiber neuropathy, a theory that is accepted . . . it's not accepted with respect to the Hepatitis B vaccine."

Reviewing the evidence on balance, the undersigned finds preponderant evidence of a "medical theory causally connecting the vaccination and the injury." To be sure, such evidence in this case is not scientifically certain—as respondent points out—the medical literature does not specifically link the Hepatitis B vaccination or any vaccination to the injury of small fiber neuropathy. However, petitioner has provided a sound "medical or scientific explanation that pertains specifically to the petitioner's case . . . that is 'legally probably,' even if not medically or scientifically certain."

The undersigned will next examine the third prong of the *Althen* test—the temporal relationship between Mr. Shaw's vaccination and his injury—as this evidence is pivotal to the undersigned's analysis of the second *Althen* prong.

The Temporal Relationship between the Vaccination and the Injury: Petitioner must show more than a proximate temporal relationship between the vaccination and the injury to satisfy the burden of showing actual causation.

The contemporaneous medical records indicate that petitioner's symptoms began six days after the receipt of his second Hepatitis B vaccination. Dr. Morgan testified that six days is appropriate for onset of an immune related disorder. Respondent's expert, Dr. Leist, agreed that the "temporal relationship between the administration of the vaccine and the onset of symptoms was appropriate." It is within a period of time that would be acceptable. . . for an immune response to appear at all." Because symptoms of petitioner's injury occurred within an appropriate medical time frame for an immune-mediated injury, petitioner has satisfied the third prong of the *Althen* standard.

The undersigned turns now to address petitioner's proposed sequence of cause and effect.

The Sequence of Cause and Effect: The Federal Circuit has observed that an offered medical theory is persuasive when accompanied by proof of a logical sequence of cause and effect showing that the vaccination was the reason for the injury, the logical sequence being supported by reputable medical or scientific explanation, i.e., evidence in the form of scientific studies or expert medical testimony. The Federal Circuit has found the opinions of treating physicians to be particularly probative in evaluating the second prong of *Althen*, particularly "if a claimant satisfies the first and third prongs of the *Althen* standard" as "treating physicians are likely to be in the best position to determine whether a logical sequence of cause and effect shows that the vaccination was the reason for the injury."

As discussed above, Mr. Shaw has satisfied the first and third prongs of the *Althen* standard. In considering whether Mr. Shaw has demonstrated a logical sequence of cause and effect, the undersigned turns to the opinions of his treating physicians. As an initial matter, the undersigned notes that it is undisputed that the "leading cause" of small fiber neuropathy is idiopathic— it cannot be identified. However, progress is being made toward identifying potential causes of small fiber neuropathy, to include the possibility of infections or autoimmune causes.

Petitioner has been evaluated and/or treated by a substantial number of physicians since his symptoms began in 1999. A remarkable number, although not all, of these treating doctors have either postulated or ascribed vaccine causation to his injury. Particularly persuasive to the undersigned was the opinion of vaccine-related causation expressed by petitioner's treating neurologists. Dr. Lin, an examining neurologist, recorded that petitioner was suffering a post-inflammatory neuropathy related to immunizations. It was Dr. Lomen-Hoerth's, Mr. Shaw's primary neurologist, early impression that petitioner had a progressive small fiber neuropathy rather than a static neuropathy related to his vaccinations. A consulting neurologist, Dr. Dresser recorded his impression in 2002 that petitioner suffers from diffuse dysesthetic pain following remote vaccinations. Dr. Martin, a rheumatologist, indicated that petitioner suffered from an idiopathic syndrome associated with chronic fatigue and . . . is possibly related to a vaccine exposure or possibly a toxin. Dr. Chiu, an internist, observed that because petitioner's neurologic changes seem to have arisen after his immunization in 1999, there is a question as to whether there is some type of autoimmune or other reaction to this vaccination." Dr. Berkenblit, an internist, maintained that while there is no clear link between Hepatitis B vaccination and progressive neuropathic pain, if Mr. Shaw did develop symptoms of a sensory neuropathy as a consequence of the vaccine, it would most likely be an autoimmune type mechanism. Dr. Roberts, petitioner's primary care physician, wrote a letter in 2002 indicating his belief that the temporal relationship between the received vaccination and the onset of petitioner's symptoms strongly correlated with the hypothesis that the symptoms were caused by the vaccination. Dr. Allen, who evaluated petitioner in connection with his worker's compensation claim, believed that petitioner's injury "may have developed as a result of the June 1999 vaccinations." Dr. Buttram, an internist, maintained the opinion that Mr. Shaw's "peripheral neuropathy is directly related to (was caused by) a series of two Hepatitis B vaccines. "Vaccine-induced neuroimmune dysfunction" was the diagnosis of Dr. Natali, a general practitioner. Dr. Cullen, an anesthesiologist, described petitioner in 2006 as "a 46-year-old man who suffered an intense adverse reaction to a Hepatitis B vaccine in 1999, developing a small fiber neuropathy." Dr. Palmer, another anesthesiologist, assessed petitioner as "a 46-year-old gentleman with six years of diffuse pain after vaccination, consistent with a diffuse small-fiber neuropathy . . . ." Dr. Sullivan found in February 2007 that petitioner's "chronic polyneuropathy persists, secondary to a Hepatitis B adverse reaction." In a report following a neuropsychological evaluation conducted at the request of petitioner's disability attorney, Dr. Scopp concluded that petitioner suffered from a "progressive peripheral neuropathy subsequent to Hepatitis B inoculation." Requesting reinstatement of petitioner's disability benefits, Dr. Julian, a primary care physician, wrote, "Specialists believe the cause of petitioner's neuropathy is likely due to a vaccine he received in the late 1990's."

Respondent points out that some of petitioner's treaters subsequently modified their early opinions of vaccine causation or failed to ascribe his injury to vaccine-related causation. For example, Dr. Chiu noted the temporal relationship to the vaccine, but did not opine as to causation. Dr. Villanueva doubted vaccine causation, and Dr. Lin later altered her initial diagnosis of vaccine-related post inflammatory neuropathy. The undersigned takes note of these observations; but the record indicates that a number of the petitioner's treating physicians postulated that petitioner's condition was vaccine-mediated, informed—in part—by the temporal relationship between Mr. Shaw's vaccinations and the onset of his injury.

Respondent further argues that Dr. Morgan's theory of a post-vaccine immune response causing a demyelinating injury must fail because the evidence does not support a finding that Mr. Shaw experienced an immune response to his vaccination. Respondent bases this assertion on the finding that petitioner's September 26, 2001 antibody testing was negative for IgG antibodies, the class of antibodies that assist in fighting against infection. Dr. Leist testified that while IgM antibodies initially mount a response to vaccination (or any other presented antigen), these antibodies are normally converted to IgG antibodies starting at day seven or eight. It was Dr. Allen's view that petitioner was suffering from fibromyalgia.

However, on cross-examination, Dr. Leist conceded that IgM antibodies may "play a role" in demyelinating disorders that petitioner may have had a significant IgM response that never converted to an IgG response, and that petitioner was never tested for IgM antibodies. However, Dr. Leist maintained that while these were "theoretical" possibilities, he found them to be "exceedingly improbable."

On balance, the undersigned is persuaded that petitioner has demonstrated a logical sequence of cause and effect. Petitioner has presented sound scientific testimony from a medical expert, well qualified in the field of neurology, that offers a cogent explanation of how petitioner's Hepatitis B vaccination more likely than not caused him to develop a small fiber neuropathy by way of molecular mimicry. Petitioner has presented uncontested evidence of a proximate temporal relationship between the vaccination and the injury. And, finally, a number of petitioner's treating physicians attributed Mr. Shaw's injury to the Hepatitis B vaccines he received.

CONCLUSION

As discussed above, the undersigned finds that petitioner has established by preponderant evidence in this close case that his Hepatitis B vaccination was the legal cause of his small fiber neuropathy. The undersigned further finds that there is not a preponderance of the evidence that the legal cause of Mr. Shaw's injury was due to factors unrelated to his Hepatitis B vaccination. Accordingly, the undersigned finds Mr. Shaw is entitled to compensation under the Vaccine Act. A separate damages order will issue.

IT IS SO ORDERED.

Anita Roberts and Gary Roberts, Co-petitioners, as Next Friends, Parents acting on behalf of Amber D. Roberts their minor child, Petitioners v. Secretary of Health and Human Services, Respondent

Summary: In this decision following a hearing, Special Master Zane rules that the victim suffered transverse myelitis after receiving a tetanus-diptheria-acellular pertussis vaccine.

Compensated Vaccine Injury: Transverse Myelitis

According to the National Institute of Neurological Disorders and Stroke, transverse myelitis is a neurological disorder caused by inflammation across both sides of one level, or segment, of the spinal cord. The term myelitis refers to inflammation of the spinal cord; transverse simply describes the position of the inflammation, that is, across the width of the spinal cord. Attacks of inflammation can damage or destroy myelin, the fatty insulating substance that covers nerve cell fibers. This damage causes nervous system scars that interrupt communications between the nerves in the spinal cord and the rest of the body.

Symptoms of transverse myelitis include a loss of spinal cord function over several hours to several weeks. What usually begins as a sudden onset of lower back pain, muscle weakness, or abnormal sensations in the toes and feet can rapidly progress to more severe symptoms, including paralysis, urinary retention, and loss of bowel control. Although some patients recover from transverse myelitis with minor or no residual problems, others suffer permanent impairments that affect their ability to perform ordinary tasks of daily living. Most patients will have only one episode of transverse myelitis; a small percentage may have a recurrence.

The segment of the spinal cord at which the damage occurs determines which parts of the body are affected. Nerves in the cervical (neck) region control signals to the neck, arms, hands, and muscles of breathing (the diaphragm). Nerves in the thoracic (upper back) region relay signals to the torso and some parts of the arms. Nerves at the lumbar (mid-back) level control signals to the hips and legs. Finally, sacral nerves, located within the lowest segment of the spinal cord, relay signals to the groin, toes, and some parts of the legs. Damage at one segment will affect function at that segment and segments below it. In patients with transverse myelitis, demyelination usually occurs at the thoracic level, causing problems with leg movement and bowel and bladder control, which require signals from the lower segments of the spinal cord.

Transverse myelitis occurs in adults and children, in both genders, and in all races. No familial predisposition is apparent. A peak in incidence rates (the number of new cases per year) appears to occur between 10 and 19 years and 30 and 39 years. Although only a few studies have examined incidence rates, it is estimated that about 1,400 new cases of transverse myelitis are diagnosed each year in the United States, and approximately 33,000 Americans have some type of disability resulting from the disorder.

Researchers are uncertain of the exact causes of transverse myelitis. The inflammation that causes such extensive damage to nerve fibers of the spinal cord may result from viral infections or abnormal immune reactions. Transverse myelitis also may occur as a complication of syphilis, measles, Lyme disease, and some vaccinations, including those for chickenpox and rabies. Cases in which a cause cannot be identified are called idiopathic.

Transverse myelitis often develops following viral infections. Infectious agents suspected of causing transverse myelitis include varicella zoster (the virus that causes chickenpox and shingles), herpes simplex, cytomegalovirus, Epstein-Barr, influenza, echovirus, human immunodeficiency virus (HIV), hepatitis A, and rubella. Bacterial skin infections, middle-ear infections (otitis media), and Mycoplasma pneumoniae (bacterial pneumonia) have also been associated with the condition.

In post-infectious cases of transverse myelitis, immune system mechanisms, rather than active viral or bacterial infections, appear to play an important role in causing damage to spinal nerves. Although researchers have not yet identified the precise mechanisms of spinal cord injury in these cases, stimulation of the immune system in response to infection indicates that an autoimmune reaction may be responsible. In autoimmune diseases, the immune system, which normally protects the body from foreign organisms, mistakenly attacks the body's own tissue, causing inflammation and, in some cases, damage to myelin within the spinal cord.

Because some affected individuals also have autoimmune diseases such as systemic lupus erythematosus, Sjogren's syndrome, and sarcoidosis, some scientists suggest that transverse myelitis may also be an autoimmune disorder. In addition, some cancers may trigger an abnormal immune response that may lead to transverse myelitis.

In some people, transverse myeltis represents the first symptom of an underlying demyelinating disease of the central nervous system such as multiple sclerosis (MS) *or neuromyelitis optica (NMO). A form of transverse myelitis known as "partial" myelitis—because it affects only a portion of the cross-sectional area of the spinal cord—is more characteristic of MS. Neuromyelitis optica typically causes both transverse myelitis and optic neuritis (inflammation of the optic nerve that results in visual loss), but not necessarily at the same time. All patients with transverse myelitis should be evaluated for MS or NMO because patients with these diagnoses may require different treatments, especially therapies to prevent future attacks.*

Transverse myelitis may be either acute (developing over hours to several days) or subacute (usually developing over 1 to 4 weeks). Initial symptoms usually include localized lower back pain, sudden paresthesias (abnormal sensations such as burning, tickling, pricking, or tingling) in the legs, sensory loss, and paraparesis (partial paralysis of the legs). Paraparesis may progress to paraplegia (paralysis of the legs and lower part of the trunk). Urinary bladder and bowel dysfunction is common. Many patients also report experiencing muscle spasms, a general feeling of discomfort, headache, fever, and loss of appetite. Depending on which segment of the spinal cord is involved, some patients may experience respiratory problems as well.

From this wide array of symptoms, four classic features of transverse myelitis emerge: (1) weakness of the legs and arms, (2) pain, (3) sensory alteration, and (4) bowel and bladder dysfunction. Most patients will experience weakness of varying degrees in their legs; some also experience it in their arms. Initially, people with transverse myelitis may notice that they are stumbling or dragging one foot or that their legs seem heavier than normal. Coordination of hand and arm movements, as well as arm and hand strength may also be compromised. Progression of the disease leads to full paralysis of the legs, requiring the patient to use a wheelchair.

Pain is the primary presenting symptom of transverse myelitis in approximately one-third to one-half of all patients. The pain may be localized in the lower back or may consist of sharp, shooting sensations that radiate down the legs or arms or around the torso.

Patients who experience sensory disturbances often use terms such as numbness, tingling, coldness, or burning to describe their symptoms. Up to 80 percent of those with transverse myelitis report areas of heightened sensitivity to touch, such that clothing or a light touch with a finger causes significant discomfort or pain (a condition called allodynia). Many also experience heightened sensitivity to changes in temperature or to extreme heat or cold.

Bladder and bowel problems may involve increased frequency of the urge to urinate or have bowel movements, incontinence, difficulty voiding, the sensation of incomplete evacuation, and constipation. Over the course of the disease, the majority of people with transverse myelitis will experience one or several of these symptoms.

Entitlement; tetanus-diptheria-accellular pertussis vaccination ("Tdap"); transverse myelitis ("TM"); oligoclonal banding; infarction; fibrocartilaginous embolism ("FCE")

Case No: 09-427V

Date Filed: August 29, 2013

Anita Roberts and Gary Roberts, Co-petitioners, as Next Friends, Parents acting on behalf of Amber D. Roberts their minor child, Petitioners v. Secretary of Health and Human Services, Respondent

RULING

Special Master Zane

Petitioners, Anita Roberts and Gary Roberts ("Petitioners"), on behalf of their daughter, Amber Roberts ("A.R."), filed a petition alleging that the tetanus-diptheria-acellular pertussisvaccine ("Tdap") caused A.R. to suffer transverse myelitis. Petitioners seek compensation pursuant to the National Childhood Vaccine Injury Act. As explained below, upon consideration of the record as a whole, the special master concludes that Petitioners have satisfied their burden of showing by preponderant evidence that the vaccine was a substantial factor in causing A.R.'s autoimmune problem, transverse myelitis ("TM"). As explained below, there is ample evidence to satisfy *Althen*'s Prong 1. Petitioners rely on the well-recognized theory of molecular mimicry as the plausible medical theory that explains how the vaccine could have caused A.R.'s injuries. And, there is no dispute regarding *Althen*'s Prong 3. The parties' experts agree that the time between vaccination and onset, approximately four weeks, is a medically appropriate temporal relationship.

The parties' primary disagreement relates to *Althen* Prong 2 and whether Petitioners made a sufficient showing that there was a logical sequence of cause and effect between the vaccine and A.R.'s injuries. With regard to this issue, both parties have presented detailed evidence regarding the proper diagnosis of A.R.'s injury, the permanent paralysis of her lower extremities, and whether it was due to an inflammation caused by an autoimmune response, TM, or was the result of an infarction, embolism or FCE. As set forth below, the record, in particular, the clinical evidence and the results of the objective diagnostic tests with supporting medical literature in the record, sufficiently supports Petitioners' claim as to *Althen*'s Prong 2. As such, Petitioners have satisfied all three *Althen* Prongs and have satisfied their burden.

FACTS

A.R. was born on July 2, 1995. P's Ex. 1. During the first 11 years of her life A.R. was generally healthy. On July 06, 2006, A.R. visited her pediatrician for a sixth grade check-up. Although she complained of back pain at that time, the records noted she was generally healthy. She received a Tdap vaccine. After receiving the vaccine, A.R. noticed a knot under the skin where she received the shot and her skin was slightly swollen. About a week after receiving the vaccine, A.R. felt her feet tingled a bit while she was riding in her father's truck. The tingling was not like the sensation of her legs falling asleep, which she had experienced before. Petitioner reported sitting in the back of her father's truck with her legs crossed for 30 to 45 minutes prior to feeling the tingling in her legs. Petitioner also reported never experiencing this type of tingling before.

On August 4, 2006, A.R. went to the county fair with her mother, brother, and some of her brother's friends. While at the fair, A.R. rode some rides, denied having any back or hip pain. Her mother said A.R. did not tell her about any pains. The next morning A.R.'s mother recalled A.R. complaining of a slight back ache. At some point on August 5, 2006, A.R. went to the bathroom. On the way to the bathroom, her feet felt a little heavy although she was still able to walk to the bathroom. In addition, she had some slight incontinence. A.R. sat down on the toilet and her legs got heavy and she could not get back up. She fell to the bathroom floor. She still had some feeling in her legs but then it started to go away and eventually she felt nothing. Her mother and brother helped her up, and they went to the hospital.

At the hospital, the initial impression was an acute onset of being unable to feel or move her legs. The notes from A.R's neurologic exam recorded A.R. as having "abnormal proprioception of the right and left lower extremities."

The symptoms were consistent with a central lesion leading to a sensory defect affecting both sides of the body. An x-ray of the thoracic spine was taken, which showed no evidence of an acute fracture. The primary diagnosis was acute paraplegia. A.R. was transferred by ambulance to the Cincinnati Children's Hospital. The impression recorded at the time A.R. presented at the emergency department of Cincinnati Children's Hospital was acute onset lower extremity paralysis, afebrile, and without any previous illness. Magnetic Resonance Imaging ("MRI") of A.R.'s cervical spine and a lumbar puncture were performed. Cerebral spinal fluid ("CSF") results indicated a protein of 60 and red blood cell count of 8. It was noted that although the CSF study was considered normal, it was to be repeated because it was still very early after presentation. The initial MRI report noted "mild central cord high T2 signal from T10 to the conus." The impression was that this might represent myelitis, viral infection, or less likely cord ischemia or Guillain-Barré. Additionally, disc desiccation was observed at L2/L3, L3/L4, L4/L5, and L5/S1 and there was no evidence of cord compression. A subsequent addendum note in the report observed an abnormal T2 signal within the cord appeared to extend to the T7 level, although axial T2-weighted images demonstrated motion artifact. A.R. was admitted to the hospital in stable condition with an ER diagnosis of paraplegia.

The hospital admission records reflect in the medical history that A.R. complained of bilateral hip pain the night of the fair. A.R. disputed this, testifying that the source of this statement was her father who had not been at home with her to have any knowledge of that.

On August 6, 2006, the attending physician noted the MRI findings with the T2 signal on at least the T10-T12 segments. P's Ex. 11 a 146. He also noted bilateral flaccid paralysis of the lower extremities. His impression was that A.R. had transverse myelitis. On August 10, 2006, repeat CSF studies were performed. The repeat studies showed a white blood cell count of six [reference range: 0-4] and CSF protein at 58 mg/dL [reference range: 12-60 mg/dL]. Testing of the CSF obtained during the lumbar puncture on August 10, 2006, revealed oligoclonal bands, with the bands also present in A.R.'s serum sample, which had not been present previously. Additionally, the IgG levels had increased from the levels of August 6, 2006.

A.R.'s condition did not improve, and she subsequently began intravenous gamma globulin treatment on August 11, 2006, followed by a prednisone taper treatment started on August 12, 2006. A.R.'s condition, however, still did not change. On August 14, 2006, it was noted that A.R. had "slightly improved sensation" and she was transferred to the inpatient rehabilitation floor with a formal diagnosis of transverse myelitis. Over the next month, A.R. received occupational, recreational, and physical therapy. A.R.'s condition, however, did not improve further, and she was discharged on September 15, 2006.

After the discharge, A.R. was seen by pediatric neurologist, Lois Krousgrill, for a follow up on September 27, 2006. Dr. Krousgrill noted that A.R. had no recovery from motor or sensory function. Dr. Krousgrill's impression was idiopathic TM.

A second MRI was performed on November 1, 2006 which showed a subtle hyperintense T2 signal "centrally within the cord at the T6-T7 level." The report continued: "Hyperintense T2 signal to a greater degree is noted with the cord from the T8-T9 level to the L1 level." The radiologist noted that the signal at the T8-T9 level "likely represents myelomalacia." "Significant atrophy" from T8-T9 to the tip of the conus was also observed. In addition, the image was remarkable for mild disc desiccation from L2-3 to L5-S1 level, as well as subtle disc bulges at L2-L3, L3-L4, and L4-L5.

A.R. was readmitted to Cincinnati Children's hospital for initial plasmapheresis treatments on October 30, 2006 and November 2, 2006. She received further plasmapheresis treatments three times per week over the next two weeks. Unfortunately, Amber did not improve upon the treatment and no marked recovery was observed. Despite treatment and therapy, A.R. continued to have a neurogenic bladder/bowel, period decubitis ulcers, multiple UTIs, incontinence, vaginal candidiasis, joint contractures, and constipation since the onset of the acute paralysis symptom. At the time of hearing, A.R. was in 11th grade, was still in a wheelchair and could not stand or walk. There were ten treatments originally scheduled, but the ninth and tenth were abandoned when A.R. had no recovery after the first eight treatments.

PROCEDURAL HISTORY
On July 1, 2009, Petitioners, Gary Roberts and Anita Roberts filed a petition for compensation under the National Vaccine Injury Act if 1986 on behalf of her daughter, A.R. Petitioners alleged that A.R. suffered from TM as a result of her receipt of a Tdap vaccine on July 06, 2006. Subsequently, the parties filed expert

reports. On October 14, 2010, pursuant to order of the previously assigned Special Master, supplemental expert reports were filed.

On March 26 and 27, 2012, an entitlement hearing was held in Cincinnati, OH One of the petitioners, Anita Roberts, and A.R. testified. Three expert witnesses testified on behalf of Petitioners. First, Dr. Lois Krousgrill, a neurologist, who had examined A.R. at and near the time of the onset of A.R.'s injuries, testified. She opined that A.R. had TM, not an embolism or infarction or fibrocartilaginous embolism ("FCE") based on her clinical picture and the results of diagnostic tests. She further testified that she believed there was a relationship between the vaccine and A.R.'s TM. Second, Dr. Sidney Houff, a neurologist, testified. Dr. Houff opined that A.R. had suffered from an autoimmune reaction to the vaccine she received which caused her to have transverse myelitis. Third and finally, Dr. Mary Edwards-Brown, a neuroradiologist, testified that this was an unusual case of TM. She further concluded that the TM was due to the vaccine.

Two experts testified on behalf of Respondent. First, Dr. John Sladky, a neurologist, testified. He opined that he believed that A.R.'s clinical features were more indicative of a spinal cord infarction, an embolism or FCE than TM, an inflammatory condition. He further opined that even if A.R. had TM, he did not think there was enough evidence to conclude the vaccine caused it. Second, Dr. Louis Vezina, a neuroradiologist, testified. Dr. Vezina opined that based on the imaging studies, the findings were consistent with those of a lower spinal cord infarction; embolism and FCE are described in various places in the record and the terms are used interchangeably. In essence, they refer to an event that abruptly stops the blood flow to the spinal cord, i.e., a stroke in the spinal cord. Infarction is a blood clot in the spine; an embolism was described as a blockage that caused a cut off of blood flow down the spine. Transverse myelitis (TM) is an acute "inflammatory" disorder of the spinal cord resulting in bilateral motor, sensory, and sphincter deficits below the level of the lesion.

APPLICABLE LEGAL STANDARDS

The Vaccine Act provides two means of recovery: Table claims and off-Table claims. In an off-Table, or causation-in-fact, case, such as this one, a petitioner must prove actual causation by a preponderance of the evidence. To prove actual causation, a petitioner must "show that the vaccine was not only a but-for cause of the injury but also a substantial factor in bringing about the injury." Causation is determined on a case-by-case basis. A petitioner satisfies this burden if he or she provides: (1) a medical theory causally connecting the vaccination and the injury; (2) a logical sequence of cause and effect showing that the vaccination was the reason for the injury; and (3) a showing of proximate temporal relationship between vaccination and injury. A petitioner must satisfy the three *Althen* prongs by preponderant evidence. This preponderant-evidence standard "simply requires the trier of fact to believe that the existence of a fact is more probable than its nonexistence" (noting the standard requires that a petitioner demonstrate the existence of the element is "more probable than not"). Evidence used to satisfy one of the *Althen* prongs can overlap and be used to satisfy another prong. There are no "hard and fast per se scientific or medical rules" for finding causation under the Vaccine Act. The Vaccine Act does provide that a claimant may satisfy the preponderant evidence standard by producing "medical records or a medical opinion." A petitioner must provide a reputable medical or scientific explanation that pertains specifically to the petitioner's case. However, the explanation need only be "legally probable, not medically or scientifically certain." Along these lines, a special master may not require "epidemiologic studies . . . or general acceptance in the scientific or medical communities. . . ." At the same time, special masters are "entitled to require some indicia of reliability to support the assertion of the expert witness." In determining reliability, in a Table case, unlike the present case, a claimant who shows that he or she received a vaccination listed in the Vaccine Injury Table, 42 U.S.C. § 300aa–14, and suffered an injury listed in the Table within a prescribed period is afforded a presumption of causation.

When a party relies upon expert testimony, that testimony must have a reliable scientific basis. Although a party need not produce medical literature to establish causation, where such evidence is submitted, the special master can consider it in reaching an informed judgment as to whether a particular vaccination likely caused a particular injury. Causation can be supported by a treating physician's opinion that a vaccination was causally linked to the vaccinee's injury if the special master finds the opinion to be both reliable and persuasive. At the same time, in cases in which a petitioner relies upon expert testimony to prove causation, the expert testimony must rest upon an objective and reliable scientific basis and must prove causation to a degree of legal certainty, but not to a medical or scientific certainty. "A petitioner must provide a reputable medical or scientific explanation that pertains specifically to the petitioner's case, although the explanation need only be legally probable, not medically or scientifically certain." Although a petitioner may rely solely on expert testimony, "an expert opinion is no better than the soundness of the reasons supporting it." Therefore, a special master does not need to credit "expert opinion testimony that is connected to the existing data or methodology 'only by the *ipse dixit* of the expert,' or where 'there is simply too great an analytical gap between the data and the opinion proffered." With regard to alternative causes, the respondent bears the burden of proving by preponderant evidence that an alternative cause, or factor unrelated, was the sole cause of the injury. But, neither 42 U.S.C. § 300aa-13 nor the decisions limit what evidence the special master may consider in deciding whether a prima facie case has been established. As a result, the government may also present and the special master may consider evidence of alternative causes on the issue of the adequacy of the petitioner's evidence regarding the petitioner's case-in-chief. In this regard, there are two particular points that the decisions make clear. First, a special master may not require the petitioner to shoulder the burden of eliminating all possible alternative causes in order to establish a *prima facie* case. Second, a special master may find that a factor other than a vaccine caused the injury in question only if that finding is supported by a preponderance of the evidence. The petitioner does not bear the burden of eliminating alternative independent potential causes, and the respondent has the burden of proving an alternative cause as the sole, unrelated factor that caused the injury by a preponderance of evidence. It is established that a special master is entitled to, and should, consider the record as a whole in determining causation. In considering the record, the Vaccine Act does not contemplate full blown tort litigation. A petitioner may use circumstantial evidence to prove the case, and "close calls" regarding causation must be resolved in favor of the petitioner. Indeed, "the purpose of the Vaccine Act's preponderance standard is to allow the finding of causation in a field bereft of complete and direct proof of how vaccines affect the human body."

DISCUSSION

Having considered the record as a whole and discussed below, the special master concludes that Petitioners have satisfied their burden of establishing by preponderant evidence that they are entitled to compensation.

Petitioners Have Presented a Plausible Medical Theory, Molecular Mimicry, Along With Supporting Literature That the Vaccine Can Cause A.R.'s Injuries, Thereby Satisfying *Althen* Prong

Petitioners have satisfied *Althen*'s Prong 1 by presenting a plausible medical theory. In support of Prong 1, Petitioners' expert, Dr. Houff, described the process of molecular mimicry as a mechanism whereby the vaccine could cause an autoimmune response that could result in TM, what he had concluded A.R. experienced. This was also discussed in the article submitted, *Transverse Myelitis and Vaccines: A Multi-analysis*. Petitioners also submitted a number of other articles from various medical journals. The medical literature submitted provided further support that it has been recognized that Tdap could cause TM. Those articles are evidence supportive of Petitioners' theory.

Respondent's expert, Dr. Sladky, did not deny that vaccines might cause autoimmune responses such as TM. In commenting on Petitioners' theory, without providing any particular reasoning, Dr. Sladky merely said, in a conclusory fashion, that he was not sure there was sufficient evidence on which to base Petitioners' conclusion regarding a theory.

Respondent's expert did admit that Petitioners had certainly submitted literature in support of their theory. Dr. Sladky expressed that the articles were not that persuasive because they showed the rarity of TM post-vaccine. Nonetheless, Dr. Sladky admitted that there were case reports that supported the theory of TM as a complication of vaccinations, including Tdap. For purposes of the Vaccine Program, Petitioners are not required to establish that there is epidemiological evidence to support their theory.

Rather, the Vaccine Program acknowledges the rarity of vaccine-caused injuries, and, nonetheless, recognizes that compensation for such injuries is appropriate. The purpose of the Vaccine Act's preponderance standard is to allow the finding of causation in a field bereft of complete and direct proof of how vaccines affect the human body, explaining that "to require identification and proof of specific biological mechanisms would be inconsistent with the purpose and nature of the vaccine compensation program."

Considering the evidence with these standards in mind, Petitioners have presented sufficient evidence to demonstrate a plausible medical theory by which the vaccine could have caused the condition with which Petitioners claim A.R. suffers, TM. Petitioners have satisfied *Althen*'s Prong 1.

Petitioners Have Presented Preponderant Evidence That There Is a Logical Sequence of Cause and Effect Between the Vaccine and A.R.'s Injuries By Showing That A.R.'s Injuries Were Caused by an Autoimmune Response and Not an Embolism and That the Vaccine Was a Substantial Factor in Causing the Injury

Petitioners claimed that A.R. suffered from transverse myelitis, an inflammatory demylinating condition in the central nervous system that was caused by an autoimmune response. Respondent, on the other hand, while not claiming to present an alternative cause or factor unrelated as a defense, nonetheless, argued that there was evidence that A.R.'s injury was more likely caused by an embolism obstructing blood from flowing down the spine. As such, according to Respondent, Petitioners had not satisfied their burden as to Prong 2.

The record demonstrates that there was evidence that A.R.'s clinical picture along with the diagnostic tests support that A.R.'s injuries were caused by an inflammation of the central nervous system that was caused by an autoimmune response. The record also demonstrates that there is preponderant evidence that the vaccine caused that injury.

Petitioners Have Shown by Preponderant Evidence That A.R. Experienced an Autoimmune Response Petitioners have presented sufficient evidence that A.R.'s symptoms were caused by an autoimmune response. First, Dr. Krousgrill, one of A.R.'s treating physicians, concluded that A.R. had TM, a condition caused by an autoimmune response. In reaching her conclusion, Dr. Krousgrill relied on her examination of A.R., her review of medical records and her medical knowledge. One factor that Dr. Krousgrill considered was the progression of A.R.'s symptoms. Dr. Krousgrill noted that A.R.'s symptoms began with A.R. experiencing tingling in her legs shortly after receipt of the vaccination. The tingling in her legs was different than that she had experienced in the past. And, A.R. had also explained that for several hours before she went to the bathroom on August 5, 2006, A.R. had experienced tingling. This indicated that the onset was not the abrupt onset that occurred over a matter of minutes, a conclusion upon which Respondent's experts had relied in formulating their opinions. Instead, it was consistent with an autoimmune response, TM. Dr. Krousgrill also looked at the temporal relation and the MRI findings that indicated a focal inflammatory process in the central portion of the cord that involved the entire cord. In addition, although the CSF proteins were steadily high between the first and second lumbar punctures, the fact is that A.R. did not have many white blood counts. Finally, the appearance of oligoclonal bands in the central nervous system indicated an active infection or inflammation. The location of the lesion and broad extent of it shown on the MRI findings indicated that it was more likely this was a transverse process.

Dr. Houff testified that he concluded that A.R. suffered an autoimmune response. He based his conclusion on A.R.'s picture as a whole, i.e., the clinical picture, the exam, the radiology, her spinal fluid and all the studies. In particular, the signal on the MRI findings from that indicated a widespread effect, from T-2 through T-7, the evidence of oligoclonal banding after the second tap, the elevated complement, her high level of C-1 inhibitor, and the emergency room finding some sensation above the knee but no sensation below the knees and a mild sensation above the knees to T-12 and her poor rectal tone and incontinence all indicated that A.R. experienced a progressive, autoimmune response. Additionally, Dr. Houff explained that A.R. met four of the criteria for TM as established by the Transverse Myelitis Working Group. The four "inflammation" criteria that were present included abnormal godlinlim enhancement of the spinal cord, "a CSF pleocytosis," and "elevated CSF IgG index." Id. at 4. Those inflammatory markers within the spinal cord are critical factors to distinguish TM, a type of inflammatory myelopathy, from other non-inflammatory myelopathy, like "ischemia, radiation, epidural lipomatosis or fibrocartilagenous embolism."

Petitioners' evidence shows that the presence of the majority of the criteria as well as the results of the independent evaluations support Petitioner's request. There is ample evidence to support Petitioners.

Respondent's Argument That the Cause of A.R.'s Injuries Is Likely an Embolism, Infarction or FCE Versus TM Is Unreliable and Unsupported by the Facts. Respondent's claims that there is evidence that A.R.'s injuries are more likely caused by an embolism are unsupported by the objective clinical and diagnostic evidence, and her expert's conclusions are unreliable. Whereas both of Petitioners' expert neurologists, Dr. Krousgill and Dr. Houff, presented logically reliable testimony, Respondent's expert's, Dr. Sladky's, testimony did not present the same level of reliability.

First, Dr. Sladky admitted that the theory that this is an infarction cannot necessarily be shown. For instance, he admitted there was no evidence as to how an infarct might have happened because there is no evidence of any trauma. In part his conclusion is simply based on the fact that he "doesn't think that TM would behave in the fashion it did. And, he admitted that there was no evidence of severe back pain, something indicative of FCE. And, the objective evidence indicated that A.R.'s conditions are unlikely due to an embolism. As Dr. Brown explained, based on the view of the MRI, this was not an infarction because there is not a focal lesion that one would expect to see in an infarction. Rather, the lesion is quite widespread, consistent with an autoimmune response. And, the injury about which Respondent theorizes is also inconsistent with the anatomy of the blood supply to the spinal cord. For this theory to actually occur this disk material would have had to enter one of the lumbar arterials and somehow communicated with a vessel coming off the aorta, but that's not the way the arterial anatomy works. One has a small artery at each lumbar vertebral level supplying a small amount of the blood supply to the cauda equine, and there's not even a spinal cord at that level, but just nerve roots. One can somehow have an embolism in one artery and have it somehow get to another part of the spinal cord. That's not the way the arterial anatomy is constructed.

Dr. Krousgrill testified that it was significant that the entire cord was affected and that inidicated this was TM versus an embolism. The two primary avenues for circulation to the cord are the anterior spinal artery. It would be unusual to have an ischemia in all 3 vessels simultaneously all at the same level. Unlike A.R.'s situation, when a spinal artery is involved it is typically an anterior or lateral cord syndrome with mild or mixed sensory results. The clinical progression is not consistent with an infarction or embolism.

Additionally, Dr. Brown also reiterated that which Petitioners' other experts, Dr. Krousgrill and Dr. Houff, had already stated in connection with their conclusions of the lumbar punctures or spinal taps performed on August 6 as compared to those performed on August 10. It was significant that in the first tap there was not evidence of oligoclonal banding, whereas in the section one there was, because an inflammatory response in the spinal cord does not look full blown immediately. It takes some time.

This objective, diagnostic evidence shows that there is a lack of support for Respondent's claimed cause and support for Petitioners' claim that A.R. experienced an autoimmune response. Second, Respondent's expert, Dr. Sladky, acknowledged that there was a basis for a conclusion that A.R. had an auto-immune response. He admitted that some of the accepted criteria for TM were definitely present. He also admitted that there is respected literature that includes TM as a complication of vaccinations, including Tdap vaccinations. And he admitted that oligoclonal bands are indicative of an immune response. In fact, Dr. Sladky's explanation for the oligoclonal bands being in the serum and spinal fluid is not logical in light of the facts. He testified that the presence of oligoclonal banding in serum and the spinal fluid even if it was infarction could be explained because IgG was produced originally in the serum as a result of immunization and was leaked into the spinal fluid through broken blood barrier resulting from infarction. But, Dr. Vezina disagreed that the banding would appear just in the course after a vaccine, saying it was clearly an abnormal response. Finally, a last factor in considering the reliability of his testimony that the special master must consider is the information that was revealed relative to Dr. Sladky's status at the time of his work on this case and testimony. In May 2013, it was revealed that Dr. Sladky's medical license had agreed not to practice medicine from August 2008 to March 2009 and then had agreed to a suspension of his license that lasted from June 2009 to March 2010. At that time his license was restored on a probationary basis, the probation finally terminating on July 2011. At the time he submitted his expert reports in this case, he was on probation. And, in discussing his qualifications at the hearing, no mention was made of these circumstances and such information was glossed over. In fact, in his testimony, Dr. Sladky said he was the Chief of the Pediatric Dept. at Emory University until 2009. But, given that he was not practicing medicine after August 2008, it is questionable whether that could be the case. Certainly, this leads the special master to pause when weighing the experts' opinions. For all the foregoing reasons, the special master does not find Dr. Sladky's testimony as reliable and persuasive as the testimony of Dr. Houff and Dr. Krousgill.

Dr. Vezina, Respondent's neuroradiologist, admitted in his testimony that although he thought TM was less likely, based on the MRI findings, A.R.'s injuries could be either spinal cord infarction or TM. He also testified that with regard to an infarction there would have to be some sort of trauma. He deferred to the neurologist on this but admitted that he needed more information before he could state that such trauma had occurred. He also acknowledged that A.R. had four of the recognized diagnostic criteria for TM, i.e., (1) development of sensory, motor, or autonomic dysfunction attributable to the spinal cord; (2)

bilateral signs and/or symptoms; (3) clearly defined sensory level (*assumes* we have this but doesn't have the medical records); (4) inflammation within the spinal cord demonstrated by CSF, or elevated IgG indexed. Dr. Vezina also testified that he had no direct evidence to prove that that Amber suffered an infarct from FCE. Finally, Dr. Vezina admitted that this was a close call and "it's not a clear vascular thing" because it's a focal lesion and on the whole cord. In many ways, Dr. Vezina's testimony was consistent with Dr. Brown's testimony as well as Petitioners' other experts. He acknowledged that there was clearly clinical and diagnostic evidence that A.R. suffered from TM. As he stated this is a close call. In the Vaccine Program, Petitioners are accorded the benefit of close calls.

There Is Preponderant Evidence Showing the Vaccine to Be a Substantial Factor in Causing the Autoimmune Response

There is also preponderant evidence that the Tdap vaccine was a substantial factor in causing A.R.'s TM. Dr. Krousgrill, the treating physician, concluded that having looked at a number of potential etiologies, the vaccine was significant. Admittedly, she could not make this a definitive diagnosis based upon a standard of reasonable degree of medical certainty, but she certainly believed there was a relationship between the vaccine and A.R.'s TM. (treating physicians' opinions should be considered). Dr. Houff also explained that in this case he felt there was enough data to conclude within a reasonable degree of medical probability that the vaccine caused A.R.'s injuries. In so doing, he explained that it's very hard to conclude that vaccines cause injuries. He acknowledged the importance of vaccines. At the same time, based on his assessment of the clinical picture in this case, including (1) the progression of her illness, (2) the temporal association, and (3) the lack of indication of another infection, the data was enough to conclude that the vaccine caused A.R. an aberrant immune response that attacked her nervous system, her spinal cord. And, Dr. Brown also discussed how she had concluded that the vaccine caused A.R.'s injuries. She relied on the classic appearance of TM on the imaging study, the time frame and A.R.'s history up to that point.

Respondent's expert, Dr. Sladky, did not definitively rule out the vaccine as a cause. Instead, in his expert report he simply stated he did not think Dr. Houff provided a compelling argument to support this position. Weighing the testimony as presented, the special master finds that Petitioners' experts were more persuasive. They explained logically and methodically their reasoning for concluding the vaccine was a substantial factor. At the same time, they did not overstate their positions, instead acknowledging that it would be difficult, if not impossible, to prove the vaccine was the cause as a matter of medical certainty. On the other hand, Respondent's expert primarily presented a conclusory statement that he did not believe Petitioners had satisfied their burden. In addition to that, the special master must also look at the cumulative evidence on all three prongs in that evidence that satisfies Prongs 1 and 3 can overlap and be used to satisfy Prong 2. Here, there is sufficient evidence to satisfy Prong 1.

There is no question that Prong 3 has been satisfied. The treating physician, Dr. Krousgrill, having considered the clinical picture of A.R. at or near the time of the onset of symptoms, looked for other potential causes and considered them but found none. Tr. at 8-9. Similarly, with regard to temporal relationship, there is not much question that it is satisfied. That evidence also overlaps and supports the evidence in the record relating to Prong 2. In sum, Petitioners have presented sufficient proof to demonstrate satisfy their burden as to Prong 2. In particular, the MRI at the time of the onset of A.R.'s condition indicated a lesion with the entire spinal cord being involved, which is consistent with inflammation versus embolism. Additionally, the presence of oligoclonal banding, which was not present initially, and the fact that the CSF protein levels increased, are indicators that the cause was an immune mediated process, which would eliminate FCE as a potential cause. The fact that A.R. reported having heaviness in her legs for some time and even up to hours before her trip to the bathroom when she was unable to move and still had some feeling for a period afterwards indicates that this was not an abrupt onset as Respondent contends and upon which her expert bases his conclusions. And Petitioners have also presented preponderant evidence that the Tdap vaccine A.R. received was a substantial factor in causing that autoimmune response. Petitioners' experts carefully examined the record for other possible explanations, [and] researched the medical literature.

In weighing the Petitioners' experts versus Respondent's experts, the special master concludes that Petitioners' experts' opinions are more reliable. In particular, A.R.'s treating physician, Dr. Krousgrill, testified for Petitioners that she had concluded A.R. had TM. Dr. Houff gave a reasoned explanation that A.R. had TM and that the vaccine caused it. On the other hand, Dr. Sladky, Respondent's expert, admitted that embolisms were more rare than TM.

Respondent's claims that the evidence of inflammation was unlikely does not seem consistent with the appearance of oligoclonal bands. Dr. Vezina said that the appearance of banding would not occur merely because someone had a vaccine. Rather, it was clearly an abnormal response.

Considering the supporting literature, the strong evidence of the temporal relation, the evidence of an autoimmune response and lack of any other possible etiology, there is sufficient evidence to show a logical sequence of cause and effect. Petitioners have satisfied *Althen*'s Prong 2.

There Is No Dispute as to *Althen* Prong 3

Finally, that there is a medically appropriate temporal relationship is not disputed. The parties agreed that the time frame between the receipt of the vaccine on July 6, 2006 and the onset of the injuries on August 5, 2006, is medially appropriate.

CONCLUSION

Upon review of the evidence and an assessment of the reliability of the opinions of the various expert witnesses, the special master concludes that Petitioners have established by preponderant evidence that they are entitled to compensation. The matter shall now proceed to consideration of damages.

IT IS SO ORDERED.

Doug Paluck and Rhonda Paluck, as parents and natural guardians on behalf of their minor son, Karl Paluck, Petitioners v. Secretary of Health and Human Services, Respondent

Summary: In this case, Judge Lettow rules on appeal after a hearing that a Special Master erred in earlier decisions and that the victim's pre-existing underlying mitochondrial disease or dysfunction was aggravated by administration of MMR, varicella, and Prevnar vaccines.

Compensated Vaccine Injury: Aggravation of a Pre-existing Mitochondrial Defect Leading to Neurologic Injury

Vaccine case; petitioners' challenge to a special master's decision on remand; off-Table claim stemming from neurological damage allegedly caused or aggravated by administration of MMR, varicella, and Prevnar vaccines to a child with a genetic mitochondrial defect; claim asserting an aggravation of a pre-existing condition; *Loving* causation framework; entitlement; remand

Case No: 07-889V

Date Filed: October 29, 2013

Doug Paluck and Rhonda Paluck, as parents and natural guardians on behalf of their minor son, Karl Paluck, Petitioners v. Secretary of Health and Human Services, Respondent

OPINION AND ORDER

Charles F. Lettow, Judge

Petitioners, Rhonda and Doug Paluck, on behalf of their son Karl Paluck, seek review of a decision on remand by a special master dated May 10, 2013, denying them compensation under the National Childhood Vaccine Injury Act of 1986. Petitioners filed in accord with the Rules of the Court of Federal Claims. This opinion and order will remain sealed for fourteen days, within which time the parties may propose redactions.

Their claim on December 21, 2007, alleging that Karl's receipt of the measles-mumps-rubella ("MMR"), varicella, and Prevnar vaccines on January 19, 2005 caused him either to develop an impairment or to exacerbate a preexisting condition, resulting in severe neurological damage. The Secretary of Health and Human Services acknowledges Karl's injury but contends that its cause is unrelated to the vaccines. Petitioners' claim is an off-Table injury claim, requiring proof of causation in fact by a preponderance of the evidence. The special master assigned to the case initially denied petitioners' claim for compensation on December 14, 2011, finding that the Palucks failed to meet the three-part causation test established in *Althen*. In response to a motion by petitioners for review, this court rendered a decision on April 18, 2012, vacating the special master's findings under all three *Althen* prongs and remanding the case to the special master, while "making no affirmative findings of its own." In its decision ordering remand, the court directed the special master and the parties first to reassess whether petitioners' claim was a significant-aggravation claim that had to be analyzed under the six-part test explicated in *Loving v. Secretary of Dep't of Health & Human Servs.*, which the special master had not applied. The *Loving* test combines the three causation factors from *Althen* with three additional factors that consider a claimant's health before and after the vaccination. The court also directed the special master to reconsider the record as a whole before making new findings regarding causation in fact.

In the remanded proceedings before the special master, no new evidence was submitted by either party. Supplemental briefing regarding Karl's developmental delays before and after the vaccine was completed by September 19, 2012. The statutory period for decision after the remand expired without a resolution, and on January 30, 2013, petitioners again moved for review by this court because of the delay. On May 3, 2013, the court denied the motion, but directed the special master to issue a decision within 120 days. The special master issued a decision a week thereafter, on May 10, 2013, again denying petitioners' claim.

Petitioners renewed their motion for review of the special master's decision by this court, contending that the special master's findings of fact and conclusions of law are arbitrary and capricious, an abuse of discretion, and not in accord with the law. The Palucks ask this court to make its own findings of fact and issue a decision on entitlement in their favor.

The government argues that the special master's decision was premised on adequate findings of fact and conclusions of law and should be left undisturbed. The Palucks' motion for review, filed June 10, 2013, has been fully briefed, and a hearing was held on September 18, 2013.

FACTS

Karl Paluck currently suffers from an unspecified mitochondrial disorder that was most likely present at birth. At the time of the vaccinations, that disorder had not been detected. After the vaccinations, Karl became severely disabled, but the parties disagree as to the cause.

Karl was born on January 15, 2004 and showed no apparent signs of disability from birth through about the first eight months of life. A concern about developmental delay was first recorded on September 27, 2004 by Ms. Heather Ernst during developmental screening at Karl's daycare provider, as part of the North Dakota Right Track Program. She observed delays in his gross and fine motor skills and referred him to an infant development service, K.I.D.S. K.I.D.S. evaluated Karl on October 21, 2004. The evaluation examined areas of fine motor skills, gross motor skills, speech and language skills, cognition, and adaptive behavior. Four test protocols were used: Bayley Scales of Infant Development ("Bayley Scales"), PDMS-2 Developmental Motor Scales—gross and fine motor scales ("PDMS-2"), Preschool Language Scale-3 ("PLS-3"), and Vineland Adaptive Behavior Scales ("Vineland").

The Bayley Scales protocol is generally used to test a child's cognitive skills (i.e., ability to remember, problem solve, use and understand language, and identify early number concepts). Karl scored "within normal limits" and was found to have an 11% delay.

Testing with PDMS-2's gross motor scales evaluated Karl's ability to use his large muscles, and testing with PDMS-2's fine motor scales evaluated Karl's ability to use his small muscles. Karl showed significant delay in his gross motor skills: 44% delay in stationary skills (i.e., head and trunk control, sitting), 67% delay in locomotion skills (i.e., rolling/crawling and object manipulation), and 67% delay in reflexes (i.e., ability to stay upright.

The special master wrongly attributed the referral to K.I.D.S. as having been prompted by a visit to Karl's pediatrician, Dr. Stephen McDonough, as a result of an examination at eight months. In actuality, Karl was not examined at eight months of age by Dr. McDonough. Rather, he was examined at four months, six months, and one year by Dr. McDonough. Overall, he ranked in the first percentile for gross motor skills. He showed less delay in his fine motor skills: 11% delay in grasping and 22% delay in visual motor integration (i.e., hand-eye control), ranking in the eighth percentile. Karl could roll over, but he could not sit without support or crawl. He could not lift his legs off of the floor while lying on his back. He was, however, using a "wide variety" of fine motor skills. The evaluators could not determine with certainty the reason for his gross motor delays, but ultimately believed that low muscle tone was the underlying cause of Karl's inability to sit and crawl. The evaluators believed that Karl presented with elevated tone in his legs because he was using them to compensate for the instability he felt in his arms and trunk. PLS-3 was employed to evaluate Karl's ability to use and understand language. Karl showed moderate delays: 33% delay in auditory comprehension and 22% delay in expressive communication, ranking in the 32nd percentile. He was able to combine sounds and produce four different consonant sounds, but he was not imitating others' sounds or responding to "no, no, Karl." Lastly, the Vineland protocol tested Karl's ability to care for his needs. It looked to his communication skills, daily living skills, socialization, and motor skills. Overall, Karl was evaluated as 14% delayed. He was 22% behind in communication skills, 11% behind in daily living skills, 0% behind in socialization skills, and 33% behind in motor skills, ranking in the thirtieth percentile overall. Ultimately, K.I.D.S. determined that Karl presented a "mixed picture" and recommended that he "receive infant development services from the K.I.D.S. program targeting his speech/language, gross motor, and the delays in fine motor related to low muscle tone."

Both parties' experts agreed that the K.I.D.S. evaluation was "good and extensive," but they disagreed as to the significance of the findings relative to Karl's neurological health. At the time Karl underwent his first evaluation for his developmental delays, he was experiencing recurrent bouts of otitis media and rashes that were later identified as erythema multiforme. The erythema multiforme was first noticed on October 14. Tone is a measurement of the muscles' ability to maintain the body in proper posture in different positions, such as sitting, standing, or being held. Normal tone means the muscles are maintaining the body in proper posture. Low tone means the muscles do not sufficiently function to maintain the body in proper posture. Otitis media is "inflammation of the middle ear," commonly known as an ear infection. Biopsy results from December 28, 2004 confirmed that the rash was consistent with erythema multiforme. Erythema multiforme, which has rash-like symptoms, is "either of two conditions characterized by sudden eruption of erythematous papules, some of which evolve into target 2004, a week before the K.I.D.S. testing. Thereafter, the record is replete with visits and telephone calls to the Dickinson Clinic between October 2004 and January 2005 regarding Karl's otitis media and erythema multiforme, documenting no fewer than eleven visits and telephone calls during those few months. Dr. Robert Snodgrass, respondent's expert, sees significance in Karl's erythema multiforme, not because children with rashes are rare, but because erythema multiforme is relatively uncommon. It is a hypersensitivity reaction, and in Karl's case, it persisted for months.

Moreover, both Dr. Snodgrass and Dr. Richard Frye, petitioners' expert, testified that it is evidence of immune activation. It suggests that Karl was under some immune stress in the months leading up to the vaccinations on January 19, 2005. Notably, the erythema multiforme improved after a physician, Dr. Amy Oksa, prescribed Orapred, an immune suppressant drug, but recurred when Karl stopped taking it. Most of Karl's medical record in November and

December 2004 centers on treating Karl's otitis media and erythema multi-forme. On December 27, 2004, Karl saw Dr. McDonough for an ear check. The record of the visit states that Karl's recent medical history, as reported by his parents, was "positive for a fever." At that time, Dr. McDonough also lesions consisting of a central papule surrounded by a discolored ring or rings. Both represent reactions of the skin and mucous membranes to factors such as viral skin infections . . . agents (including drugs) that are ingested or irritate the skin; [or] malignancy."

For its arguments, the government relies upon the testimony and reports submitted to the special master by its expert, Dr. Robert Snodgrass. Dr. Snodgrass is a professor of pediatrics and neurology at the University of California, Los Angeles School of Medicine. He received a bachelor's degree in social relations from Harvard College and an M.D., magna cum laude, from Harvard Medical School. Dr. Snodgrass is board-certified in neurology, with special competence in child neurology. He has written dozens of articles and has held professorships at medical institutions associated with Harvard University, Cambridge University, the University of Southern California, Stanford University, the University of Mississippi, and the University of California, Los Angeles.

To support their contentions, the Palucks rely upon the testimony and reports submitted to the special master by their expert, Dr. Richard Frye. Dr. Frye is an assistant professor of pediatrics and neurology at the University of Texas Houston Health Science Center. He received a bachelor's degree in psychobiology from C.W. Post of Long Island University, a master's degree in biomedical science/biostatistics from Drexel University, and both a Ph.D. in physiology and biophysics and an M.D. from Georgetown University. Dr. Frye is board-certified in general pediatrics and in neurology with special competence in child neurology. He has published numerous articles and has held residencies or professorships affiliated with Harvard University, Boston University, the University of Miami, the University of Florida, and the University of Texas.

On January 6, 2005, the daycare noted that the K.I.D.S. Program worked with Karl for thirty minutes, that Karl cried during "tummy time," and that he seemed very tired that day. The next day, the daycare recorded that he was "crabby" in the afternoon. There are no other daycare notes describing Karl before the vaccinations.

On January 19, 2005, Karl saw Dr. McDonough for his one year well-child checkup. Dr. McDonough administered DENVER II, a common developmental screening test. The evaluation is recorded on a standardized form on which the doctor notes whether a child "passes" or "fails" certain developmental skills appropriate for his or her chronological age. On January 19, Karl passed "imitate activities," "play ball with examiner," "indicate wants," "bang 2 cubes held by hands," "thumb finger grasp," "jabber," say "dada/mama specific," say "single syllables," "pull to stand," and "stand holding on." Karl failed "get to sitting," "stand 2 [seconds]," "stand alone," say "one word," "wave bye-bye," and "play pat a cake."

Dr. Frye testified that Dr. McDonough incorrectly scored the DENVER II screening for some skills. Petitioners provided a standard DENVER II chart, which shows that there is a shaded box behind each skill listed on the form. Dr. Frye explained that only when that shaded box ends before reaching the child's chronological age should the child be considered to have "failed" the skill. The shaded box indicates what percentage of children have developed a skill at a certain chronological age. For example, the skill of saying "one word" is accompanied by a shaded box that extends from about ten months to fifteen months. Only when a child turns 15 months and still cannot speak one word, should a child be noted as having "failed" the skill. Thus, according to Dr. Frye's testimony, Karl's only true failed skills should have been "get to sitting," "stand 2 [seconds]," and "play pat-a-cake." Dr. Frye also noted that some of the skills Karl passed were fairly advanced for his age, such as "imitate activities," which less than 75% of children can do at that age. Dr. Frye testified that Karl showed less of a delay at twelve months than he did at nine months. He estimated that Karl was about four or five months delayed in October based on the results of the K.I.D.S. evaluation, and about three months delayed in January based on the DENVER II evaluation.

At this same appointment, Dr. McDonough made additional findings regarding Karl. On a chart labeled "physical examination," Dr. McDonough marked the category "neuromuscular" as abnormal, noting "muscle tone ↑ . . . upper . . . extremities . . . beats clonus [right ankle]." Dr. McDonough checked the category "hips" as normal and wrote next to it some word or words followed by "ROM," meaning range of motion. Dr. McDonough also wrote on the same chart that Karl "doesn't hold cup well," circled the word "babbles," and next to

"1-3 words," he wrote "no words." He also circled the word "crawl" and wrote next to it "4 point" (i.e., hands and knees). Finally, at this same appointment, Karl was given the MMR, varicella, and Prevnar vaccines.

Within two days of receiving the vaccinations, Karl showed signs of irritability, fever, and fatigue. His daycare recorded that he had a temperature of 101.5 degrees on January 21, 2005, and recorded a temperature of 101.3 degrees seven days later on January 28, 2005. Dr. Frye and Dr. Snodgrass disagree over whether the vaccinations caused Karl's subsequent and persistent fever. The daycare records in the two weeks following the vaccination reveal that Karl was often fussy, did not eat or nap well, and was tired. The only positive note occurred on February 3, 2005, when the daycare recorded that "Shiela from the K.I.D.S. [text missing]." There is some confusion over precisely what Dr. McDonough wrote on the "neuromuscular" line of the chart. Dr. Snodgrass testified as follows on cross-examination:

Q. If you look at that handwritten note of Dr. McDonough, he's noting muscle tone increase positive upper. He doesn't say upper and lower, does he?

A. I think he does. It's kind of hard to read. Now I wouldn't criticize anybody who has trouble reading it, but if you look along that line it says muscle tone and there's an arrow pointing up and a plus. Then it says upper and then you go down to the next line and you see L-O-W-E-R. To the left of the L-O-W-E-R is something that I think is an ampersand sign, meaning upper and lower, and then I think you can clearly read extremities after you see lower.

Frye maintained in testimony that the writing preceding "ROM" is the word "full," meaning Karl's hips showed a full range of motion. In contrast, Dr. Snodgrass stated that the writing preceding "ROM" indicated decreased range of motion. The word could also possibly be "good." Based on other medical records, Dr. McDonough's notation likely does not mean that Karl could successfully complete full cross-crawl movements.

On February 8, 2005, the daycare noted that Karl was trying to crawl by "pulling his body." On February 7, 2005, the Palucks first took Karl to a chiropractor to address his problems sitting, crawling, and walking. On February 9, 2005, the chiropractor recorded some abnormalities with Karl's hips on cross crawl. Karl's chiropractic record contains an entry for February 11, 2005 in which is written the word "spastic." There is significant disagreement between the parties over whether the chiropractic records suggest decline or improvement through February and March 2005. The subjective assessments noted in later entries are variable:

- February 14—"better mood,"
- February 16—"less rigid—more comfortable on all 4s"
- February 18—"less rigid—'happier'"
- February 20—"stiff Mid + T—'happy—moving around—til last nite & today'"
- February 21—"Mid T tite & SOP—irritable"
- February 24—"Spastic Mid T's & ↓ Ts"
- March 1—"No BM yesterday"
- March 4—"BMs better—less fussy"
- March 8—"less hypertonicity—[illegible] ↑ on all fours/BMs more regular"
- March 10—"Not sleeping last night/2AM-5AM/irritable/good day yesterday"
- March 17— "Upper [illegible] skin blotches—back pain." On this day the chiropractor also noted, "palpation of spine [painful] baby cries loud when touched."
- March 27—"rigid lower extreme. Palp. [illegible]—'doing well 'til yesterday' 'took a few crawl steps'"
- March 30 (record of a phone conversation)—"Phone convers. w/ Brenda [Erie] SCSS Re. poss. abuse alleg. I responded—No—discussed poss. Adverse Rx/vaccine, CP [cerebral palsy], Cerebellar Tumor."

Although these entries are variable, they do not show any significant improvement. Many of the comments in the records are written in quotes or describe Karl's behavior outside his appointment, suggesting that they are descriptions of his mood and behavior at home, given to the chiropractor by the Karl's parents. For example, February 18: "happier," February 20: "happy," March 27: "doing well 'til yesterday," "took a few crawl steps," April 2: "good mood this week" "seeing improvement." A telephone conversation record with Dr. McDonough's office dated March 22, 2005 documents the Palucks' report that Karl had "some brief crawling" and is "babbling more," but is "not sitting on his own," "leans to one side."

On January 19, 2005, Dr. McDonough had referred Karl to physical and occupational therapy. Dr. Frye described spasticity as "being the extreme for increased tone."

Dr. Snodgrass found that the notations of Karl's "brief crawling" and "babbling more" were signs of progress since Karl's December 27, 2004, visit with Dr. McDonough. This conclusion by the government's expert was contrary to that reached contemporaneously by Karl's treating physician, Dr. McDonough, who noted on the same telephone record that he would make a referral to Dr. Siriwan Kriengkrairut, a pediatric neurologist. On March 24, 2005, Dr. McDonough wrote the consultation request, citing Karl's "gross motor delay, global developmental delay, and hypertonicity" as the reasons. Global developmental delay is broader than isolated gross motor delay. "Global developmental delay is when you're affected in several areas." (Frye). Dr. McDonough wrote that he "would appreciate [Dr. Kreingkrairut's] evaluation and medical investigations into the etiology of [Karl's] developmental delay and hypertonicity."

In mid to late March, Karl developed a cold. On March 28, 2005, he saw Dr. Gary Peterson at the Dickinson Clinic for "four days of [a] wheezy cough" and a "runny nose for two weeks." The doctor noted early bilateral otitis media and bronchiolitis. He provided a SVN (nebulizer) treatment in the office and also prescribed one for use at home. He noted that Mrs. Paluck preferred "no antibiotics be written as yet since he has had the trouble with erythema multiforme in the past."

By mid-April, Karl's health was significantly worse than it was in January 2005. He continued to suffer from recurrences of otitis media. Karl saw Dr. McDonough on April 13, 2005 for a Pre-Anesthesia Evaluation for a magnetic resonance imaging ("MRI") test that was to be performed on Karl. He noted "global developmental delay," including problems with "speech and fine and gross motor development." Dr. McDonough also wrote that Karl's "hips are tight with decreased hip flexion to about 70 degrees bilaterally with increased [a word appears to be absent, probably "tone"] in the lower extremities. This is a change of hip movement over the last couple of months." Karl had not had any evidence of erythema within the past three weeks.

The neurologist, Dr. Kriengkrairut, examined Karl on April 19, 2005. She documented a brief history of the onset of Karl's problems. "According to the

Culu i ainee [the onset of erythema multiforme in October 2004] the child has regressed. . . . In December of 2004 his condition got worse. His hands and feet were swelled up. He was given medications. This has markedly improved from a month ago when he seemed back to his normal. Father reported that since he has been improving with the skin lesions, he also made progress in terms of development, but overall he is still behind." Following the physical examination, she reported "truncal hypotonia with marked spasticity of the extremities. The baby has tendency to do cortical thumb bilaterally, worse on the right compared to the left. . . . Baby does not babble. . . . Delayed development as well as hypotonia of the extremities may be secondary to central nervous system pathology." Overall, she labeled Karl as having "global delayed development."

Dr. Frye testified that this report by Dr. Kriengrairut suggests a substantial neurological regression in Karl since January 2005. Dr. Snodgrass disagreed that the problems observed by Dr. Kriengkrairut differed substantially from the problems observed by Dr. McDonough in January.

A chiropractic record entry from April 25, 2005, reports decreased range of motion. Dr. McDonough saw Karl the next day, on April 26, 2005, and wrote that Karl "rolls over but does not sit without support. He does not crawl and does not say any words. . . . Hips are tight on range of motion." Dr. McDonough again described Karl as suffering from global developmental delay.

Dr. Kriengkrairut had recommended an MRI of Karl's brain, which was performed on April 27, 2005. The results were initially interpreted as normal, but a reexamination of the results from April 2005 following a more apparently abnormal MRI in July 2005 discerned evidence of a then-existing brain abnormality—thinning of the corporal callosum. The parties' experts disagreed as to when the thinning most likely began. Dr. Frye opined that it occurred "recent to the MRI, after January 2005" (Frye), whereas Dr. Snodgrass testified that he has "seen similar scans in people who had prenatal infections."

Karl declined further in the ensuing months. While the special master found isolated instances of slight improvement, these events contrasted with a general trend of deterioration from April 2005 to July 2005. On May 4, 2005, Karl was evaluated by a speech therapist, Ms. Trisha Getz. At that time, Karl had fewer language skills than he had in October 2004, and his total language score was in the first percentile (Frye). In October 2004, he could produce at least four consonant sounds, but by May 2005, he could no longer produce any consonant sounds, although he could still produce a couple vowel sounds. By May, Karl's only gesture was reaching for objects. Ms. Getz noted, "Karl's parents report he had an MRI last week, which has 'wiped him out' and they report a decrease in many skills since undergoing the anesthesia. . . . Mom reports he has had a decrease in speech production in the last few months." Her reports through September 8, 2005 indicate little to no improvement. ("very little progress" and "no goals met"). Karl continued to be unable to approximate sounds or produce any consonants.

Karl suffered a seizure on July 12, 2005, followed by additional seizures over the next two days. Dr. McDonough examined Karl on July 16, 2005 and assessed him as having "global developmental delay with seizure disorder, possible deteriorating neurologic status in that he is unable to do some things that he was able to do previously." On July 19, 2005, Karl was admitted to Children's Hospital in St. Paul, Minnesota by Dr. Michael Frost. While there, MRI results showed furthering thinning of the corporal callosum, strongly suggesting that Karl was suffering from neurodegeneration. On October 27, 2005, Karl had another MRI, which showed no significant change in Karl's brain since the July 2005 MRI. "The progression of signal changes between [4/27/05 and 7/22/05] may have represented evolution of one toxic/metabolic or hypotoxic ischemic event."

Since July 2005, Karl has lived in a state of severe neurological disability. Earlier in 2013, he was in dire health. "There is a 'do not resuscitate order now in place' for him, and 'he is bedridden or wheelchair-ridden, has a tracheotomy tube, and is on a ventilator to breathe for him.'"

PRIOR DECISIONS

Paluck I

The Palucks filed their petition for compensation on December 21, 2007, alleging that Karl "sustained a permanent injury to his brain and central nervous system as a result of receipt of his childhood vaccines . . . [and] that the exposure to childhood vaccines caused and/or aggravated a mitochondrial disorder in Karl." Three hearings in the case were held over the course of 2010. At the hearings, the parties disagreed as to whether Karl's vaccines caused or aggravated his neurodegenerative course. Dr. Frye testified that the vaccines either caused Karl's injury, or aggravated his condition, according to the following theory:

[V]accines, by intention, activate the immune system; this in turn leads to the th oo lnpuon m of proo nntially uoxic clomonts within the body, namely reactive oxygen species (ROS) and reactive nitrogen species (RNS); ROS and RNS are usually balanced under normal conditions by the (antioxidant) systems of the body; however, if certain parts of the body, namely the mitochondria, are not working properly, more toxic elements will be produced and will be unchecked by antioxidants, resulting in oxidative stress, leading to a cascade of intracellular events leading to apoptosis or cellular death. Brain cells are more vulnerable to this process and with death of brain cells, neurodegeneration and developmental regression are likely.

Applying the theory to Karl's case, Dr. Frye testified that Karl had an underlying mitochondrial disorder that prevented him from coping with the oxidative stress of the vaccines. This led to "decompensation" within his cells and eventually cellular death, resulting in neurodegeneration.

Dr. Snodgrass disagreed, testifying that "there are problems with [Dr. Frye's] theory in general and there are problems with its specific application to the case of Karl Paluck." He criticized Dr. Frye's theory generally on the ground of lack of published peer-reviewed literature demonstrating that vaccines cause oxidative stress in humans, although he acknowledged supporting animal-model data. In his view also, Karl's medical history did not support the idea that vaccines caused or aggravated his condition. Dr. Snodgrass stated that Karl manifested developmental delays before his vaccinations on January 19, 2005. Dr. Snodgrass additionally stated that between January and April 2005, Karl's condition fluctuated, but did not worsen, as would be expected had the vaccines caused Karl's injury.

The special master issued a decision denying compensation on December 14, 2011, concluding that petitioners had failed to prove by a preponderance of the evidence that the vaccines administered to Karl on January 19, 2005 caused his injury or significantly aggravated a preexisting condition. In so holding, the special master applied the three-prong causation framework set out in *Althen*, which requires a petitioner to show by preponderant evidence that the vaccination brought about [the] injury by providing: (1) a medical theory causally connecting the vaccination and the injury; (2) a logical sequence of cause and effect showing that the vaccination was the reason for the injury; and (3) a showing of a proximate temporal relationship between vaccination and injury.

The special master found that the Palucks had failed to carry their burden as to any of the three prongs.

Regarding *Althen*'s first prong, the special master was not convinced by the evidence presented that vaccines produce oxidative stress generally or oxidative damage particularly in persons with mitochondrial disorders. Regarding *Althen*'s second prong, the special master found that Karl's history did not demonstrate a logical sequence of cause and effect between the vaccinations and Karl's injury. According to the special master, Dr. Frye's theory required that Karl's medical history evidence a continuous downward trajectory, which "did not match what actually happened to Karl." Instead, the special master credited Dr. Snodgrass's testimony that Karl's development fluctuated between September 2004 and April 2005, with Karl actually improving between the time of his January 2005 vaccinations and late March 2005. Regarding *Althen*'s third prong, the special master concluded that oxidative damage would have occurred in Karl within fourteen days, and that Karl's immediate post-vaccination symptoms—fever, irritability, and, according to his chiropractor, spasticity and hypertonicity—did not evidence such damage. Finding that Karl did not manifest further neurological regression until April 2005, the special master determined that Karl's injury fell outside the medically acceptable time-frame for vaccine injury.

Paluck II

Petitioners filed a motion for review of the special master's decision in *Paluck I* on January 13, 2012, arguing that the special master's conclusions on all three *Althen* prongs were "arbitrary and capricious, an abuse of discretion, or not otherwise in accord with the law." The government urged affirmance.

Oral argument was held on March 21, 2012. On April 18, 2012, this court vacated the special master's findings of fact and conclusions of law, and remanded the case to the special master for further proceedings. The court expressly did not make any affirmative findings of fact of its own. The court reviewed the special master's determinations of law *de novo*, and his findings of fact for clear error.

First, the court directed the special master to reconsider whether petitioners' claim should be analyzed as a significant aggravation claim or a new injury claim. The special master had analyzed it using the standards applicable to a new injury claim without discussion of whether those standards were most appropriate.

Second, the court addressed the special master's findings under each of the three *Althen* prongs. Regarding *Althen*'s first prong, a medical theory causally connecting the vaccination and the injury, the court held that the special master required a higher level of proof, i.e., a higher level of scientific certainty, than is demanded by the Vaccine Act. The Vaccine Act does not require that "evidence be medically or scientifically certain." To support his theory, Dr. Frye relied on a peer-reviewed study published in a well-respected medical journal, various studies showing oxidative stress in animals as a result of vaccines, and a case study. While the special master correctly determined that none of the evidence was definitive proof of the medical validity of Dr. Frye's theory, it was arbitrary and capricious for him to discard it as completely as he did. The court also noted that Dr. Snodgrass did not dispute the reputability of the theory but only noted the dearth of human studies establishing it as fact. The court vacated the special master's finding that petitioners failed to show by a preponderance of the evidence that vaccines can cause oxidative stress and that children with mitochondrial disorders are particularly vulnerable to oxidative stress and directed the special master to reconsider the evidence in the record under the correct legal standard. The court also vacated the special master's finding under *Althen*'s second prong that petitioners failed to demonstrate, by a preponderance of the evidence, a logical sequence of cause and effect showing that the vaccinations caused Karl's injury. The special master had given considerable weight to unexplained notations throughout the record that Karl was progressing in his ability to prepare to crawl through the months of February, March, and April, which was something he could not do at the critical appointment on January 19, 2005 with Dr. McDonough, when he was vaccinated. Karl was never formally evaluated as being able to crawl. At most, there was evidence that he was making some preparatory crawl motions at times. Similarly, the special master concluded that notations of babbling suggested development throughout the same months, despite evidence that Karl actually lost language abilities. Moreover, the court opined that the special master failed fully to consider the chiropractor's records from February and

March and Dr. McDonough's referral to a pediatric neurologist in March. The court held that the special master's finding that Karl's efforts to crawl and babbling signaled improvement, therefore negating a logical sequence of cause and effect between Karl's vaccines and injury, should be vacated due to a failure to consider all of the salient evidence.

Lastly, the court vacated the special master's finding regarding *Althen*'s third prong, a proximate temporal relationship between the vaccination and injury. According to the special master, the medical literature suggested that the medically acceptable interval between vaccination and the onset of symptoms of neurological injury would be two weeks. The court rejected this conclusion. Given the medical literature relied upon by Dr. Frye, including a case study demonstrating neurodegeneration occurring post-vaccination over a period of several months and a published study showing neurodegeneration occurring following infection in patients with mitochondrial disorders over a period extending to nineteen days, it was arbitrary and capricious for the special master to set a "hard and fast limit of two weeks." The court also held that the special master's finding that Karl did not manifest any symptoms of neurologic injury within a medically acceptable interval after the vaccination was arbitrary and capricious because it failed to consider the record as a whole.

Paluck IV

Before deciding the case on remand, the special master requested supplemental briefing and any additional evidence from the parties regarding the classification of Karl's injury as a new injury or a significant aggravation claim. If the claim were found to be a significant aggravation claim, then the *Loving* factors would apply, which combine the three *Althen* causation factors with three additional factors that inquire into the claimant's condition before and after the vaccination. Both parties submitted supplemental briefs, but neither submitted additional evidence. The special master determined that Karl's claim is one of significant aggravation and must be analyzed under the six *Loving* factors because Karl's developmental delays in the autumn of 2005 strongly suggested pre-existing problems with his central nervous system.

The first prong of *Loving* requires addressing Karl's condition prior to vaccination. The parties agreed that Karl's mitochondrial defect was likely affecting his health before the vaccinations. The parties disagreed over the extent of delay in Karl's language skills and the cause of Karl's gross motor delays. The special master found that the "preponderant weight of the evidence favors finding that Karl's language development was delayed prior to his vaccination." He also found that Karl's gross motor delays and language delays, in existence before the vaccinations, were caused by abnormalities in his central nervous system. He further determined that Karl's gross motor skill delays had worsened between December 27, 2004 and January 19, 2005.

The second prong concerns Karl's condition following the vaccination. The special master extensively summarized Karl's records in the months following the vaccination. He looked to Karl's daycare records, Karl's chiropractic record, Dr. McDonough's referral to the pediatric neurologist, Dr. Kriengkrairut's neurological exam, Karl's MRI in April 2005, Karl's speech therapy records, the seizures and hospitalization in July 2005, and Karl's other medical visits and mitochondrial testing.

The third prong of *Loving* asks whether Karl's current condition constitutes a significant aggravation of his condition prior to the vaccine. Without elaboration, the special master found that "by virtually any metric, Karl was worse" after receiving the vaccines.

The fourth prong of *Loving*, which correlates to the first prong of *Althen,* addresses whether there is a medical theory causally connecting the worsened condition to the vaccine. In response to this court's opinion in *Paluck II*, "both parties essentially agreed that the Palucks' evidence met the standard for medical plausibility as defined by the court." The special master accepted this apparent concession by the government without discussion, noting only that this concession does not lessen the petitioners' burden of proof under *Loving* prongs five and six.

The fifth prong of *Loving* requires petitioners to establish, by a preponderance of the evidence, a logical sequence of cause and effect showing that the vaccination significantly aggravated Karl's condition. The special master determined that Dr. Frye's theory "was predicated on a downhill trajectory." Thus, the special master looked for evidence that Karl's health declined without any improvement from one day to the next following the vaccinations on January 19, 2005. In accordance with this court's order on remand, the special master considered in detail "Karl's chiropractic records, Karl's treating doctors' statements regarding the cause of Karl's decline, and Dr. McDonough's referral to a pediatric neurologist." In considering the chiropractor's notations from February and March, the special master found that it was "difficult to glean much significance from them." Ultimately, he found that the evidence of decline was too variable to suggest a linear decline, as he considered Dr. Frye's theory to require.

The final prong of *Loving* requires the special master to determine a medically acceptable temporal relationship between the vaccine and the significant aggravation and then determine whether the claimant's injuries occurred within that time frame. Upon reconsideration of an article by Dr. Joseph L. Edmonds, the special master lengthened the medically acceptable temporal interval from two weeks, which he had specified in *Paluck I*, to three weeks. Accordingly, the special master looked for evidence of neurodegeneration, defined as the loss of a skill, within three weeks following January 19, 2005, which extended to February 10, 2005. Karl's daycare records and chiropractic records were the only records contemporaneously created during that period. The special master was persuaded by the government's expert that Karl's fevers and irritability in the ten days following the vaccinations did not constitute encephalopathy, as Dr. Frye had opined. Additionally, the special master was unconvinced by Dr. Frye's testimony that the chiropractor's notation describing Karl as "spastic" on February 11, 2005 was evidence of "a very severe neurological event suggesting a very rapid change in his central nervous system."

The special master posited three reasons for not relying on the chiropractor's notation: in his view, (1) spasticity is closely related to hypertonia, which Dr. McDonough noticed on January 19, 2005, (2) chiropractors are not sufficiently well trained to recognize clinical spasticity in infants, and (3) the variability of the chiropractor's records rendered them unreliable. The special master also placed emphasis on the fact that Karl did not appear to stay home from daycare in February, nor did he see doctors with the same frequency he had in December, although he saw the chiropractor frequently.

Overall, the special master concluded that Karl had not been as sick in February as he was in December. The special master concluded that the petitioners could not show by a preponderance of the evidence that Karl manifested evidence of neurological degeneration within the three-week "bound of the appropriate temporal limit."

Based upon a failure of proof respecting the fifth and sixth prongs of *Loving*, the special master denied entitlement to compensation.

STANDARDS FOR REVIEW

Under the Vaccine Act, the court may "set aside any findings of fact or conclusions of law of the special master found to be arbitrary, capricious, an abuse of discretion, or otherwise not in accordance with law and issue its own findings of fact and conclusions of law." The special master's determinations of law are reviewed *de novo*. The special master's findings of fact are reviewed for clear error. "We uphold the special master's findings of fact unless they are arbitrary or capricious" (citing *Capizzano v. Secretary of Health & Human Servs.*).

Under Vaccine Rule 8(b) (1), the special master must "consider all relevant and reliable evidence." Vaccine Rule 8(b) (1); *see also* 42 U.S.C. § 300aa-13(b) (1) "The special master or court shall consider the entire record and the cause of the injury, disability, illness, or condition until the date of the judgment of the special master or court." A special master's findings regarding the probative value of the evidence and the credibility of witnesses will not be disturbed so long as they are "supported by substantial evidence." *Doe v. Secretary of Health & Human Servs.* (citing *Whitecotton*).

As this court stated previously, a deferential standard of review "is not a rubber stamp." The special master must "consider the relevant evidence of record, draw plausible inferences and articulate a rational basis for the decision." And, while the special master need not address every snippet of evidence adduced in the case, he cannot dismiss so much contrary evidence that it appears that he "simply failed to consider genuinely the evidentiary record before him" (*Campbell v. Secretary of Health & Human Servs.*).

ANALYSIS

There is no dispute that Karl's claim involves an "off-Table" injury, i.e., an injury or aggravated condition that is not listed on the Vaccine Injury Table set out at 42 U.S.C. § 300aa-14(a). Accordingly, petitioners must prove causation in fact. The special master concluded that petitioners' claim is most appropriately analyzed as a significant-aggravation claim governed by the *Loving* factors. Petitioners continue to contest classification of the claim as a significant-aggravation claim rather than a new-injury claim, notwithstanding the circumstance that the special master found that the factors related specifically to significant aggravation had been satisfied. Petitioners also contest the special master's conclusions primarily respecting *Loving* prongs five and six, i.e., logical sequence of cause and effect and medically acceptable temporal interval, respectively. The government urges affirmance of the special master's findings.

New Injury or Significant Aggravation

The Vaccine Act defines "significant aggravation" as "any change for the worse in a preexisting condition which results in markedly greater disability, pain, or illness accompanied by substantial deterioration of health." After giving the parties an opportunity to file supplemental briefs and giving them an opportunity to present more evidence, the special master concluded that the preponderance of the evidence weighed in favor of finding that petitioners' claim should be analyzed as a significant-aggravation claim. Petitioners maintain that Karl's neurodegeneration constitutes a new injury, distinct from any delays he might have been experiencing in the months before the vaccination. The government avers that Karl's neurodegeneration can only be properly analyzed as a significant-aggravation claim because he already showed signs of developmental delay before the vaccination. Whether petitioners' claim should be classified as a new injury or significant-aggravation claim rests on the "the precise definition of Karl's injury, which is a precondition to identifying the timing of its symptoms" and "whether indicia of Karl's neurodegeneration followed the typical course of a person that suffers from his type of mitochondrial defect." In its remand opinion, this court sought elucidation of whether developmental delays were the best indicator of neurological injury in someone with a mitochondrial defect. The special master, on remand, specifically asked the parties to address Karl's "neurological, not mitochondrial, symptoms" before the vaccination.

The government responded that "one cannot separate 'mitochondrial symptoms' from the symptoms related to mitochondrial disorder-affected organs, including the central nervous system."

Petitioners, however, pointed to pieces of evidence in the record to show that Karl first exhibited neurological symptoms after the vaccinations, including the chiropractor's records from February and March 2005, the K.I.D.S. evaluation, the April 2005 MRI, and the April 2005 neurological assessment.

The experts disagree about the significance each of these pieces of evidence.

Petitioners emphasized the October 2004 K.I.D.S. evaluation which found "Karl's brain to be functioning within normal limits" and attributed Karl's gross motor delay to low muscle tone. Dr. Frye testified that the K.I.D.S. evaluation was significant because it showed that Karl's cognitive abilities were unimpaired in October 2004. In his view, the concern was Karl's low muscle tone, not his central nervous system. He further explained that this low muscle tone was most likely due to Karl's then-undiagnosed mitochondrial disorder. Dr. Frye testified that although Karl's language skills were below average according to the PLS-3 test, the delay was minimal. His combined standard score for the PLS-3 was 96, and Dr. Frye testified that the average is 100. "Ninety-six is very close to 100 on these scales." According to Dr. Frye, "Karl's delays were most prominently gross motor delays, maybe a little bit of fine motor delays, but cognition, language was absolutely normal…His ability to make language sounds and to interact with others, to be attentive to what was going on in the room, this was all very important and shows that his brain and cognition were working."

Dr. Snodgrass disagreed without elaboration. He opined that describing Karl as "right at the average" was not accurate and that the K.I.D.S. evaluation did not show Karl's cognition and language as "absolutely normal," as Dr. Frye described.

In turning to the chiropractor's notation of spasticity in February 2005, the cortical thumbing noted in April 2005, and the MRI results from April 2005, the experts disagreed over the significance of all three of these. In short, Dr. Frye found all three to be evidence of sudden neurological regression after the vaccinations, and Dr. Snodgrass found them to be either a continuation of the same problems that existed before the vaccinations or insignificant.

The experts disputed the value of the chiropractic records in determining Karl's neurological state in February and March. In particular, they disagreed over the significance of the chiropractor's notation of "spastic" on February 11, 2005. Dr. Frye testified that the chiropractor's finding of spasticity "suggests a very severe neurological event, and that suggests . . . that there was very rapid change in his central nervous system." Dr. Snodgrass saw no special significance in that record, testifying that "they [the chiropractic clinic] often say spastic, stiff, et cetera. So they are reporting on the same general phenomenon which first became evident to Dr. McDonough in January . . . I think that a chiropractor would have some idea of what spastic means, but not necessarily the same that a physician would. And I think when you're talking about a 13- or 14-month-old child, I don't think chiropractors are in a position to make any nuanced statements about them. . . . I don't believe they are trained to evaluate infants."

The experts also disputed the importance of Dr. Kriengkrairut's finding of cortical thumbing in April 2005. Dr. Frye called it a "significant sign of advanced upper motor neuron lesions and something that you don't see with just some type of change in tone or even mild spasticity; that is a very significant finding." He considered that the cortical thumbing, in addition to being a sign of neurological change, demonstrated an impairment occurring since December 2004, when Karl was able to open his hands and grab wrapping paper at Christmas (Frye). Dr. Snodgrass disagreed that the problems observed by Dr. Kriengkrairut differed substantially from the problems observed by Dr. McDonough in January 2005. "The function recorded in January by Dr. McDonough is the same function that was recorded by Dr. Kriengkrairut in April and by Dr. McDonough when he again saw Karl in April." Dr. Snodgrass testified that cortical thumbing is not a significant finding and is not one he would have expected Dr. McDonough, a pediatrician, to note. Upon further questioning by the special master, Dr. Snodgrass stated that thumbing is abnormal in a one-year-old, but in the context of also seeing increased tone, it is insignificant. He further stated that the thumbing was not necessarily "cortical," and thus was not necessarily representative of a brain abnormality.

Lastly, regarding the April 2005 MRI, Dr. Snodgrass and Dr. Frye both concede that it showed evidence of thinning of the corporal callosum, but Dr. Snodgrass testified that that thinning could have been present since birth, whereas Dr. Frye testified that it most likely occurred close in time to the MRI, after the January 2005 vaccinations.

Whether Karl's severe neurodegeneration would have eventually resulted from his mitochondrial defect without the vaccinations posed a vexing issue. The government and petitioners appear to agree that mitochondrial disorders are "a heterogeneous group of disorders characterized by impaired energy production due to genetically based oxidative phosphorylation dysfunction." They also agree that manifestations of mitochondrial diseases are variable. The government maintains that "the aggravation of symptoms as Karl aged stemmed from the natural progression of the disease."

The special master asked Dr. Frye what he would think if a hypothetical child, with Karl's same genetic makeup and medical history, experienced the same neurodegeneration as Karl, without having received any vaccinations. Dr. Frye responded that he would immediately look for some other trigger, such as a bad infection or a bad viral illness because it would be very puzzling to see such a regression with no identifiable cause.

Dr. Snodgrass stated that "mitochrondrial problems are heterogeneous. . . . They vary enormously."

The evidentiary record is bereft of any basis for a natural progression of a mitochrondrial condition to the severely debilitating point Karl experienced. The special master acknowledged that it was possible that Karl's gross motor delays were purely related to low muscle tone and not his central nervous system, but he believed three reasons supported finding that Karl had preexisting neurodegeneration allegedly significantly aggravated by the vaccines. First, it is generally accepted that there is a connection between muscle tone and the nervous system. Second, Karl showed delay in his expressive language according to the K.I.D.S. evaluation in October 2004. Third, the special master pointed to the Palucks' Amended Petition, filed October 17, 2008, stating that they allege that the vaccines "caused a 'significant aggravation' of Karl's underlying mitochondrial disorder, leading to . . . subsequent neurodevelopmental regression."

The special master's reasoning in finding evident neurodegeneration prior to the vaccinations is partially but not fully supported by the record. The parties accepted that the central nervous system helps maintain muscle tone, but the experts did not agree that low muscle tone is necessarily a result of a problem in the central nervous system. Dr. Frye testified that Karl's gross motor delays were attributable to "problems with muscle development, and energy that the muscle needs, because of his [then-undiagnosed] mitochondrial disorder." This testimony is corroborated by the contemporaneous finding by the K.I.D.S. evaluators that Karl's delays were likely a result of low muscle tone. It is also corroborated by the fact that Dr. McDonough did not recommend that Karl see a neurologist until late March. If low muscle tone was necessarily caused by a problem in the central nervous system, that would have been evidence that the K.I.D.S. evaluators and Dr. McDonough should have been and actually were concerned about neurological causes from October 2004 onwards. Contrastingly, Dr. Snodgrass nonetheless opined that Karl's gross motor delays and observed low muscle tone were secondary to undiagnosed problems in his central nervous system. Although Dr. Snodgrass's opinion is plausible, it is supported by the contemporaneous medical records only insofar as Dr. McDonough's examination of Karl on January 19, 2005 indicated "two beats clonus [right ankle]."

The special master's emphasis on Karl's language delay as evidence of pre-vaccination neurodegeneration is minimally supported by the record. There is evidence of delay, but the delay is moderate at most. Petitioners assert there was absolutely no cognitive or language delay. Karl tested within normal limits on the Bayley Scales and tested slightly below average on the PLS-3 scales. Karl was, however, referred to speech therapy by the K.I.D.S. program evaluators. There is room for debate over whether Karl's language skills were actually "delayed," and the special master could have reasonably concluded that being below average, even just slightly, constitutes delay, but to label that delay as evidence of then-existing problems in the central nervous system stretches inference from the evidence too far. In stating that "expressive language tends, at least in the absence of other identified causes, to be considered a Central Nervous System problem," the special master only cites Dr. Snodgrass's testimony that "alludes" to such a connection between expressive language and CNS. Any cognitive and language delays that Karl had were mild prior to the vaccination and were not of strong concern. To find that these delays definitively represented a "CNS problem" is not supported by substantial evidence.

The special master commented that "special masters 'can always rule on a factual issue no matter how scanty the evidence is,'" but that recitation is not a license to ignore the record. In this instance, substantial contemporaneous medical records exist. The four-month and six-month evaluations by Dr. McDonough, the records of illness with otitis media and erytherma multiforme, and especially the K.I.D.S. evaluative results provide significant information about Karl's condition pre-vaccination. These records suggest that no one believed or even suspected Karl's problems were neurological in nature until after the vaccinations. The special master is not free to decide otherwise in the face of this evidence.

Despite these flaws, the special master's conclusion that petitioners' claim is one of significant aggravation and not new injury will not be disturbed. It is evident that Karl faced a multitude of setbacks in the fall. He was not a completely healthy child when he received the vaccinations. He had an undiagnosed mito-chondrial disorder that was causing developmental delays in some areas, and he was experiencing repeated stresses to his immune system in the form of persistent otitis media and erythema multiforme. Given this, the ankle clonus might, but does not necessarily, represent neurological injury. On cross-examination, Dr. Snodgrass explained that a severely agitated child "who is screaming his head off" might have clonus. Petitioners' counsel asked Dr. Snodgrass whether two beats of clonus is "mild clonus." Dr. Snodgrass replied, "I think that depends on the circumstance. I think the basic issue is it's clonus, which was not present before." Upon further questioning, Dr. Snodgrass responded, "Well, it's—two beats of clonus is less than say five. But it's still not normal."

Evidence that Karl's immune system was not functioning optimally, the court concurs that petitioners' claim is more appropriately analyzed as one of significant aggravation. It is not necessary to find with specificity that Karl's gross motor delays were neurological rather than musculoskeletal in nature prior to the vaccinations. If Karl's problems prior to the vaccinations on January 19, 2005, were neurological, the impairment was small and not evident to the treating physicians. Given petitioners' claim that the vaccine overwhelmed Karl's immune system, causing cell death, it is enough to find that Karl's body was under immune stress in the months leading up to the vaccinations and that his underlying mitochondrial defect made his body less able to respond to immune stressors. Thus, petitioners' claim is properly analyzed as one of significant aggravation and not new injury.

Loving Factors
After determining that petitioners' claim is more properly analyzed as a significant aggravation claim, the special master applied the *Loving* test. The court concurs that the *Loving* test applies and requires preponderant proof of: (1) the person's condition prior to administration of the vaccine, (2) the person's current condition (or the condition following the vaccination if that is also pertinent), (3) whether the person's current condition constitutes a 'significant aggravation' of the person's condition prior to vaccination, (4) a medical theory causally connecting such a significantly worsened condition to the vaccination, (5) a logical sequence of cause and effect showing that the vaccination was the reason for the significant aggravation, and (6) a showing of a proximate temporal relationship between the vaccination and the significant aggravation.

Loving Prong 1—Condition Prior to the Vaccinations: The special master found that "overall, by January 19, 2005, Karl had problems in his CNS. His pediatrician diagnosed him with gross motor delays, which had worsened in the preceding three weeks. Karl was also having problems with his language. Finally, Karl was recovering from the most recent episode of erythema multiforme."

Petitioners contest the special master's findings regarding Karl's condition before the vaccinations as arbitrary and capricious and not in accord with the law. First, they challenge the special master's interpretation of Dr. Snodgrass's testimony as meaning that the erythema multiforme was another possible cause of the neurodegeneration. Second, they dispute the special master's finding that Karl had expressive language delay that, "in the absence of other identified causes, is to be considered a CNS problem." Third, petitioners question the special master's finding that Karl's developmental delays worsened between December 2004 and January 2005, contending that the special master ignored Dr. Frye's testimony to the contrary.

The government asserts that the special master's conclusions of fact, including his conclusion that Karl's delays prior to January 2005 represented a problem with his central nervous system, are supported by appropriate evidence.

The special master recounted the evidentiary record in his analysis of Karl's condition prior to the vaccinations. He considered both the contemporaneous medical records and the expert testimony regarding Karl's recurrent erythema multiforme, finding that it was evidence of chronic activation of Karl's immune system.

The dispute over whether Karl's language abilities were delayed poses a different type of issue. As discussed *supra*, reasonable minds could differ over whether Karl could or should be classified as having had a speech delay before the vaccinations. Consequently, the special master could properly conclude that Karl had speech delays. On the other hand, there is no evidence that those speech delays were necessarily a result of neurological problems. As discussed *supra* regarding the propriety of a significant-aggravation analysis, the contemporaneous records do not suggest that Karl's treating physicians and therapists believed that any extant pre-vaccination speech delay was neurological in nature.

Regarding Karl's gross motor delays, the special master found that they represented problems in his central nervous system before the January 19, 2005 vaccinations. In support, the special master compares Dr. McDonough's findings in December 2004, that Karl had normal muscle tone and no ankle clonus, to his findings in January 2005, that Karl had increased tone and two beats of clonus in his right ankle. This evidence supports the special master's conclusion that Karl's physical condition had worsened between December 2004 and January 2005. A report by the same doctor that Karl went from normal muscle tone to increased muscle tone and from no ankle clonus to two beats of ankle clonus is compelling. Again, however, the special master's conclusion that this worsening is necessarily a result of problems with Karl's central nervous system steps beyond the inferences that can permissibly be drawn from the medical evidence. Although Karl's medical problems make this case a significant-aggravation claim rather than a new-injury claim, there is very little direct evidence.

The special master questioned whether the erytherma multiforme could have caused Karl's eventual neurodegeneration but determined that "resolution of this question is not necessary because . . . Karl did not significantly decline in the weeks immediately following January 19, 2005, when he both received a set of vaccinations and suffered another bout of erythema multiforme." This latter observation foreshadows the special master's analysis of *Loving* prong six, addressed.

December 27, 2004, Dr. McDonough saw Karl when his parents brought him into the clinic for otitis media and possible erythema multiforme. Under "Developmental History" Dr. McDonough recorded, possibly based upon discussion with Karl's parents that "he has several words that he says." On January 19, 2005, however, he recorded that Karl had no words, except for "mama" and "dada." No other evidence suggests that Karl ever had any words beyond "mama" and "dada," and, as such, the descriptive statement in Dr. McDonough's report of December 27, 2004 is uncorroborated that Karl's condition before the vaccinations had a neurological foundation. Certainly his treating medical providers did not think it was neurological at the time. Thus, the evidence shows that Karl had gross motor delays and speech delays, but it does not support finding that those delays were caused by a significant impairment of his central nervous system. If his central nervous system was adversely affected, any such disability was not a major one.

Loving Prong 2—Condition Following the Vaccinations: *Loving* prong two inquires into the claimant's current condition or condition following the vaccinations. As the special master noted, because Karl's current condition is not at issue, the focus turns to his condition in the six months following receipt of the vaccines. Two days after the vaccinations, Karl's daycare recorded that he had a temperature of 101.5 degrees. For the next week, Karl reportedly acted tired and fussy. On January 28, nine days after the vaccinations, Karl still had a fever of 101.3, as recorded by his daycare. The experts disagree as to the cause of the fever. Dr. Frye testified that the fever was a symptom of immune activation caused by the vaccinations on January 19, 2005. Dr. Frye also opined that Karl's symptoms in late January and early February indicated the first signs of the biological processes that eventually led to Karl's neurological regression (describing Karl's post-vaccination symptoms as manifesting encephalopathy). Dr. Snodgrass disagreed, stating that the fever on January 21 manifested too quickly to be attributed to the vaccines, that the continued fever on January 28 was more likely due to an outbreak of Karl's erythema multiforme, and that the fevers in any event were not related to Karl's neurological decline. Karl's daycare records, which extend through February 8th, largely describe him as being tired, irritable, and fussy. Karl's chiropractic records, which begin on February 7, 2005, describe Karl as "irritable" on February 9th and then "spastic" on February 11, 2005. The next three visits suggest some slight progress, but the chiropractor's assessment of Karl's condition remained the same. The following visits noted increased stiffening and spasticity, with the assessment of Karl's condition remaining the same. The first visits of March again indicated some slight progress, but the remaining three visits in March showed a decline and decreased range of motion. In April, Karl's condition continued to be variable. The K.I.D.S. evaluation pointed specifically to low muscle tone, and Dr. McDonough did not refer Karl to a neurologist until late March 2005, two months after the vaccination, following reports that Karl was deteriorating further. Dr. Snodgrass testified that the MMR vaccine introduces a virus into the body that grows with time. Those viruses "will present a larger stimulus at seven to ten days than they do on day 1, 2, or 3." This is unlike a killed bacteria vaccine, which does not multiply in the body and causes reactions more quickly. Karl's daycare noted the reappearance of spots on his arms and legs on January 31, 2005. The chiropractor's records document a decline, albeit not a linear one. The observation by the chiropractor that he was "spastic" is significant. That Karl was a little less spastic or stiff some days than others does not mean that Karl's condition improved beyond his initial appointments in early February. This is consistent with Dr. Frye's theory that Karl was likely experiencing changes at the cellular level that would take time to appear at the clinical observation level. Moreover, there was a phone conversation between Brenda Erie of Stark County Social Services and the chiropractor on March 30, 2005, reproduced below, where the chiropractor discussed possible causes for Karl's condition, including abuse, adverse reaction to medication or a vaccine, cerebral palsy, or a cerebellar tumor. The special master read this record as indicating that "the chiropractor answered 'No'" to the possibility that an adverse reaction to the vaccination might have caused Karl's deteriorating condition. In the hearing held by the court on September 18, 2013, the government acknowledged that the special master misread this record. The chiropractor said "No" to child abuse allegations, not to the possibility of an adverse reaction to a medication, cerebral palsy, or a cerebellar tumor.

On March 24, 2005, Dr. McDonough referred Karl to a neurologist. This occurred two days after a phone call between Dr. McDonough and the Palucks, during which the Palucks reported that Karl had some brief crawling, was not sitting on his own, leans to one side, is babbling more, and has an intermittent rash. This is the first time in the record that anyone recommended Karl see a neurologist. At that point, Dr. McDonough could not have thought Karl had improved since the January vaccinations.

On March 28, 2005, Karl had a bout of otitis media and bronchiolitis, documented by Dr. Gary Peterson. A week later, Karl's symptoms were improving in that regard and the doctor recommended weaning him off the nebulizer that he had been using to treat the bronchiolitis. On April 13, Karl saw Dr. McDonough for a pre-anesthesia appointment in preparation for his planned MRI. At that point, Dr. McDonough noted "increased tone in the upper and lower extremities," no clonus, "decreased hip flexion to about 70 degrees bilaterally," no speech, and "global developmental delay with resolving otitis media." Dr. McDonough described the decreased hip flexion as "a change in hip movement over the last couple months." He also documented his hope that "the parents would agree to evaluation for congenital infections, metabolic disorders, and other tests requested by Dr. Kriengkrairut for his global developmental delay."

Dr. Frye testified that this examination represented a neurological decline in Karl "because now he has increased tone in the upper and lower extremities, so—and he says, 'Global developmental delay with resolving otitis media.' So here his concerns are that his neurological exam has gotten worse" since January 2005. Dr. Frye further opined that Dr. McDonough's suspicion of a metabolic disorder was consistent with a finding of increased tone. Increased tone suggested damage to the cortex of the brain, which can be seen in white-matter abnormalities in an MRI.

Dr. Snodgrass disagreed that the examination on April 13th evidenced significant change, stating that while the hip flexion is more severely limited, it was present in January in any case.

On April 19, 2005, Karl saw the pediatric neurologist, Dr. Kriengkrairut. She reported "truncal hypotonia with marked spasticity of the extremities. The baby has tendency to do cortical thumb bilaterally, worse on the right compared to the left. . . . Baby does not babble. . . . Delayed development as well as hypotonia of the extremities may be secondary to central nervous system pathology."

Dr. Frye testified that this report by Dr. Kriengkrairut suggests substantial worsening in Karl. "This is a third medical provider talking about spasticity, not just some subtle increases in tone. She actually says on the motor exam 'marked spasticity.' This is very, very different than just a subtle change in tone." Dr. Frye also explained that hypotonia, cortical thumbing, and cessation of babbling all represent neurological regression. Dr. Snodgrass disagreed. He considered that Dr. Kriengkrairut's exam revealed no new neurological problems in Karl. In his view, cortical thumbing was not a significant finding. He also stated that the thumbing was not necessarily "cortical" and thus was not necessarily representative of a brain abnormality. Dr. Snodgrass's critical commentary on Dr. Kriengkrairut's findings appears to have had two objectives, first, to suggest that Karl's neurological condition in April 2005 was not substantially different from his condition before the vaccinations, and, second, to suggest that Karl's neurological condition was not deteriorating. Both implications have no support in the contemporaneous medical records. Karl's pediatrician, Dr. McDonough, in March had referred Karl to Dr. Kriengkrairut for a detailed neurological examination because of perceived neurological abnormalities. Dr. Kriengkrairut found multiple indicia of "central nervous system pathology." What Dr. McDonough had suspected was in fact borne out by Dr. Kriengkrairut. The spasticity first observed by the chiropractor in early mid-February, shortly after the vaccinations, was still evident, along with other neurological abnormalities. By April, Karl was regressing markedly.

In summary, the court finds that Karl had significant signs of neurodegeneration by the end of April, as evidenced by the marked spasticity, cortical thumbing, and lack of babbling observed by Dr. Kriengkrairut, the decreased hip flexion and "global developmental delay" noted by Dr. McDonough, and the belatedly diagnosed abnormal MRI exam from April 27, 2005.

In May 2005, Karl saw a speech therapist. Karl made no progress throughout May regarding his speech, and the therapist's records show that Karl had lost skills since October 2004. He could no longer produce consonant sounds, but continued to be able to reach for desired toys. Karl's evaluation in September 2005 stated, "No goals met."

On July 12, 2005, Karl experienced his first seizure. Upon discharge from the Med Center One Hospital in Bismarck, Dr. McDonough noted that he had "global developmental delay with seizure disorder, possible deteriorating neurologic status in that he is unable to do some things that he was able to do previously." On July 19, 2005, Karl saw Dr. Michael Frost at St. Paul Children's Hospital in Minnesota. His medical history from that appointment notes that Karl "has been receiving therapies with some intermittent decreased tone but overall he is declining in all areas." It also notes that by fourteen months, i.e, March 15, 2005, Karl showed no signs of significant developmental progress. Dr. Frost noted that Karl was being admitted for a determination of what the etiology might be for his deteriorating neurological status. Dr. Frost believed, after a second MRI in July, that Karl was experiencing neurodegeneration. A third MRI performed in October 2005 showed that the thinning of Karl's corporal callosum had stabilized, suggesting that there may have been a toxic or metabolic event he experienced that had also stabilized. In short, Karl's condition following the vaccinations reflected marked neurodegeneration.

Loving Prong 3—Whether the post-vaccination condition constitutes a significant aggravation of the pre-vaccination condition: By October 2005, Karl had "no purposeful movements. He had increased tone throughout and increased deep tendon reflexes throughout with multiple beats of clonus at the ankles." He had no specific smiling or distinctive eye contact. This condition starkly contrasts to the previously "very happy" child, that was "aware and tuned into faces" and who "enjoyed interactive play." The special master properly concluded that substantial evidence showed that Karl was indisputably worse in the months following his vaccination. The parties do not dispute this finding, and the court concurs that substantial evidence supports the special master's conclusion.

Loving Prong 4 (*Althen* Prong 1)—Whether there is a medical theory causally connecting the significantly worsened condition to the vaccination: The special master found that petitioners satisfied their burden of proof as to *Loving* prong four (Althern prong one), i.e., in showing that a medical theory causally connected Karl's worsened condition to the vaccination. The special master succinctly stated that "in briefing after the court's Opinion and Order, the parties essentially agreed that the Palucks' evidence met the standard as defined by the court." In that connection, the special master quoted the government's interpretation of *Paluck II* as having "hamstrung the special master from denying compensation under prong one of *Althen*."

On this second review, the government contends that the court in *Paluck II* "inappropriately relaxed the Vaccine Act's requirements." Respondent's opinion (referring to the court's observation in *Paluck II*), is "that Dr. Frye's theory is, while not scientifically certain, under active, continuing scientific investigation by a range of researchers, showing that it is sufficiently worthy and reliable to merit that extensive scientific injury." The government's criticism is misplaced. The Federal Circuit has repeatedly emphasized that preponderant proof of causation does not require scientific certainty, but rather a showing that the vaccine more likely than not caused the injury.

"While this case involves . . . a sequence hitherto unproven in medicine, the purpose of the Vaccine Act's preponderance standard is to allow the finding of causation in a field bereft of complete and direct proof of how vaccines affect the human body. A petitioner must provide a reputable medical or scientific explanation that pertains specifically to the petitioner's case, although the explanation need only be 'legally probable, not medically or scientifically certain.'" "Requiring 'epidemiologic studies . . . or general acceptance in the scientific or medical communities . . . impermissibly raises a claimant's burden under the Vaccine Act.'" Even so, the preponderance standard for causation is not to be confused with a standard requiring only "possible" or "plausible" causation.

Mitochondrial disorders are only incompletely understood in biomedical science, although basic mechanisms are known. Those with normally functioning mitochondria have better antioxidant defenses that allow them to "convert . . . reactive oxygen species to harmless compounds." This is because mitochondria are responsible for the creation of the energy-carrying molecule, adenosine triphosphate ("ATP"), which is required for the synthesis of the primary antioxidant, glutathione. Contrastingly, defective mitochondria can have an opposite effect, themselves producing abnormally high amounts of reactive oxygen species, which can cause damage. Thus, people with mitochondrial defects are more vulnerable to oxidative stress.

Dr. Snodgrass did not disagree with the basic premises behind Dr. Frye's theory, but he disagreed that there was evidence, i.e., published peer-reviewed studies, that normal vaccines given to humans cause oxidative stress. "I would say that if you have a mitochondrial abnormality, your ability to recover from excessive reactive oxygen species or reactive nitrogen species may be less." Vaccines can affect children with mitochondrial disorders. Dr. Snodgrass stated that of his about twenty patients with a mitochondrial disorder, none of them have worsened with immunization, but he admitted that because mitochondrial disorders are heterogeneous, it is difficult to predict how the same stressor would affect different people. On cross-examination, Dr. Snodgrass conceded that, in theory, Karl's otitis media, erythema multiforme, and the vaccines administered in January 2005 could have "all worked together and been a substantial factor in bringing about his neurodegeneration." He maintained, however, that that the theoretical postulate was not established in this case because Karl did not get worse in January and February after the immunizations. Nonetheless, whether Karl got worse in January and February after the vaccinations does not relate to the legal acceptability of Dr. Frye's theory under *Loving* prong four, but instead bears on *Loving* prongs five and six, i.e., the logical sequence of cause and effect and a medically acceptable approximate temporal relationship.

Contrary to the government's reading of this court's articulation of a standard for *Loving* prong four (*Althen* prong one) in *Paluck II*, it is not solely because a theory is under active scientific investigation that it is reputable, worthy, and reliable. The court instead was stating that the special master could not wholly discount animal studies showing oxidative stress resulting from vaccinations *plus* ongoing, continuing scientific investigation into whether humans also can experience similar oxidative stress resulting from vaccinations. Nor could the special master discredit a peer-reviewed study that suggested oxidative stress in humans resulted from receipt of the flu vaccine, solely because the researcher used a different biomarker than he did in a prior study. (Michael Phillips et al., *Effect of Influenza Vaccination on Oxidative Stress Products in Breath*, J. Breath Research, June 2010). The court was not relaxing the standard for reliability, but rather was applying the pertinent and appropriate standard where research was underway testing reputable theories that were supported by basic knowledge.

Loving Prong 5 (*Althen* Prong 2)—Whether there is a logical sequence of cause and effect showing that the vaccination caused the significant aggravation: Accepting Dr. Frye's theory of causation that vaccines can activate an over-whelming immune response in children with mitochondrial defects and lead to neurodegeneration, the next inquiry is whether, in Karl's particular case, that process occurred. Similar to the level of proof required in establishing a medical theory, the sequence of cause and effect must be "logical and legally probable, not medically or scientifically certain."

Petitioners contend that the special master put aside expert testimony and con-temporaneous medical records in favor of drawing his own medical conclu-sions from the evidence. Specifically, petitioners challenge his reading of the chiropractic records, Dr. McDonough's referral to the neurologist in March 2005, and testimony regarding the various MRIs.

First, the special master determined that Dr. Frye's theory requires a linear, downward decline without any periodic improvements. Both the government and the special master cite this court's opinion in *Paluck II* for the proposi-tion that this court approved of the special master's prior conclusion that "peti-tioners' medical theory predicted a steady, downward decline in health after vaccination." The court did not disturb the finding that Dr. Frye's theory was predicated on a downhill trajectory." The citation provided by both the respondent and the special master misapprehends the court's prior action. This court did not address the special master's determination in *Paluck I* that Karl's regression could only fit Dr. Frye's theory if Karl experienced a "continuous downward slope" of injury. The decision to require a linear, downward slope is unfounded in the testimony. The special master in *Paluck I* interpreted Dr. Frye's phrase that "Karl's progress looked like it was just a progressive hill downward for about six months," to mean "a continuous downward slope." The special master maintained this interpretation in *Paluck IV* ("the special master again concludes that Karl's deterioration was non-linear"). Dr. Frye, however, never suggested that a child experiencing neurodegeneration could not have periods of remission or improvement. His use of the word "progressive" does not mean a continuous linear decline. As a general matter, when used in describing a disease, progressive means "increasing in extent or severity." *Merriam-Webster's Tenth Collegiate Dictionary* 932 (1998); *see also New Oxford American Dictionary* 1396 (2010) ("(of a disease or ailment) increasing in severity or extent"). This standard medical usage allows for a non-linear decline. To fall within Dr. Frye's theory and the applicable medical literature, it is sufficient if Karl's medical records show a decline in condition over time, notwithstanding periods of remission or modest improvement.

Second, the special master considered the chiropractic records and statements by his treating physicians regarding Karl's decline. In the remand, the court ordered the special master to reconsider the importance of these particular pieces of the record, in conjunction with other pieces of the record. Accordingly, this court will consider the entire record in determining whether petitioners have met their burden of proof under *Loving* prong five.

Karl had a fever on January 21, 2005, two days after the vaccinations that continued to be evident on January 28, 2005, nine days after the vaccinations. Daycare notes from the intervening days consistently show that Karl was tired, irritable, and not eating well. According to Dr. Frye, these are all systemic signs of being sick, that is, signs of immune activation. Dr. Frye testified that a fever any time within two weeks of a vaccination could reasonably be attributed to the vaccination.

Dr. Snodgrass disagreed that Karl's fever could have been caused by the vaccines. He explained that the MMR and varicella vaccines do cause fever in some children, but fever would not usually appear until the seventh or eighth day. On cross-examination, petitioners' counsel asked Dr. Snodgrass whether he was familiar with the packaging insert accompanying the Prevnar vaccine, which states that "15% of children who receive PCV-7 report fever of greater than 38 degrees centigrade within two days following vaccination." He responded that he was, but that the packaging insert does not truly prove causation as a scientific matter. He referred to a study about the MMR vaccine, one of the other vaccines Karl received, which took 500 sets of identical twins, giving one twin the vaccine and the other a placebo. In his view, this type of study better proves that a vaccine causes fevers. In short, Dr. Snodgrass again looked for medical certainty where none is required. It is sufficiently logical that Karl had a reaction to the Prevnar vaccine, manifesting as a fever within two days. He additionally did not explain why the fever on day nine could not be attributed to the vaccinations, stating only that Karl's fevers could have been due to an outbreak of his erythema multiforme, which reappeared on January 31st. He testified further that fever is very common among children in daycare and may not specifically indicate oxidative stress. Similarly, in his view, while irritability might be an indication of something serious, it is not specific.

Several points of common ground exist. A fever is usually a symptom of immune activation; that much was acknowledged by both experts. And, the daycare records contemporaneously documented that Karl had lethargy and irritability along with the fever in the days following the vaccinations. While fever, lethargy, and irritability might possibly have been caused by something besides the vaccinations, sufficient evidence exists to indicate that they were in fact caused by the vaccinations. That at least one of the five vaccines that Karl received, or a combination thereof, caused him to have a fever due to immune activation is logical and legally probable. A *prima facie* case to that effect was established. Accordingly, the burden shifted to the respondent to show another, alternative, cause. That shifted burden was not met, nor did the respondent attempt to meet it.

Dr. Frye's theory postulates that immune activation can cause the development of potentially toxic reactive oxygen species and reactive nitrogen species that, if left unchecked by the body's antioxidants, can lead to oxidative stress and cell death. Thus, one would look for evidence of whether Karl experienced cell death. In this case, petitioners contend that Karl's neurodegeneration is evidence of brain cell death.

Karl's health deteriorated in February 2005. The chiropractor noted he was spastic on February 11, 2005. As detailed previously, Karl's later chiropractic records reflect varying levels of rigidity and tone. Regardless of whether Karl had days in the subsequent weeks where he was more or less rigid, Karl never appeared to improve above his initial assessment, and he was still reported as spastic in April by the pediatric neurologist, Dr. Kriengkrairut. Upon questioning by the special master regarding the chiropractic treatment Karl received, Dr. Frye testified that spasticity can be improved by "pulling the muscles and loosening the muscles so that they have full range of motion." This does not solve the upper neuron problem causing the spasticity, but it can mitigate the symptoms. "By manipulating the muscles you're resetting the feedback mechanism that sets the tone of the muscles. . . . When neurons from the brain aren't there the feedback loop becomes or is set too high and the muscles have too much tone. . . . By using physical therapy we start to stretch out the muscles and that can try to reset the feedback loop that we have in the muscles." That Karl's tone fluctuated while he was seeing the chiropractor and the K.I.D.S. therapists would be expected.

In asserting that Karl did not decline between January and February, Dr. Snodgrass stated that "the single most important thing is that we had a lot of calls and doctor visits in November and December. If Karl had a precipitous decline in January and February, these parents who seem to be responsible parents would have been calling and visiting the doctor, that's number one." Dr. Snodgrass's inference and the special master's reliance on it are not supported by substantial evidence. Karl's parents actually *were* taking him frequently to a medical provider, i.e., the chiropractor. They took him to the chiropractor nine times in a three week period in February alone, apparently believing that Karl had a pinched nerve preventing his development. Dr. Snodgrass can disagree with their course of action, implicitly being critical of treatment by a chiropractor rather than a physician, but his testimony implying that the Palucks thought medical treatment unnecessary for Karl is not supported by evidence.

Contrary to the special master's conclusion, the fact that Karl had few visible signs of injury other than fever immediately following the vaccinations is in keeping with Dr. Frye's theory ("part of the *Althen* prong 2 analysis may consider whether the expert's 'theory accounted for the vaccinee's injury'" (quoting *Hibbard v. Secretary of Health & Human Servs.*). Dr. Frye testified that changes at the cellular level would occur first and would take time to become clinically visible. That the MRI from April 2005 was initially interpreted as normal and only later reinterpreted as abnormal upon re-examination in July 2005 suggests that the changes were indeed small at first, but they had been initiated. Because the changes were likely occurring at a cellular level at first, Karl was probably worsening in February and March even if it was not linearly progressive. The rate at which that process would occur would depend on the type and severity of the person's mitochondrial disorder. As an example, Dr. Frye pointed to the Hannah Poling case study (referring to R. Ex. 21q, Jon S. Poling, Richard E.

Frye, John Shoffner & Andrew W. Zimmerman, *Developmental Regression and Mitochondrial Dysfunction in a Child with Autism*, 21 J. Child Neurology 170 (2006)). Hannah was a developmentally normal nineteen-month-old girl who, within 48 hours of receiving several vaccinations, developed a high fever, inconsolable crying, irritability, and lethargy, and refused to walk. Four days later, she could not walk up stairs. She had a low-grade intermittent fever during the next twelve days. She continued to decline over the next three months, developing autistic behaviors and losing all speech. Previously she had been able to say at least twenty words. It was later discovered that she had a mitochondrial disorder. In 2006, at the time of publication of the case study, Hannah was six and had greatly improved in her language functions and sociability, although she still exhibited mild autism. This case study did not prove causation with any medical certainty, but it hypothesized that "if mitochondrial dysfunction is present at the time of infections and immunizations in young children, the added oxidative stresses from immune activation on cellular energy metabolism are likely to be especially critical for the central nervous system, which is highly dependent on mitochondrial function." Dr. Frye pointed to similarities between Hannah and Karl. First, they have similar mitochondrial abnormalities. Both received MMR and varicella vaccinations, developed a fever around 48 hours later, became noticeably irritable, and eventually experienced neurological regression. Hannah's decline occurred more quickly in some ways, but her regression, like Karl's, appeared to continue over a number of months. Her appetite remained poor for six months, but she began saying a few words again about four months after the vaccinations. In contrast, Karl has experienced complete neurodegeneration and is not expected to improve. Dr. Frye opined that Karl's pre-existing chronic immune activation may have impaired his ability to recover as Hannah did.

Dr. Frye also pointed to a peer-reviewed article by Dr. John Shoffner and others. The researchers found in a retrospective study that autistic regression occurred twice as often in a subset of autistic children with mitochondrial disorders after a fever than it did in the general population of autistic children (referring to John Shoffner *et al.*, *Fever Plus Mitochondrial Diseases Could Be Risk Factors for Autistic Regression*, 25 J. Child Neurology, 2010). Approximately 25% of children with autism will experience autistic regression before the age of three. The researchers defined autistic regression to mean "a loss of developmental skills that included speech, receptive skills, eye contact, and social interests in individuals." A relationship between fever and regression was defined as "regression beginning within two weeks of a febrile episode without the suggestion of infection, meningitis, or encephalitis." In the study, 60.7% of the children experienced autistic regression, which was a "statistically significant increase" over the estimated 25% reported in the general autistic population. A high percentage, 70.6%, of those who experienced autistic regression did so following a fever. In 33.3% of those who experienced autistic regression following fever, the fever was associated with response to a vaccination. The specific vaccine schedule leading to fever in the subjects was not available. The study acknowledged that "due to the complexities in mitochondrial disease pathogenesis, oxidative phosphorylation enzyme defects are highly variable even among groups of individuals who harbor identical mutations." According to Dr. Frye, this study, combined with the Poling case study, strongly suggested that vaccinations in children with mitochondrial diseases can cause fever followed by regressive loss of skills.

Dr. Snodgrass cited a number of differences between Karl's case and Hannah's case. First, Hannah's clinical worsening was much more dramatic than Karl's. She refused to walk within 48 hours of receiving the vaccination, a more notable loss of skill than anything Karl experienced. Second, there is no evidence that Karl suffered encephalopathy, and it was agreed that Hannah did. "In Karl's case we really don't see that. In this retrospective study, researchers examined the charts of 28 children who they knew to have autism and mitochondrial disease. They used the charts to determine whether the children experienced fever followed by autistic regression.

(Phosphorylation is defined as "the metabolic process of introducing a phosphate group into an organic molecule." Oxidative phosphorylation, specifically, is defined as "the formation of high energy phosphate bonds by phosphorylation of ADP to ATP coupled to the transfer of electrons from reduced coenzymes (NADH or FADH2) to molecular oxygen via the electron transport chain. . . . Three molecules of ATP per NADH and two per FADH2 are produced as a result of a proton gradient created across the mitochondrial inner membrane by the electron transport chain." Thus, "oxidative phosphorylation enzyme defects" can be understood as defects in ATP production.)

"Yes, he was irritable. Irritability is not encephalopathy. He was not kept home from day care, he was not taken to the doctor. So we do not see evidence that Karl had encephalopathy." As for Dr. Frye's reliance on the Shoffner paper,

Dr. Snodgrass criticized its simplicity, questioning how researchers could have known that any particular fever that a child experienced caused the regression.

Dr. Snodgrass's critiques might provide valid points of departure for further scientific study in this area of medicine, but they do not negate the evidentiary value provided by the Poling case report or the Shoffner study. Dr. Snodgrass and Dr. Frye agreed that case studies do not prove causation. But Dr. Frye correctly pointed out that "that's where science starts is with case reports." Dr. Frye testified that this particular area of medicine is "emerging and evolving." Mitochondrial diseases themselves are difficult to identify, and their courses of progression are not easily predicted. The effect of fevers on those with a mitochondrial disorder is even more difficult to assess. The Poling case report and the Shoffner study nonetheless provide indicia for this case.

In considering the opinions of Karl's treating doctors as to the cause of Karl's decline, the special master considered the chiropractor's opinion, Dr. McDonough's referral to the neurologist, and the MRI reports. First, as discussed *supra*, the special master's statement that the chiropractor did not believe Karl had an adverse reaction to a vaccine simply misread a handwritten entry in the medical record. Rather, the chiropractor believed it *was* possible Karl had an adverse reaction to a vaccine. Second, in reviewing Dr. McDonough's referral to Dr. Kriengkrairut, the pediatric neurologist, the special master inquired into Dr. McDonough's motivations. Aside from desiring more complete testing of Karl's neurological system, the special master opined that Dr. McDonough made the referral because he was "frustrated the Palucks were not following his recommendations for physical therapy, occupational therapy, and a stimulation program for Karl." The special master criticized petitioners for not raising the argument that Dr. McDonough made the referral because he believed Karl was getting worse. The special master apparently ignored Dr. Frye's testimony on direct examination that the referral is "the first indication that we have that the pediatrician is now concerned to such a level that Karl needs to see a neurologist." There simply is no evidentiary support for the special master's hypothesis that Dr. McDonough made the referral out of frustration with the Palucks. Third, regarding the MRI reports, the special master concluded that "the Palucks have not established that Dr. Frye's conclusion that Karl's corpus callosum started to thin after the vaccination is more likely than Dr. Snodgrass's conclusion that the corpus callosum could have been thin before the vaccination." Accordingly, the special master used his finding that Karl had problems in his central nervous system before the vaccination as the tie breaker to determine that the thinning occurred before the vaccinations. This court has overturned the special master's finding that Karl definitively had neurological problems before. Evidence of causation need not be proven to a medical certainty; it need only be "logical and legally probable." The subtlety of the thinning in April, and the clarity of the thinning in July, suggests that the thinning had only begun in April or shortly before then. Petitioners have presented sufficient evidence to show that Karl regressed after receiving the vaccines, and they have provided medical records and medical literature to establish, by a preponderance of the evidence, that Karl's pre-existing medical problems were significantly aggravated by the vaccinations. Karl had a fever shortly after receiving the vaccinations, was described as "spastic" for the first time on February 11, was referred to a neurologist in March, and by April had a negative neurological evaluation and an abnormal MRI. Petitioners presented a peer-reviewed study showing increased regression in children with mitochondrial diseases following fever. They also presented a case study demonstrating that a young girl with an underlying mitochondrial disorder lost previously developed skills over the course of months after experiencing a fever within 48 hours of vaccinations. Petitioners have carried their burden of proof on this prong.

Loving Prong 6 (*Althen* Prong 3)—Whether a medically acceptable proximate temporal relationship exists between the vaccination and the significant aggravation: The final prong of the *Loving* analysis requires the court to determine the time frame for which it is medically acceptable to infer causation and whether the onset of the claimant's injury occurred within that time frame.

Petitioners contend that the special master ignored the record in concluding that Karl exhibited no evidence of neurodegeneration within an acceptable time frame. Specifically, they argue that he ignored Dr. Frye's testimony that evidence of neurodegeneration occurred within a medically acceptable time.

Respondent maintains that the special master carefully considered all of the evidence and found respondent's expert more persuasive than petitioners', an approach and result that is well within the special master's role as a finder of fact.

In *Paluck IV*, the special master found that the medically acceptable temporal interval is three weeks. He based this determination largely on an article by Dr. Edmonds entitled *The Otolaryngological Manifestations of Mitochondrial Disease and the Risk of Neurodegeneration with Infection*. The Edmonds article collected information about 40 patients with mitochondrial diseases. Of these forty patients, eighteen experienced neurodegenerative events. Intercurrent infection was recognized as a precipitant of neurodegenerative events in thirteen of these eighteen patients. The article graphically depicts the timing of the onset of neurodegenerative events after the onset of infection as ranging until nineteen days after infection. While the Edmonds article looked for neurodegeneration after infection, not reaction to a vaccination, both experts agree that it provides a reasonable guideline for neurodegeneration following immune activation.

The special master also relied on the Shoffner study, which found that a relationship between fever and autistic regression existed, but this reliance is somewhat misplaced because the Shoffner study *defined* a relationship between fever and regression as occurring within two weeks, excluding later sequelae. Therefore, by definition, the study could not have found a relationship between fever and regression more attenuated than two weeks. Thus, while the Shoffner article supports a statement that autistic regression following fever can occur within two weeks, it cannot equally support a statement that autistic regression following fever must occur within two weeks. The special master also relied on the Hannah Poling case study, noting that she had a fever within 48 hours, could not climb the stairs within seven days, and developed a rash within two weeks.

The Edmonds article is the most enlightening regarding an acceptable medical time frame for the onset of neurodegenerative events following immune system activation. The Edmonds article, however, acknowledges the severe dearth of medical literature in this area: "Because of the relative novelty of mitochondrial disorders, no reports in the literature have quantified the risk for neurodegenerative events triggered by infections in patients with mitochondrial disease." Dr. Bob Naviaux, Co-Director of the Mitochondrial and Metabolic Disease Center at the University of California, San Diego, expressed a similar sentiment in commenting on the Shoffner study—"*Commentary on* John Shoffner *et al., Fever Plus Mitochondrial Disease Could Be Risk Factors for Autistic Regression, published in* J. Child Neurology (2010)." According to Dr. Naviaux, the temporal relationship between the triggering event and neurodegeneration is unsettled. There appears to be a more rapid "flare" response and a more delayed "fade" response. He credited the Shoffner study with providing a touchstone for new questions, such as "which kinds of mitochondrial defects lead to rapid, high-grade fevers in response to infection or vaccination" and "which defects lead to a failed fever response, or to a low-grade fever, or to a reduced immune response to vaccination?"

Dr. Frye accepted the premises of these articles, testifying that the temporal link requires much further study. He did testify, however, that an adverse reaction to a vaccine is likely to appear within a week of receiving it. He further stated that the adverse reaction can peak several days after the vaccination, and then "lead to . . . metabolic decompensation, which is an ongoing process . . . that will continue until it burns itself out," if it is not interrupted. Dr. Snodgrass and Dr. Frye disagree whether Karl's first fever, within two days of the vaccination, could have been caused by the vaccination, but they apparently agree that any fever around one week following Karl's vaccinations could have been caused by the vaccines. Thus, at least Karl's continuing fever is safely within any type of medically accepted time frame for Karl's injury.

The special master appeared determined to establish a definitive bound for neurodegeneration, but the court disagrees that such a bound can be sharply delineated in this specific area. Neither the medical literature nor the expert testimony stated with any certainty when neurodegeneration can be expected to begin in all cases. Dr. Snodgrass based his testimony that a change would have to begin "within a few weeks" on the Edmonds article. As previously discussed, the Edmonds article is the first of its kind and cannot be read to suggest a definitive temporal interval for neurodegeneration in response to all triggering events for any type of mitochondrial disorder. In response to questioning from the special master, Dr. Frye testified that the timing for neurodegenerative changes to appear clinically in a child would depend on the severity and type of mitochondrial disorder. This is consistent with Dr. Naviaux's commentary on the Shoffner study.

In this instance, Dr. Frye pinpointed the chiropractor's notation that Karl was "spastic" on February 11, 2005 as an identifiable neurodegenerative event. To Dr. Frye, the neurodegenerative process must have begun by then. This event occurred within the general time frame suggested by both the special master and Dr. Snodgrass. ("The change should come within a few weeks.") Starting with this chiropractic notation, the record shows Karl experienced a general decline. His chiropractic assessment remained the same throughout all of February, even if the subjective descriptions of Karl's day-to-day behaviors varied. Karl was losing language throughout this period, and by late March, Dr. McDonough saw a need for him to be evaluated by a neurologist.

In conclusion, setting a hard and fast time frame in an uncertain area undergoing sustained scientific investigation is contrary to the precepts governing the Vaccine Act. Karl had a fever within 48 hours of the vaccinations, accompanied by a week of lethargy, irritability, more fever, and disrupted sleeping and eating cycles. This prompt reaction is consistent with an adverse immune reaction to the vaccines. An observation of spasticity followed within a time that all agreed would have been appropriate for a neurodegenerative event. Karl experienced total decline within six months, and he did not continue to develop in any way after the vaccinations. These facts combined with his febrile reaction to the vaccine show, by a preponderance of the evidence, that Karl's existing medical setbacks were significantly aggravated by his receipt of the vaccinations within a medically acceptable time.

CONCLUSION

For the reasons stated, the Palucks' motion for review is GRANTED, the special master's decision of May 10, 2013 denying compensation is VACATED, and the court acts in accord with 42 U.S.C. § 300aa-12(e)(2)(B) to find that petitioners have satisfied each of the six *Loving* elements and are entitled to compensation under the Act. The case is remanded to the special master to determine compensation.

IT IS SO ORDERED.

12

SELECTED UNREPORTED CASES: 2013

From www.uscfc.uscourts.gov

Bryan Comeaux and Kelly Comeaux, parents of Caroline Comeaux, a minor child, Petitioners v. Secretary of Health and Human Services, Respondent

Summary: In this decision, the special master accepts a settlement stipulation between the parties in which compensation is awarded for intussusception.

Compensated Vaccine Injury: Intussusception

Stipulation; rotavirus vaccine; intussusception.

Case No: 12-348V

Date Filed: December 19, 2013

Bryan Comeaux and Kelly Comeaux, parents of Caroline Comeaux, a minor child, Petitioners v Secretary of Health and Human Services, Respondent

DECISION

Special Master Christian J. Moran

On December 18, 2013, respondent filed a stipulation concerning the petition for compensation filed by Bryan and Kelly Comeaux, on behalf of their daughter, Caroline Comeaux, on June 1, 2012. In their petition, the Comeauxs alleged that the rotavirus vaccine, which is contained in the Vaccine Injury Table (the "Table"), 42 C.F.R. §100.3(a), and which Caroline received on July 22, 2011, caused her to suffer intussusception. Petitioners further allege that Caroline suffered the residual effects of this injury for more than six months. Petitioners represent that there has been no prior award or settlement of a civil action for damages on their behalf as a result of Caroline's condition.

Respondent denies that the rotavirus vaccine caused Caroline to suffer intussusception, or any other injury.

Nevertheless, the parties agree to the joint stipulation, attached hereto as Appendix A. The undersigned finds said stipulation reasonable and adopts it as the decision of the Court in awarding damages, on the terms set forth therein.

Damages awarded in that stipulation include:

A lump sum of $150,000.00 in the form of a check payable to petitioners, Bryan and Kelly Comeaux, as guardians/conservators of Caroline's estate. This amount represents compensation for all damages that would be available under 42 U.S.C. §300aa-l 5(a).

IT IS SO ORDERED.

Lorin Forcine and Blaise Forcine, legal representatives of minor child William Forcine, Petitioners v. Secretary of Health and Human Services, Respondent

Summary: In this decision, the special master accepts a settlement stipulation between the parties in which compensation is awarded for anaphylaxis.

Anaphylaxis is a severe, whole-body allergic reaction to a chemical that has become an allergen. After being exposed to a substance such as bee sting venom, the person's immune system becomes sensitized to it.

When the person is exposed to that allergen again, an allergic reaction may occur. Anaphylaxis happens quickly after the exposure, is severe, and involves the whole body.

Tissues in different parts of the body release histamine and other substances. This causes the airways to tighten and leads to other symptoms.

Proffer; Damages; Table Injury MMR

Case No: 13-167V

Date Filed: December 16, 2013

Lorin Forcine and Blaise Forcine, legal representatives of minor child William Forcine, Petitioners v. Secretary of Health and Human Services, Respondent

DECISION AWARDING DAMAGES

Vowell, Chief Special Master

On March 5, 2013, Lorin Forcine and Blaise Forcine, legal representatives of minor child, William Forcine, filed a petition for compensation under the National Vaccine Injury Compensation Program, 42 U.S.C. § 300aa-10, et seq. [the "Vaccine Act" or "Program"] alleging that William Forcine received the measles mumps rubella [MMR] vaccine on March 5, 2010 and thereafter suffered the "Table Injury" known as anaphylaxis within four hours, which was caused in fact by the above stated vaccination.

Respondent filed her Rule 4(c) Report on November 18, 2013, concluding that William's injury met the Table requirements for the presumptive injury of anaphylaxis and that compensation should be awarded for that injury and its sequela. Respondent's Report at 4. On November 18, 2013, I issued a decision finding petitioners entitled to compensation, concluding that in view of respondent's concession and the evidence before me petitioners were entitled to compensation based on a Vaccine Table injury.

On December 16, 2013, respondent filed her Proffer on Award of Compensation. Pursuant to the terms stated in the attached Proffer, I award petitioners:

1. A lump sum payment of $146,815.56, representing the discounted present value of William's projected vaccine-related injury expenses ($12,275.76), and pain and suffering ($134,539.80), in the form of a check payable to petitioners, Lorin and Blaise Forcine, as guardian(s)/conservator(s) of the estate of William Forcine, for the benefit of William Forcine. No payments shall be made until petitioners provide respondent with documentation establishing

that they have been appointed as guardian(s)/conservator(s) of William Forcine's estate.

2. A lump sum payment of $3,387.87, representing compensation for past unreimbursable expenses, payable to Lorin and Blaise Forcine, petitioners.

These amounts represent compensation for all damages that would be available under § 300aa-15(a).

IT IS SO ORDERED.

William Blatt, Petitioner v. Secretary of Health and Human Services, Respondent

Summary: In this decision, the special master accepts a settlement stipulation between the parties in which compensation is awarded for Kleine-Levin Syndrome.

Compensated Vaccine Injury: Kleine-Levin Syndrome (KLS)

Kleine-Levin syndrome is a rare disorder that primarily affects adolescent males (approximately 70 percent of those with Kleine-Levin syndrome are male). It is characterized by recurring but reversible periods of excessive sleep (up to 20 hours per day). Symptoms occur as "episodes," typically lasting a few days to a few weeks. Episode onset is often abrupt, and may be associated with flu-like symptoms. Excessive food intake, irritability, childishness, disorientation, hallucinations, and an abnormally uninhibited sex drive may be observed during episodes. Mood can be depressed as a consequence, but not a cause, of the disorder. Affected individuals are completely normal between episodes, although they may not be able to remember afterwards everything that happened during the episode. It may be weeks or more before symptoms reappear. Symptoms may be related to malfunction of the hypothalamus and thalamus, parts of the brain that govern appetite and sleep.

There is no definitive treatment for Kleine-Levin syndrome and watchful waiting at home, rather than pharmacotherapy, is most often advised. Stimulant pills, including amphetamines, methylphenidate, and modafinil, are used to treat sleepiness but may increase irritability and will not improve cognitive abnormalities. Because of similarities between Kleine-Levin syndrome and certain mood disorders, lithium and carbamazepine may be prescribed and, in some cases, have been shown to prevent further episodes. This disorder should be differentiated from cyclic re-occurrence of sleepiness during the premenstrual period in teen-aged girls, which may be controlled with birth control pills. It also should be differentiated from encephalopathy, recurrent depression, or psychosis.

Episodes eventually decrease in frequency and intensity over the course of eight to 12 years.

Damages decision based on stipulation; Kleine-Levin Syndrome; Varicella vaccine

Case No: 10-526V

Date Filed: November 25, 2013

William Blatt, Petitioner v. Secretary of Health and Human Services, Respondent

DECISION AWARDING DAMAGES

Millman, Special Master

On November 25, 2013, the parties filed the attached stipulation in which they agreed to settle this case and described the settlement terms. Petitioner alleges his receipt of Varicella vaccine on December 12, 2007, caused him to suffer Kleine-Levin syndrome ("KLS"). He further alleges that he experienced the residual effects of this injury for more than six months.

Respondent denies that Varicella vaccine caused petitioner's KLS, any other injury, or his current condition, and denies that petitioner experienced the residual effects of his injury for more than six months. Nonetheless, the parties agreed to resolve this matter informally.

The undersigned finds the terms of the stipulation to be reasonable. The court hereby adopts the parties' said stipulation, attached hereto, and awards compensation in the amount and on the terms set forth therein. Pursuant to the stipulation, the court awards a lump sum of $450,000.00, representing compensation for all damages that would be available under 42 U.S.C. § 300aa-15(a)

(2012). The award shall be in the form of a check for $450,000.00 made payable to petitioner.

IT IS SO ORDERED.

Julie A. Coddington, Petitioner v. Secretary of Health and Human Services, Respondent

Summary: In the next four (4) decisions, the Special Master accepts settlement stipulations between the parties in which compensation is awarded for acute disseminated encephalomyelitis (ADEM). Compensation for ADEM is fairly common within the unreported case settlements.

Compensated Vaccine Injury: Acute Disseminated Encephalomyelitis (ADEM)

Acute disseminated encephalomyelitis (ADEM) is characterized by a brief but widespread attack of inflammation in the brain and spinal cord that damages myelin—the protective covering of nerve fibers. ADEM often follows viral or bacterial infections, or less often, vaccination for measles, mumps, or rubella. The symptoms of ADEM appear rapidly, beginning with encephalitis-like symptoms such as fever, fatigue, headache, nausea and vomiting, and in the most severe cases, seizures and coma.

ADEM typically damages white matter (brain tissue that takes its name from the white color of myelin), leading to neurological symptoms such as visual loss (due to inflammation of the optic nerve) in one or both eyes, weakness even to the point of paralysis, and difficulty coordinating voluntary muscle movements (such as those used in walking). ADEM is sometimes misdiagnosed as a severe first attack of multiple sclerosis (MS), since the symptoms and the appearance of the white matter injury on brain imaging may be similar. However, ADEM has several features which differentiate it from MS. First, unlike MS patients, persons with ADEM will have rapid onset of fever, a history of recent infection or immunization, and some degree of impairment of consciousness, perhaps even coma; these features are not typically seen in MS.

Children are more likely than adults to have ADEM, whereas MS is a rare diagnosis in children. In addition, ADEM usually consists of a single episode or attack of widespread myelin damage, while MS features many attacks over the course of time. Doctors will often use imaging techniques, such as MRI (magnetic resonance imaging), to search for old and new lesions (areas of damage) on the brain. The presence of older brain lesions on MRI suggest that the condition may be MS rather than ADEM, since MS can cause brain lesions before symptoms become obvious. In rare situations, a brain biopsy may be necessary to differentiate between ADEM and some other diseases that involve inflammation and damage to myelin.

Treatment for ADEM is targeted at suppressing inflammation in the brain using anti-inflammatory drugs. Most individuals respond to several days of intravenous corticosteroids such as methylprednisolone, followed by oral corticosteroid treatment.

When corticosteroids fail to work, plasmapheresis or intravenous immunoglobulin therapy are possible secondary treatment options that are reported to help in some severe cases. Additional treatment is symptomatic and supportive.

Corticosteroid therapy typically helps hasten recovery from most ADEM symptoms. The long-term prognosis for individuals with ADEM is generally favorable. For most individuals, recovery begins within days, and within six months the majority of ADEM patients will have total or near total recoveries. Others may have mild to moderate lifelong impairment ranging from cognitive difficulties, weakness, loss of vision, or numbness. Severe cases of ADEM can be fatal but this is a very rare occurrence. ADEM can recur, usually within months of the initial diagnosis, and is treated by restarting corticosteroids. A small fraction of individuals who are initially diagnosed as having ADEM can go on to develop MS, but there is currently no method or known risk factors to predict whom those individuals will be.

Joint Stipulation on Damages; Trivalent Influenza (Flu) Vaccine; Acute Disseminated Encephalomyelitis (ADEM).

Case No: 10-245V

Date Filed: April 11, 2013

Julie A. Coddington, Petitioner v. Secretary of Health and Human Services, Respondent

DECISION

Special Master Dorsey

On April 16, 2010, Julie Coddington (petitioner), filed a petition pursuant to the National Vaccine Injury Compensation Program.2 42 U.S.C. §§ 300aa-1 to -34 (2006). Petitioner alleged that a trivalent influenza vaccine she received on October 9, 2008, caused or significantly aggravated her acute disseminated encephalomyelitis (ADEM). She also alleged that she experienced the residual effects of her injuries for more than six months. On April 10, 2013, the parties filed a stipulation, stating that a decision should be entered awarding compensation.

Respondent denies that the influenza vaccine caused or significantly aggravated petitioner's alleged ADEM and residual effects, or any other injury.

Nevertheless, the parties agree to the joint stipulation. The undersigned finds the stipulation reasonable and adopts it as the decision of the Court in awarding damages, on the terms set forth therein. The parties stipulated that petitioner shall receive the following compensation:

A lump sum of $500,000.00, in the form of a check payable to petitioner. This amount represents compensation for all damages that would be available under 42 U.S.C. §300aa-15(a).

IT IS SO ORDERED.

Jessica Mura, Petitioner v. Secretary of Health and Human Services, Respondent

Damages Decision Based on Proffer; Influenza Vaccine; Acute Disseminated Encephalomyelitis; ADEM.

Case No: 08-819V

Date Filed: December 18, 2013

Jessica Mura, Petitioner v. Secretary of Health and Human Services, Respondent

DECISION AWARDING DAMAGES

Vowell, Chief Special Master

On November 18, 2008, Jessica Mura filed a petition for compensation under the National Vaccine Injury Compensation Program, 42 U.S.C. § 300aa-10, et seq.2 [the "Vaccine Act" or "Program"], alleging that she developed acute disseminated encephalomyelitis ("ADEM") as a result of the influenza vaccine she received on November 19, 2006.

On May 30, 2012, the special master previously assigned to this case issued a ruling on entitlement, finding petitioner entitled to compensation. This case was reassigned to me on September 5, 2013. On December 17, 2013, respondent filed a proffer on award of compensation ("Proffer") detailing compensation for life care items, lost future earnings, pain and suffering, past unreimbursed expenses, and a Medicaid lien. According to respondent's Proffer, petitioner agrees to the proposed award of compensation. Pursuant to the terms stated in the attached Proffer, I award petitioner:

1. A lump sum payment of $1,648,817.90 in the form of a check payable to petitioner, Jessica Mura, representing life care expenses for Year 1 ($152,773.00), compensation for lost future earnings ($1,254,833.00), compensation for past unreimbursed expenses ($1,008.90), and pain and suffering ($240,203.00);

2. A lump sum payment of $618,582.67, representing compensation for satisfaction of the State of New York Medicaid lien, payable jointly to Jessica Mura, and Erie County Department of Social Services 95 Franklin Street, 7th Floor, Buffalo, New York 14202

These amounts represent compensation for all damages that would be available under §300aa-15(a).

IT IS SO ORDERED.

Diane Froelick, Petitioner v. Secretary of Health and Human Services, Respondent

Stipulation; trivalent influenza; multiple sclerosis ("MS"); acute disseminated encephalomyelitis ("ADEM").

Case No: 11-01V

Date Filed: December 18, 2013

Diane Froelick, Petitioner v. Secretary of Health and Human Services, Respondent

DECISION

Special Master Christian J. Moran

On December 17, 2013, respondent filed a stipulation concerning the petition for compensation filed by Diane Froelick on January 3, 2011. In her petition, Ms. Froelick alleged that the trivalent influenza ("flu") vaccination, which is contained in the Vaccine Injury Table (the "Table"), 42 C.F.R. §100.3(a), and which she received on November 4, 2009, caused her to suffer a "disease process" "consistent with multiple sclerosis ("MS")" with possible acute disseminated encephalomyelitis ("ADEM"). Petitioner further alleges that she suffered the residual effects of this injury for more than six months. Petitioner represents that there has been no prior award or settlement of a civil action for damages on her behalf as a result of her condition.

Respondent denies that the influenza vaccine caused petitioner to suffer MS, ADEM, or any other injury.

Nevertheless, the parties agree to the joint stipulation, attached hereto as Appendix A. The undersigned finds said stipulation reasonable and adopts it as the decision of the Court in awarding damages, on the terms set forth therein.

Damages awarded in that stipulation include:

A lump sum of $625,000.00 in the form of a check payable to petitioner, Diane Froelick. This amount represents compensation for ail damages that would be available under 42 U.S.C. §300aa-l 5(a).

IT IS SO ORDERED.

LK, Petitioner v. Secretary of Health and Human Services, Respondent

HPV Vaccination; Hypersensitivity Reaction; Acute Demyelinating Encephalomyelitis; Gastrointestinal and Menstrual Issues; Decision; Stipulation.

Case No: 12-339V

Date Filed: August 2, 2013

Reissued as Redacted: August 27, 2013

I K, Petitioner v. Secretary of Health and Human Services, Respondent

DECISION AWARDING DAMAGES

Special Master Hamilton-Fieldman

On May 30, 2012, Petitioner, LK, filed a petition seeking compensation under the National Vaccine Injury Compensation Program. Petitioner alleged that she suffered a hypersensitivity reaction, acute demyelinating encephalomyelitis ("ADEM"), and gastrointestinal and menstrual issues, as a result of receiving an HPV vaccination.

Respondent denies that Petitioner's HPV vaccination caused her hypersensitivity reaction, acute demyelinating encephalomyelitis ("ADEM"), and gastrointestinal, and menstrual issues.

Nonetheless, both parties, while maintaining their above stated positions, agreed in a stipulation, filed August 2, 2013 ("Stipulation"), that the issues before them can be settled and that a decision should be entered awarding Petitioner compensation. The undersigned finds said stipulation reasonable and adopts it as the decision of the Court in awarding damages, on the terms set forth therein. The stipulation awards:

A lump sum of $115,000.00 in the form of a check payable to Petitioner. This amount represents compensation for all damages that would be available under 42 U.S.C. §300aa-15(a) to which Petitioner would be entitled; and a lump sum of $10,000.00, in the form of a check payable to Petitioner and Petitioner's mother, AK, for past unreimbursed medical expenses; Stipulation ¶ 8(b).

The parties further stipulated that they had reached the following agreement with respect to attorneys' fees: A lump sum of $20,500.00, in the form of a check payable to Petitioner and Petitioner's attorney. The above amounts represent compensation for all damages that would be available under 42 U.S.C. ' 300aa-15(a).

IT IS SO ORDERED.

Leslie Crandall, Petitioner v. Secretary of Health and Human Services, Respondent

Summary: In this decision, the Special Master accepts settlement stipulations between the parties in which compensation is awarded for an autoimmune demyelinating condition.

Compensated Vaccine Injury: Autoimmune demyelinating condition

Decision by stipulation; influenza vaccine; autoimmune demyelinating condition.

Case No: 11-652V

Date Filed: May 3, 2013

Leslie Crandall, Petitioner v. Secretary of Health and Human Services, Respondent

DECISION

Hastings, Special Master

This is an action seeking an award under the National Vaccine Injury Compensation Program on account of an injury suffered by Leslie Crandall. On May 1, 2013, counsel for both parties filed a Stipulation, stipulating that a decision should be entered granting compensation. The parties have stipulated that petitioner shall receive the following compensation:

A lump sum of $300,000.00, in the form of a check payable to petitioner, representing compensation for all damages that would be available under 42 U.S.C. §300aa-15(a).

IT IS SO ORDERED.

Thomas Taylor, Petitioner v, Secretary of Health and Human Services, Respondent

Summary: In this decision, the Special Master accepts settlement stipulations between the parties in which compensation is awarded for a neurological demyelinating injury.

Compensated Vaccine Injury: Neurological Demyelinating Injury

Decision; Stipulation: Trivalent influenza vaccination; Neurological demyelinating injury.

Case No. 11-640V

Date Filed: May 22, 2013
Thomas Taylor, Petitioner v. Secretary of Health and Human Services, Respondent

DECISION AWARDING DAMAGES

Special Master Hamilton-Fieldman

On October 4, 2011, Petitioner, Thomas Taylor, filed a petition seeking compensation under the National Vaccine Injury Compensation Program. Petitioner alleged that he suffered a neurological demyelinating injury, as a result of receiving a trivalent influenza vaccination.

Respondent denies that Petitioner's influenza vaccination caused his neurological demyelinating injury, and/or any other injury.

Nonetheless, both parties, while maintaining their above stated positions, agreed in a Stipulation, filed May 22, 2013, that the issues before them can be settled and that a decision should be entered awarding Petitioner compensation. The undersigned finds said stipulation reasonable and adopts it as the decision of the Court in awarding damages, on the terms set forth therein. The stipulation awards:

A lump sum of $250,000.00 in the form of a check payable to Petitioner. This amount represents compensation for all damages that would be available under 42 U.S.C. §300aa-15(a) to which Petitioner would be entitled.

IT IS SO ORDERED

Zvi Fisch and Tzipora Fisch, legal representative of a minor child, Dov Fisch, Petitioners v. Secretary of Health and Human Services, Respondent

Summary: In this decision, the Special Master accepts settlement stipulations between the parties in which compensation is awarded for Encephalitis. Encephalitis is a noted on the Vaccine Injury Table.

Compensated Vaccine Injury: Encephalitis

Damages; decision based on proffer; measles-mumps-rubella vaccine; encephalitis; on-Table injury.

Case No: 10-382V

Date Filed: November 8, 2013

Zvi Fisch and Tzipora Fisch, legal representative of a minor child, Dov Fisch, Petitioners v. Secretary of Health and Human Services, Respondent

DECISION AWARDING DAMAGES

Special Master Christian J. Moran

On June 21, 2010, Zvi and Tzipora Fisch filed a petition for compensation, as legal representatives of their child, Dov Fisch (Dov), alleging that he suffered encephalitis caused by his receipt of a measles-mumps-rubella ("MMR") vaccine, which he received on June 25, 2007. The petitioners seek compensation pursuant to the National Vaccine Injury Compensation Program, 42 U.S.C. §300aa-10 et seq. (2006). On February 10, 2011, the undersigned ruled, based upon respondent's concession, see Respondent's Report, filed January 24, 2011, that petitioners are entitled to compensation.

On November 5, 2013, respondent filed a Proffer on Award of Compensation. Based upon the record as a whole, the special master finds the Proffer reasonable and that petitioners are entitled to an award as stated in the Proffer. Pursuant to the attached Proffer (Appendix A), the court awards petitioners:

A. A lump sum payment of $870,099.19, representing trust seed funds consisting of the present year cost of compensation for facility expenses in Compensation Year 2028 through Compensation Year 2030 ($613,200.00) and life care expenses in the first year after judgment ($256,899.19), in the form of a check payable to Regions Bank, as Trustee of the Reversionary Trust established for the benefit of Dov Fisch, as set forth in Appendix A: Items of Compensation for Dov Fisch;

B. A lump sum payment of $848,697.87, representing compensation for lost future earnings ($616,828.82) and pain and suffering ($231,869.05), in the form of a check payable to petitioners as guardians/conservators of Dov Fisch, for the benefit of Dov Fisch. No payments shall be made until petitioners provide respondent with documentation establishing that they have been appointed as the guardians/conservators of Dov Fisch's estate;

C. A lump sum payment of $1,590,163.70, representing compensation for satisfaction of the New York City lien, payable jointly to petitioners and:

NYC Human Resources Administration
Division of Liens and Recovery
P.O. Box 3786 - Church Street Station
New York, NY 10008-3786

Petitioners agree to endorse this payment to New York City.

D. A lump sum payment of $237,268.50, representing compensation for satisfaction of the Suffolk County lien, payable jointly to petitioners and:

County of Suffolk
Department of Social Services
P.O. Box 18100
Hauppauge, NY 11788-8900

Petitioners agree to endorse this payment to Suffolk County.

E. An amount sufficient to purchase the annuity contract, subject to the conditions described below, that will provide payments for the life care items contained in the life care plan, as illustrated by the hart at Tab A attached hereto (Appendix A), paid to the life insurance company from which the annuity will be purchased.

Compensation for Year Two (beginning on the first anniversary of the date of judgment) and all subsequent years shall be provided through respondent's purchase of an annuity, which annuity shall make payments directly to Regions Bank, as Trustee of the Reversionary Trust established for the benefit of Dov Fisch, only so long as Dov Fisch is alive at the time a particular payment is due. At the Secretary's sole discretion, the periodic payments may be provided to the Trustee of the Reversionary Trust in monthly, quarterly, annual or other installments. The "annual amounts" set forth in the chart at Tab A (Appendix A) describe only the total yearly sum to be paid to the Trustee of the Reversionary Trust and do not require that the payment be made in one annual installment.

IT IS SO ORDERED.

David Peddy and Alysia A. Peddy, legal representatives of minor child, David Pierce Peddy, Jr., Peditioners v. Secretary of Health and Human Services, Respondent

Summary: In this decision, the Special Master accepts settlement stipulations between the parties in which compensation is awarded for a vaccine injury that resulted in a seizure disorder and developmental delay.

Compensated Vaccine Injury: Seizure Disorder; Developmental Delay

Stipulation: Damages; Measles, Mumps, and Rubella (MMR) Vaccine; Pre-existing Seizure Disorder; Developmental Delay.

Case No: 08-720V

Date Filed. August 7, 2013

David Peddy and Alysia A. Peddy, legal representatives of minor child, David Pierce Peddy, Jr., Petitioners v. Secretary of Health and Human Services, Respondent

DECISION AWARDING DAMAGES

Hamilton-Feldman, Special Master

On October 19, 2008, Petitioners David and Alysia Peddy filed a petition seeking compensation under the National Vaccine Injury Compensation Program (the Vaccine Program), on behalf of their minor child David Pierce Peddy, Jr. ("David"), alleging that David suffered injuries as a result of receiving certain vaccinations.

On August 6, 2013, Respondent filed a Proffer on Award of Compensation (Proffer). The Proffer indicates that Petitioners agrees with the amounts specified therein. Based on the record as a whole, the undersigned finds that Petitioners are entitled to an award as stated in the Proffer. Pursuant to the terms stated in the attached Proffer, the court awards Petitioners:

1. A lump sum payment of $1,751,663.00, representing compensation for lost future earnings ($717,984.00), pain and suffering ($250,000.00), and life care expenses for Year One ($783,679.00), in the form of a check payable to Petitioners as guardians/conservator of David, for the benefit of David.

2. A lump sum payment of $53,938.44, representing compensation for past unreimbursable expenses, payable to Petitioners, David P. Peddy and Alysia A. Peddy.

3. A lump sum of $450,400.89, representing compensation for satisfaction of the State of Florida Medicaid lien, in the form of a check payable jointly to Petitioners and

>   Agency for Health Care Administration
>   Florida TPL Recovery Unit
>   Tallahassee, FL 32317

4. An amount sufficient to purchase the annuity contract described in section II. D. of the attached Proffer, paid to the life insurance company(ies) from which the annuity(ies) will be purchased.

IT IS SO ORDERED.

Reese Tower, a Minor, by His Next Friend, Lynda Curran, Petitioner v. Secretary of Health and Human Services, Respondent

Summary: In this decision, the Special Master accepts settlement stipulations between the parties in which compensation is awarded for a vaccine injury that resulted in developmental delay.

Compensated Vaccine Injury: Developmental Delay

According to the CDC, developmental disabilities are a group of conditions due to an impairment in physical, learning, language, or behavior areas. These conditions begin during the developmental period, may impact day-to-day functioning, and usually last throughout a person's lifetime

Damages decision based on stipulation; diphtheria-tetanus-acellular pertussis vaccine; hepatitis B vaccine; inactivated polio vaccine; Haemophilus influenzae type B vaccine; pneumococcal conjugate vaccine; rotavirus vaccine; massive gastrointestinal bleed; necrotizing enterocolitis; developmental delay.

Case No: 10-169

Date Filed: November 19, 2013

Reese Tower, a Minor, by His Next Friend, Lynda Curran, Petitioner v. Secretary of Health and Human Services, Respondent

DECISION AWARDING DAMAGES

Millman, Special Master

This petition was initially filed by Stephanie Tower, Reese Tower's mother. On December 17, 2010, Lynda Curran was appointed temporary guardian of the person for Reese Tower. On October 9, 2012, the special master granted petitioner's motion to substitute Lynda Curran as petitioner. On July 19, 2013, petitioner's counsel reported that petitioner was appointed as permanent legal guardian of Reese's estate and person.

On November 19, 2013, the parties filed the attached stipulation in which they agreed to settle this case and described the settlement terms. Petitioner alleges that Reese suffered massive gastrointestinal bleed and necrotizing enterocolitis that was caused by his March 23, 2007 receipt of diphtheria-tetanus-acellular pertussis ("DTaP"), Hepatitis B ("hep B"), inactivated polio ("IPV"), Haemophilus influenzae type B ("Hib"), pneumococcal conjugate ("PCV"), and rotavirus vaccinations. Petitioner further alleges that Reese suffered developmental delay as sequela of his injury and that he experienced residual effects of this injury for more than six months.

Respondent denies that DTaP, hep B, IPV, Hib, PCV, and rotavirus vaccines caused Reese's alleged injuries and that his current disabilities are sequelae of his alleged injury.

Nonetheless, the parties agreed to resolve this matter informally.

The undersigned finds the terms of the stipulation to be reasonable. The court hereby adopts the parties' said stipulation, attached hereto, and awards compensation in the amount and on the terms set forth therein. Pursuant to the stipulation, the court awards:

A. A lump sum of $219,251.56 (which amount includes $24,251.56 for first year life care plan expenses and $195,000.00 for pain and suffering). The award shall be in the form of a check for $219,251.56 made payable to petitioner as Guardian/Conservator of the estate of Reese Tower, for the benefit of Reese Tower;

B. A lump sum of $5,758.77 for past unreimbursed expenses. The award shall be in the form of a check for $5,758.77 made payable to petitioner;

C. A lump sum of $233,605.18, representing compensation for satisfaction of the State of California Medicaid lien. The award shall be in the form of a check for $233,605.18, made payable jointly to petitioner and

> State of California
> Recovery Section, MS 4720
> P.O. Box 997425
> Sacramento, CA 95899-7425

Petitioner agrees to endorse this check to the State of California, Recovery Section, MS 4720; and

D. An amount sufficient to purchase the annuity contract described in paragraph 10 of the attached stipulation.

IT IS SO ORDERED.

Adrea Botan, as the mother and legal representative of her minor daughter, Evelyn Botan, Petitioner v. Secretary of Health and Human, Respondent

Summary: In this decision, the special master accepts the respondent's concession that the vaccine injury resulted in an encephalopathy as stated on the Vaccine Injury Table. Compensation is awarded.

Compensated Vaccine Injury: Encephalopathy

DTaP Vaccine; Table Encephalopathy; Respondent's Concession; Finding of Entitlement; Damages Decision Based

Case No: 11-0063V

Date Filed: July 3, 2013

Adrea Botan, as the mother and legal representative of her minor daughter, Evelyn Botan, Petitioner v. Secretary of Health and Human, Respondent

DECISION AWARDING DAMAGES

Special Master Hamilton-Fieldman

On January 28, 2011, Petitioner, Andrea Botan, filed a petition on behalf of her minor child seeking compensation under the National Vaccine Injury Compensation Program (the Vaccine Program) for a vaccine-related injury. The Proffer requires that Petitioner appoint a guardian/conservator of Evelyn Botan's estate, as duly authorized under the laws of the State of Texas. As of the date of this decision, nothing in the record indicates that this requirement has been fulfilled.

Respondent has conceded that Petitioner is entitled to compensation due to Evelyn Botan suffering a diphtheria, tetanus, acellular pertussis (DTaP) Vaccine Table presumptive injury of encephalopathy. Informed by Respondent's concession that an award of damages is appropriate, the undersigned finds that Petitioner is entitled to compensation under the Vaccine Program.

On June 26, 2013, Respondent filed a Proffer detailing Respondent's recommendations of Damages (Proffer). In the Proffer Respondent represented that Petitioner had agreed to all of the terms set forth therein. Based on the record as a whole, the undersigned finds the Proffer reasonable and that Petitioner is entitled to an award as stated in the Proffer. Pursuant to the terms stated in the attached Proffer, the court awards Petitioner:

1. A lump sum payment of $551,303.00, representing the life care expenses for Year One ($321,303.00), and the net present value of a portion of the expenses for Year 2030 ($230,000.00), in the form of a check payable to The Broadway National Bank for the benefit of the Evelyn Botan U.S. Grantor Reversionary Trust;

2. A lump sum payment of $900,300.00, representing compensation for lost future earnings ($650,300.00) and pain and suffering ($250,000.00), in the form of a check payable to the guardian/conservator of Evelyn Botan's estate. No payments shall be made until Petitioner satisfies the requirements set forth in the attached proffer with respect to the guardianship/conservatorship of the estate of Evelyn Botan;

3. A lump sum payment of $7,000.00, representing compensation for past un-reimbursed expenses, in the form of a check payable to Petitioner;

4. A lump sum payment of $31,490.11, representing compensation for satis-faction of the State of Texas Medicaid lien, payable jointly to the guardian/conservator and:
> TMHP/Medicaid
> TPL/Tort Department
> P.O. Box 202948
> Austin, TX 78720-2948
> Attn: Tort Receivables

5. An amount sufficient to purchase an annuity contract(s), subject to the conditions described in Section II. E. of the attached Proffer, that will provide payments for the life care items contained in the life care plan, as illustrated by the chart at Tab A [attached hereto as Appendix A at 1-2] paid to the life insurance company(ies) from which the annuity(ies) will be purchased. Compensation for Year Two (beginning on the first anniversary of the date of judgment) and all subsequent payments shall be provided through Respondent's purchase of an annuity, which annuity will make payments directly to the Evelyn Botan U.S. Grantor Reversionary Trust, only so long as Evelyn Botan is alive at the time a particular payment is due. The "annual amounts" set forth in Tab B [attached hereto as Appendix A at 3-4] describe the total year sum to be paid to the Trust and do not require that the payment be made in one single payment.

IT IS SO ORDERED.

Terri Turnage, Natural Parent of a Minor Child, M.A.T., Petitioner v. Secretary of Health and Human Services, Respondent

Summary: In this decision, the special master accepts the parties' settlement and awards compensation for encephalopathy.

Compensated Vaccine Injury: Encephalopathy

Damages decision based on proffer; MMR vaccine; encephalopathy

Case No: 04-1225V

Date Filed: December 13, 2013

Terri Turnage, Natural Parent of a Minor Child, M.A.T., Petitioner v. Secretary of Health and Human Services, Respondent
DECISION AWARDING DAMAGES

Millman, Special Master

On July 28, 2004, petitioner filed a petition under the National Childhood Vaccine Injury Act, 42 U.S.C. § 300aa–10-34 (2012), alleging that MMR vaccine caused M.A.T.'s encephalopathy. On May 27, 2009, after a fact hearing, then-Chief Special Master Golkiewicz found the petition timely filed. See Order Resolving Statute of Limitations Issue and Order Setting Further Proceedings, May 27, 2009, ECF No. 57. On June 19, 2009, the parties filed a joint status report confirming that respondent did not contest that the MMR vaccine received in this case was the presumed cause of M.A.T.'s encephalopathy.

On December 13, 2013, respondent filed Respondent's Proffer on Award of Compensation. The undersigned finds the terms of the proffer to be reasonable. Based on the record as a whole, the undersigned finds that petitioner is entitled to the award as stated in the proffer. Pursuant to the terms stated in the attached proffer, the court awards petitioner:

A. a lump sum payment of $1,214,987.18, representing compensation for lost future earnings ($748,644.98), pain and suffering ($229,352.17), and life care expenses expected to be incurred during the first year after judgment ($236,990.03). The award shall be in the form of a check payable to petitioner as guardian/conservator of M.A.T., for the benefit of M.A.T.; and

B. a lump sum payment of $30,000.00, representing compensation for past unreimbursable expenses. The award shall be in the form of a check payable to Terri Turnage, petitioner;

C. a lump sum payment of $187,627.48, representing compensation for satisfaction of the State of Oklahoma Medicaid lien. The award shall be in the form of a check payable jointly to petitioner and

State of Oklahoma
OK Health Care Authority
2401 N.W. 23rd
Oklahoma City, OK 73107

Petitioner agrees to endorse this payment to the State of Oklahoma.

IT IS SO ORDERED.

Yanping Xu, Natural Father, and Qiuyue Yu, Natural Mother, of Kyle Xu, a minor, Petitioners v. Secretary of Health and Human Services, Respondent

Summary: In the next four cases, Special Masters accept settlements between the parties and award compensation for transverse myelitis.

Compensated Vaccine Injury: Transverse Myelitis

According to the National Institutes of Neurological Disorder and Stroke, transverse myelitis is a neurological disorder caused by inflammation across both sides of one level, or segment, of the spinal cord. The term myelitis refers to inflammation of the spinal cord; transverse simply describes the position of the inflammation, that is, across the width of the spinal cord. Attacks of inflammation can damage or destroy myelin, the fatty insulating substance that covers nerve cell fibers. This damage causes nervous system scars that interrupt communications between the nerves in the spinal cord and the rest of the body.

Symptoms of transverse myelitis include a loss of spinal cord function over several hours to several weeks. What usually begins as a sudden onset of lower back pain, muscle weakness, or abnormal sensations in the toes and feet can rapidly progress to more severe symptoms, including paralysis, urinary retention, and loss of bowel control. Although some patients recover from transverse myelitis with minor or no residual problems, others suffer permanent impairments that affect their ability to perform ordinary tasks of daily living. Most patients will have only one episode of transverse myelitis; a small percentage may have a recurrence.

The segment of the spinal cord at which the damage occurs determines which parts of the body are affected. Nerves in the cervical (neck) region control signals to the neck, arms, hands, and muscles of breathing (the diaphragm). Nerves in the thoracic (upper back) region relay signals to the torso and some parts of the arms. Nerves at the lumbar (mid-back) level control signals to the hips and legs. Finally, sacral nerves, located within the lowest segment of the spinal cord, relay signals to the groin, toes, and some parts of the legs. Damage at one segment will affect function at that segment and segments below it. In patients with trans-verse myelitis, demyelination usually occurs at the thoracic level, causing problems with leg movement and bowel and bladder control, which require signals from the lower segments of the spinal cord.

Transverse myelitis occurs in adults and children, in both genders, and in all races. No familial predisposition is apparent. A peak in incidence rates (the number of new cases per year) appears to occur between 10 and 19 years and 30 and 39 years. Although only a few studies have examined incidence rates, it is estimated that about 1,400 new cases of transverse myelitis are diagnosed each year in the United States, and approximately 33,000 Americans have some type of disability resulting from the disorder.

Researchers are uncertain of the exact causes of transverse myelitis. The inflamma-tion that causes such extensive damage to nerve fibers of the spinal cord may result from viral infections or abnormal immune reactions. Transverse myelitis also may occur as a complication of syphilis, measles, Lyme disease, and some vaccinations, including those for chickenpox and rabies. Cases in which a cause cannot be identi-fied are called idiopathic.

Transverse myelitis often develops following viral infections. Infectious agents sus-pected of causing transverse myelitis include varicella zoster (the virus that causes chickenpox and shingles), herpes simplex, cytomegalovirus, Epstein-Barr, influenza, echovirus, human immunodeficiency virus (HIV), hepatitis A, and rubella. Bac-terial skin infections, middle-ear infections (otitis media), and Mycoplasma pneu-moniae (bacterial pneumonia) have also been associated with the condition.

In post-infectious cases of transverse myelitis, immune system mechanisms, rather than active viral or bacterial infections, appear to play an important role in causing damage to spinal nerves. Although researchers have not yet identified the precise mechanisms of spinal cord injury in these cases, stimulation of the immune system in response to infection indicates that an autoimmune reaction may be responsible. In autoimmune diseases, the immune system, which normally protects the body from foreign organisms, mistakenly attacks the body's own tissue, causing inflammation and, in some cases, damage to myelin within the spinal cord.

Because some affected individuals also have autoimmune diseases such as systemic lupus erythematosus, Sjogren's syndrome, and sarcoidosis, some scientists suggest that transverse myelitis may also be an autoimmune disorder. In addition, some cancers may trigger an abnormal immune response that may lead to transverse myelitis.

In some people, transverse myeltis represents the first symptom of an underlying demyelinating disease of the central nervous system such as multiple sclerosis (MS) or neuromyelitis optica (NMO). A form of transverse myelitis known as "partial" myelitis—because it affects only a portion of the cross-sectional area of the spinal cord—is more characteristic of MS. Neuromyelitis optica typically causes both transverse myelitis and optic neuritis (inflammation of the optic nerve that results in visual loss), but not necessarily at the same time. All patients with transverse myelitis should be evaluated for MS or NMO because patients with these diagnoses may require different treatments, especially therapies to prevent future attacks.

Transverse myelitis may be either acute (developing over hours to several days) or subacute (usually developing over 1 to 4 weeks). Initial symptoms usually include localized lower back pain, sudden paresthesias (abnormal sensations such as burning, tickling, pricking, or tingling) in the legs, sensory loss, and paraparesis (partial paralysis of the legs). Paraparesis may progress to paraplegia (paralysis of the legs and lower part of the trunk). Urinary bladder and bowel dysfunction is common. Many patients also report experiencing muscle spasms, a general feeling of discomfort, headache, fever, and loss of appetite. Depending on which segment of the spinal cord is involved, some patients may experience respiratory problems as well.

From this wide array of symptoms, four classic features of transverse myelitis emerge: (1) weakness of the legs and arms, (2) pain, (3) sensory alteration, and (4) bowel and bladder dysfunction. Most patients will experience weakness of varying degrees in their legs; some also experience it in their arms. Initially, people with transverse myelitis may notice that they are stumbling or dragging one foot or that their legs seem heavier than normal. Coordination of hand and arm movements, as well as arm and hand strength, may also be compromised. Progression of the disease leads to full paralysis of the legs, requiring the patient to use a wheelchair.

Pain is the primary presenting symptom of transverse myelitis in approximately one-third to one-half of all patients. The pain may be localized in the lower back or may consist of sharp, shooting sensations that radiate down the legs or arms or around the torso.

Patients who experience sensory disturbances often use terms such as numbness, tingling, coldness, or burning to describe their symptoms. Up to 80 percent of those with transverse myelitis report areas of heightened sensitivity to touch, such that clothing or a light touch with a finger causes significant discomfort or pain (a condition called allodynia). Many also experience heightened sensitivity to changes in temperature or to extreme heat or cold.

Bladder and bowel problems may involve increased frequency of the urge to urinate or have bowel movements, incontinence, difficulty voiding, the sensation of incomplete evacuation, and constipation. Over the course of the disease, the majority of people with transverse myelitis will experience one or several of these symptoms.

Stipulation; Inactivated Polio Virus Vaccine; Diphtheria, Tetanus, and Acellular Pertussis Vaccine; Transverse Myelitis.

Case No: 11-0047V

Date Filed: August 26, 2013

Yanping Xu, Natural Father, and Qiuyue Yu, Natural Mother, of Kyle Xu, a minor, Petitioners v. Secretary of Health and Human Services, Respondent

DECISION ON JOINT STIPULATION

Vowell, Special Master

Yanping Xu and Qiuyue Yu ["petitioners"] filed a petition for compensation under the National Vaccine Injury Compensation Program on January 18, 2011. Petitioners allege that their son, Kyle Xu ["Kyle"], developed transverse myelitis as a result of the inactivated polio virus ["IPV"] and diphtheria, tetanus, and acellular pertussis ["DTaP"] vaccines he received on or about May 7, 2008. They further allege that Kyle developed neurogenic bladder, dysphagia, and dysfunction of his upper and lower extremities as sequelae of his injury, and that he experienced residual effects of this injury for more than six months.

Respondent denies that Kyle's vaccines caused his transverse myelitis and current disabilities, and denies that his current disabilities are sequelae of his alleged injury.

Nevertheless, the parties have agreed to settle the case. On August 23, 2013, the parties filed a joint stipulation agreeing to settle this case and describing the settlement terms. Respondent agrees to pay petitioner:

A. A lump sum of $100,000.00 in the form of a check payable to petitioners, as the court-appointed guardian(s)/conservator(s) of the estate of Kyle Xu for the benefit of Kyle Xu. No payments shall be made until petitioner provide respondent with documentation establishing that they have been appointed as the guardian(s)/conservator(s) of Kyle Xu's estate. This amount represents partial compensation for all damages that would be available under § 300aa-15(a).

B. An amount sufficient to purchase the annuity contract described in paragraph 10 of the attached stipulation, paid to the life insurance company from which the annuity will be purchased (the "Life Insurance Company").

The special master adopts the parties' stipulation attached hereto, and awards compensation in the amount and on the terms set forth therein.

IT IS SO ORDERED.

Camille Vega-Willard, Petitioner v. Secretary of Health and Human Services, Respondent

Compensated Vaccine Injury: Transverse Myelitis

Joint Stipulation on Damages; influenza (flu) vaccine; transverse myelitis (TM).

Case No: 09-606V

Date Filed: September 18, 2013

Camille Vega-Willard, Petitioner v. Secretary of Health and Human Services, Respondent

DECISION

Special Master Dorsey

On September 15, 2009, Camille Vega-Willard (petitioner) filed a petition pursuant to the National Vaccine Injury Compensation Program 42 U.S.C. §§ 300aa-1 to -34 (2006). Petitioner received an influenza (flu) vaccine on October 31, 2007. Petitioner alleged that she sustained the first symptom or manifestation of the onset of transverse myelitis (TM) within six days of receipt of her flu vaccine. Petitioner also alleged that she experienced the residual effects of her injuries for more than six months. On September 18, 2013, the parties filed a stipulation, stating that a decision should be entered awarding compensation.

Respondent denies that the vaccine either caused or significant aggravated petitioner's alleged symptoms, any of her ongoing symptoms, or any other injury. Nevertheless, the parties agree to the joint stipulation, attached hereto as Appendix A (the stipulation). The undersigned finds the stipulation reasonable and adopts it as the decision of the Court in awarding damages, on the terms set forth therein. The parties stipulated that petitioner shall receive the following compensation:

1. A lump sum of $550,000.00, in the form of a check payable to petitioner. This amount represents compensation for all damages that would be available under 42 U.S.C. §300aa-15(a), except as set forth below and in ¶8(b) of the stipulation, attached as Appendix A.

2. An amount sufficient to purchase an annuity contract described in paragraph 10 of the stipulation, paid to the life insurance company from which the annuity will be purchased, subject to the conditions and terms contained in the stipulation, attached as appendix A.

IT IS SO ORDERED.

Stanley Rye, Petitioner v. Secretary of Health and Human Services, Respondent

Compensated Vaccine Injury: Transverse Myelitis

Decision by Stipulation; Influenza Vaccine; Transverse Myelitis (TM)

Case No: 10-736V

Date Filed: November 14, 2013

Stanley Rye, Petitioner v. Secretary of Health and Human Services, Respondent

DECISION

Hastings, Special Master.

This is an action seeking an award under the National Vaccine Injury Compensation Program on account of an injury suffered by Stanley Rye. On November 13, 2013, counsel for both parties filed a Stipulation, stipulating that a decision should be entered granting compensation. The parties have stipulated that petitioner shall receive the following compensation:

A lump sum of $175,000, in the form of a check payable to petitioner, representing compensation for all damages that would be available under 42 U.S.C. §300aa-15(a).

I have reviewed the file, and based on that review, I conclude that the parties' stipulation appears to be an appropriate one. Accordingly, my decision is that a Program award shall be made to petitioner in the amount set forth above. In the absence of a timely-filed motion for review of this Decision, the clerk shall enter judgment in accordance herewith.

IT IS SO ORDERED.

Mitch Steinberg, Petitioner v. Secretary of Health and Human Services, Respondent

Compensated Vaccine Injury: Transverse Myelitis

Damages decision based on stipulation; flu vaccine; transverse myelitis

Case No: 12-445V

Date Filed: December 18, 2013

Mitch Steinberg, Petitioner v. Secretary of Health and Human Services, Respondent

DECISION AWARDING DAMAGES

Millman, Special Master

On December 18, 2013, the parties filed the attached stipulation in which they agreed to settle this case and described the settlement terms. Petitioner alleges that he suffered transverse myelitis that was caused by his September 15, 2009 receipt of influenza ("flu") vaccine. He further alleges that he experienced the residual effects of this injury for more than six months. Respondent denies that flu vaccine caused petitioner's transverse myelitis, any other injuries, or his current condition. Nonetheless, the parties agreed to resolve this matter informally.

The undersigned finds the terms of the stipulation to be reasonable. The court hereby adopts the parties' said stipulation, attached hereto, and awards compensation in the amount and on the terms set forth therein. Pursuant to the stipulation, the court awards a lump sum of $325,000.00, representing compensation for all damages that would be available under 42 U.S.C. § 300aa-15(a) (2012).

IT IS SO ORDERED.

Karen Doyle v. Secretary of Health and Human Services, Respondent

Summary: In the next two (2) cases, Special Master accepts settlements between parties and award compensation for Multiple Sclerosis.

Compensated Vaccine Injury: Multiple Sclerosis

Damages decision based on stipulation; influenza vaccine; chemically-induced multiple sclerosis; transverse myelitis.

Case No: 07-242V

Date Filed: September 30, 2013

Karen Doyle v. Secretary of Health and Human Services, Respondent

DECISION AWARDING DAMAGES

Millman, Special Master

On September 30, 2013, the parties filed the attached stipulation in which they agreed to settle this case and described the settlement terms. Petitioner alleges that she suffered "chemically-induced multiple sclerosis ("MS") and/or transverse myelitis ("TM") that were caused by her November 10, 2005 receipt of trivalent influenza ("flu") vaccine. Petitioner further alleges that she suffered the residual effects of these injuries for more than six months.

Respondent denies that the flu vaccine caused petitioner's alleged MS and/or TM or any other injury and further denies that her current disabilities are a sequela of a vaccine-related injury.

Nonetheless, the parties agreed to resolve this matter informally. The undersigned finds the terms of the stipulation to be reasonable. The court hereby adopts the parties' said stipulation, attached hereto, and awards compensation in the amount and on the terms set forth therein. Pursuant to the stipulation, the court awards a lump sum of $265,000.00, representing compensation for all damages that would be available under 42 U.S.C. § 300aa-15(a). The award shall be in the form of a check for $265,000.00 made payable to petitioner.

IT IS SO ORDERED.

Maria Giunta, Petitioner v. Secretary of Health and Human Services, Respondent

Compensated Vaccine Injury: Multiple Sclerosis

Stipulation; human papillovavirus quadrivalent ("HPV") vaccine; multiple sclerosis.

Case No: 11-025V

Date Filed: January 4, 2013

Maria Giunta, Petitioner v. Secretary of Health and Human Services, Respondent

UNPUBLISHED DECISION

Special Master Zane

On January 3, 2013, the parties in the above-captioned case filed a Stipulation memorializing their agreement as to the appropriate amount of compensation in this case. Petitioner alleged that she suffered from multiple sclerosis as a consequence of her receipt of the human papillovavirus quadrivalent ("HPV") vaccine, which vaccine is contained in the Vaccine Injury Table, 42 C.F.R. § 100.3(a), and which she received on or about January 30, 2008 and April 14, 2008. Petitioner alleges that she experienced the residual effects of this injury for more than six months. Petitioner also represents that there have been no prior awards or settlement of a civil action for these damages. Petitioner seeks compensation related to her injuries pursuant to the National Vaccine Injury Compensation Program, 42 U.S.C. §300aa-10 to 34.

Respondent denies that the HPV vaccine caused Petitioner's multiple sclerosis or any other injury and denies that Petitioner's current disabilities are sequelae of her alleged vaccine-related injury.

Nonetheless, the parties have agreed informally to resolve this matter. The undersigned hereby ADOPTS the parties' said Stipulation and awards compensation in the amount and on the terms set forth therein. Specifically, Petitioner is awarded:

a lump sum of $100,000.00, in the form of a check payable to Petitioner. This amount represents compensation for all damages that would be available under 42 U.S.C. § 300aa-15(a).

IT IS SO ORDERED.

Sandra J. Cort, Petitioner v. Secretary of Health and Human, Respondent

Summary: In the next three cases, special masters accept settlements between parties and award compensation for Guillain-Barré syndrome (GBS), a fairly common vaccine injury in the unreported cases.

Compensated Vaccine Injury: Guillain-Barré Syndrome (GBS)

According to the National Institute of Neurological Disorders and Stroke, Guillain-Barré syndrome (GBS) is a disorder in which the body's immune system attacks part of the peripheral nervous system. The first symptoms of this disorder include varying degrees of weakness or tingling sensations in the legs. In many instances, the weakness and abnormal sensations spread to the arms and upper body. These symptoms can increase in intensity until the muscles cannot be used at all and the patient is almost totally paralyzed. In these cases, the disorder is life-threatening and is considered a medical emergency. The patient is often put on a ventilator to assist with breathing. Most patients, however, recover from even the most severe cases of Guillain-Barré syndrome (GBS), although some continue to have some degree of weakness. Guillain-Barré syndrome is rare.

Stipulation; influenza (flu) vaccine; Guillain-Barré syndrome.

Case No: 10-727V

Date Filed: December 5, 2013

Sandra J. Cort, Petitioner v. Secretary of Health and Human, Respondent

DECISION

Special Master Christian J. Moran

On December 2, 2013, respondent filed a stipulation concerning the petition for compensation filed by Sandra J. Cort on October 27, 2010. In her petition, petitioner alleged that the influenza vaccine, which is contained in the Vaccine Injury Table (the "Table"), 42 C.F.R. §100.3(a), and which she received on

November 12, 2007, caused her to suffer Guillain-Barré syndrome ("GBS"). Respondent denies that the influenza vaccine caused petitioner to suffer GBS or any other injury.

Nevertheless, the parties agree to the joint stipulation, attached hereto as Appendix A. The undersigned finds said stipulation reasonable and adopts it as the decision of the Court in awarding damages, on the terms set forth therein.

Damages awarded in that stipulation include:

A lump sum of $300,000.00 in the form of a check payable to petitioner, Sandra J. Cort. This amount represents compensation for all damages that would be available under 42 U.S .C. § 300aa-15(a).

IT IS SO ORDERED.

Ann McClenaghan, Administrator of the Estate of Madeline Mackay, deceased, Petitioner v. Secretary of Health and Human Services, Respondent

Compensated Vaccine Injury: Guillain-Barré Syndrome

Stipulated Decision; Influenza Vaccine; Guillain-Barré Syndrome

Case No: 12-757V

Date Filed: December 2, 2013

Ann McClenaghan, Administrator of the Estate of Madeline Mackay, deceased, Petitioner v. Secretary of Health and Human Services, Respondent

DECISION

Special Master Hamilton-Fieldman

On November 5, 2012, Ann McClenaghan ("Petitioner"), as administrator of the estate of Madeline MacKay, deceased, filed a petition seeking compensation under the National Vaccine Injury Compensation Program (the "Program").

Petitioner alleges that as a result of a trivalent influenza vaccination Ms. MacKay received on October 21, 2010, Ms. Mackay developed Guillain-Barré syndrome. Petitioner further alleges that Ms. Mackay's death on November 11, 2010 was the sequela of her alleged vaccine-related injury.

Respondent denies that the flu vaccination caused Ms. MacKay's Guillain-Barré syndrome, and/or any other injury. Respondent further denies that Ms. MacKay experienced the residual effects of her alleged vaccine-related injury for more than six months, and denies that Ms. MacKay's death was vaccine related.

On December 2, 2013, counsel for both parties filed a stipulation, stating that a decision should be entered awarding compensation. The parties stipulated that Petitioner shall receive the following compensation:

A lump sum of $302,500.00 in the form of a check payable to petitioner as legal representative of the estate of Madeline MacKay. This amount represents compensation for all damages that would be available under 42 U.S.C. §300aa-15(a).

IT IS SO ORDERED.

Marc Davis, Petitioner v. Secretary of Health and Human Services, Respondent

Compensated Vaccine Injury: Guillain-Barré Syndrome

Damages decision based on stipulation; Tdap vaccine; Guillain-Barré syndrome

Case No: 13-53V

Date Filed: December 19, 2013

Marc Davis, Petitioner v. Secretary of Health and Human Services, Respondent

DECISION AWARDING DAMAGES

Millman, Special Master

On December 19, 2013, the parties filed the attached stipulation in which they agreed to settle this case and described the settlement terms. Petitioner alleges that he suffered Guillain-Barré syndrome ("GBS") that was caused by his February 20, 2012 receipt of Tetanus-diphtheria-acellular pertussis ("Tdap") vaccine. He further alleges that he experienced the residual effects of this injury for more than six months.

Respondent denies that Tdap vaccine caused petitioner's GBS, any other injuries, or his current condition. Nonetheless, the parties agreed to resolve this matter informally.

The undersigned finds the terms of the stipulation to be reasonable. The court hereby adopts the parties' said stipulation, attached hereto, and awards compensation in the amount and on the terms set forth therein. Pursuant to the stipulation, the court awards a lump sum of $175,000.00, representing compensation for all damages that would be available under 42 U.S.C. § 300aa-15(a) (2012).

IT IS SO ORDERED.

Paul W. Poling, Petitioner v. Secretary of Health and Human Services, Respondent

Summary: In the next four cases, special masters accept settlements between the parties and compensation is awarded for chronic inflammatory demyelinating polyneuropathy (CIDP), a fairly common disorder noted in unreported cases.

Compensated Vaccine Injury: Chronic Inflammatory Demyelinating Polyneuropathy (CIDP)

Decision by Stipulation; Influenza Vaccine; Guillain-Barré Syndrome (GBS); Chronic Inflammatory Demyelinating Polyneuropathy (CIDP)

Case No: 11-887V

Date Filed: November 1, 2013

Paul W. Poling, Petitioner v. Secretary of Health and Human Services, Respondent

DECISION

Hastings, Special Master

This is an action seeking an award under the National Vaccine Injury Compensation Program on account of an injury suffered by Paul W. Poling. On October 31, 2013, counsel for both parties filed a Stipulation, stipulating that a decision should be entered granting compensation. The parties have stipulated that petitioner shall receive the following compensation:

A lump sum of $100,000, in the form of a check payable to petitioner, representing compensation for all damages that would be available under 42 U.S.C. §300aa-15(a).

I have reviewed the file, and based on that review, I conclude that the parties' stipulation appears to be an appropriate one. Accordingly, my decision is that a Program award shall be made to petitioner in the amount set forth above.

IT IS SO ORDERED.

Steven Dudash, Petitioner v. Secretary of Health and Human Services, Respondent

Compensated Vaccine Injury: Chronic Inflammatory Demyelinating Polyneuropathy

Stipulation; influenza vaccine; chronic inflammatory demyelinating polyneuropathy (CIDP).

Case No: 09-646V

Date Filed: January 8, 2013

Steven Dudash, Petitioner v. Secretary of Health and Human Services, Respondent

DECISION

Special Master Christian J. Moran

On January 7, 2013, respondent filed a joint stipulation concerning the petition for compensation filed by Steven Dudash on October 1, 2009. In his petition, petitioner alleged that the influenza ("flu") vaccine, which is contained in the Vaccine Injury Table (the "Table"), 42 C.F.R. §100.3(a), and which he received on October 5, 2006, caused him to suffer chronic inflammatory demyelinating polyneuropathy ("CIDP"). Petitioner further alleges that he experienced residual effects of this injury for more than six months. Petitioner represents that there has been no prior award or settlement of a civil action for damages on his behalf as a result of his condition.

Respondent denies that the flu vaccine caused petitioner to suffer CIDP, or any other injury, and denies that his current disabilities are sequelae of a vaccine-related injury.

Nevertheless, the parties agree to the joint stipulation, attached hereto as Appendix A.

The undersigned finds said stipulation reasonable and adopts it as the decision of the Court in awarding damages, on the terms set forth therein. Damages awarded in that stipulation include:

A lump sum payment of $475,000.00 in the form of a check payable to petitioner, Steven Dudash. This amount represents compensation for all damages that would be available under 42 U.S.C. § 300aa-15(a).

IT IS SO ORDERED.

David Frost, Petitioner v. Secretary of Health and Human Services, Respondent

Compensated Vaccine Injury: Chronic Inflammatory Demyelinating Polyneuropathy

Damages decision based on stipulation; influenza vaccine; chronic inflammatory demyelinating polyneuropathy; fees and costs based on stipulation.

Case No: 12-610V

Date Filed: April 16, 2013

David Frost, Petitioner v. Secretary of Health and Human Services, Respondent

DECISION AWARDING DAMAGES

Millman, Special Master

On April 16, 2013, the parties filed the attached stipulation in which they agreed to settle this case and described the settlement terms. Petitioner alleges that he suffered from chronic inflammatory demyelinating polyneuropathy (CIDP) as a result of his receipt of influenza vaccine on September 23, 2009. Petitioner further alleges that he suffered the residual effects of this injury for more than six months.

Respondent denies that petitioner's CIDP, or any other injury, was caused in fact by the influenza vaccine.

Nonetheless, the parties agreed to resolve this matter informally. The court finds the terms to be reasonable, hereby adopts the parties' stipulation, and awards compensation in the amount and on the terms set forth therein. Pursuant to the stipulation, the court awards a lump sum of $100,000.00. The award shall be in the form of a check for $100,000.00 made payable to petitioner.

IT IS SO ORDERED.

Janice Fickett, Petitioner v. Secretary of Health and Human Services, Respondent

Compensated Vaccine Injury: Chronic Inflammatory Demyelinating Polyneuropathy

Stipulation; influenza vaccine; chronic inflammatory demyelinating polyneuropathy (CIDP).

Case No: 12-350V

Date Filed: September 18, 2013

Janice Fickett, Petitioner v. Secretary of Health and Human Services, Respondent

DECISION

Special Master Christian J. Moran

On September 9, 2013, the parties filed a joint stipulation concerning the petition for compensation filed by Janice Fickett on June 4, 2012. In her petition, petitioner alleged that the influenza vaccine, which is contained in the Vaccine Injury Table (the "Table"), 42 C.F.R. §100.3(a), and which she received on September 21, 2009, caused her to suffer chronic inflammatory demyelinating polyneuropathy ("CIDP"). Petitioner further alleges that she suffered the residual effects of this injury for more than six months. Petitioner represents that there has been no prior award or settlement of a civil action for damages on her behalf as a result of her condition.

Respondent denies that petitioner suffered a demyelinating neuropathy, CIDP, or any other injury that was caused by her flu vaccination. Respondent further denies that petitioner's current disabilities were caused by her flu vaccination.

Nevertheless, the parties agree to the joint stipulation, attached hereto as Appendix A. The undersigned finds said stipulation reasonable and adopts it as the decision of the Court in awarding damages, on the terms set forth therein. Damages awarded in that stipulation include:

A lump sum payment of $200,000.00 in the form of a check payable to petitioner, Janice Fickett. This amount represents compensation for all damages that would be available under 42 U.S.C. § 300aa-15(a).

IT IS SO ORDERED.

Judy Dodd, Petitioner v. Secretary of Health and Human Services, Respondent

Summary: In this case, the special master accepted a settlement between the parties and compensation was awarded for brachial plexopathy.

Compensated Vaccine Injury: Brachial Plexopathy/Plexitis

Stipulation; Influenza Vaccine; Brachial Plexopathy/Plexitis

Case No: 11-661V

Date Filed: February 25, 2013

Judy Dodd, Petitioner v. Secretary of Health and Human Services, Respondent

DECISION

Special Master Zane

On February 25, 2013, the parties in the above-captioned case filed a Stipulation memorializing their agreement as to the appropriate amount of compensation in this case. Petitioner, Judy Dodd, alleged that she suffered a brachial plexopathy/plexitis injury that was caused-in-fact by her receipt of an influenza ("flu") vaccine received on October 21, 2008, which is a vaccine that is contained in the Vaccine Injury Table, 42 C.F.R § 100.3(a). Petitioner alleges that she experienced the residual effects of this injury for more than six months and that she has not otherwise received compensation for such injuries. Petitioner seeks compensation related to her injuries pursuant to the National Vaccine Injury Compensation Program, 42 U.S.C. §300aa-10 to 34.

Respondent denies that the vaccine caused Petitioner's brachial plexopathy/plexitis or any other injury.

Nonetheless, the parties have agreed informally to resolve this matter. The undersigned hereby ADOPTS the parties' said Stipulation and awards compensation in the amount and on the terms set forth therein. Specifically, Petitioner is awarded a lump sum of $800,000.00, in the form of a check payable to petitioner, Judy Dodd. This amount represents compensation for all damages that would be available under 42 U.S.C. § 300aa-15(a). The Court thanks the parties for their cooperative efforts in resolving this matter.

IT IS SO ORDERED.

Melissa Biggs, Petitioner v. Secretary of Health and Human Services, Respondent

Summary: In this case, the special master accepted a settlement between the parties and compensation was awarded for brachial neuritis.

Compensated Vaccine Injury: Brachial Neuritis

Damages decision based on stipulation; influenza vaccine; bilateral brachial neuritis

Case No: 12 247 V

Date Filed: July 3, 2013

Melissa Biggs, Petitioner v. Secretary of Health and Human Services, Respondent

DECISION AWARDING DAMAGES

Millman, Special Master

On July 2, 2013, the parties filed the attached stipulation in which they agreed to settle this case and described the settlement terms. Petitioner alleges that she suffered bilateral brachial neuritis that was caused by her October 6, 2009, influenza vaccination. Petitioner further alleges that she suffered the residual effects of this injury for more than six months.

Respondent denies that petitioner's bilateral brachial neuritis or any other injury was caused by influenza vaccine.

Nonetheless, the parties agreed to resolve this matter informally. The court hereby adopts the parties' said stipulation, attached hereto, and awards compensation in the amount and on the terms set forth therein. Pursuant to the stipulation, the court awards petitioner a lump sum of $250,000.00 representing compensation for all damages that would be available under 42 U.S.C. § 300aa-15(a). The award shall be in the form of a check for $250,000.00 made payable to petitioner.

IT IS SO ORDERED.

Verda Lawellin, Petitioner v. Secretary of Health and Human Services, Respondent

Summary: In this case, the special master accepted a settlement between the parties and compensation was awarded for a vaccine injury that caused the petitioner to develop brachial neuritis and significantly aggravated her fibromyalgia.

Compensated Vaccine Injury: Fibromyalgia (with Brachial Neuritis)

Fibromyalgia syndrome is a common and chronic disorder characterized by widespread pain and a number of other symptoms.

Stipulation; tetanus-diphtheria-acellular pertussis vaccine ("Tdap"); brachial neuritis; fibromyalgia.

Case No: 12-333V

Date Filed: December 19, 2013

Verda Lawellin, Petitioner v. Secretary of Health and Human Services, Respondent
DECISION

Special Master Christian J. Moran

On December 18, 2013, respondent filed a stipulation concerning the petition for compensation filed by Verda Lawellin on May 25, 2012. In her petition, Ms. Lawellin alleged that the tetanus-diphtheria-acellular-pertussis ("Tdap") vaccine, which is contained in the Vaccine Injury Table (the "Table"), 42 C.F.R. §100.3(a), and which she received on June 17, 2009, caused her to develop brachial neuritis and significantly aggravated her fibromyalgia. Petitioner further alleged that she suffered the residual effects of these injuries for more than six months. Petitioner represents that there has been no prior award or settlement of a civil action for damages on her behalf as a result of her condition.

Respondent denies that the Tdap vaccine is the cause of petitioner's brachial neuritis, or any other injuries, or her current condition, or that it significantly aggravated her fibromyalgia.

Nevertheless, the parties agree to the joint stipulation, attached hereto as Appendix A. The undersigned finds said stipulation reasonable and adopts it as the decision of the Court in awarding damages, on the terms set forth therein.

Damages awarded in that stipulation include:

A lump sum of $100,000.00 in the form of a check payable to petitioner, Verda Lawellin. This amount represents compensation for all damages that would be available under 42 U.S.C. §300aa-15(a).

IT IS SO ORDERED.

Joseph Lerro and Brittany Lerro, Legal Representatives of the Estate of Joseph N. Lerro, deceased, Petitioners v. Secretary of Health and Human Services, Respondent

Summary: In the following six cases, the special masters have accepted settlements between the parties and awarded compensation for the estates of the deceased.

Compensated Vaccine Injury: Death

Damages decision based on stipulation; DTaP, HiB, IPV, Prevnar, rotavirus vaccines; injuries and death

Case No: 12-812V

Date Filed: July 3, 2013

Joseph Lerro and Brittany Lerro, Legal Representatives of the Estate of Joseph N. Lerro, deceased, Petitioners v. Secretary of Health and Human Services, Respondent

DECISION AWARDING DAMAGES

Millman, Special Master

On July 3, 2013, the parties filed the attached stipulation in which they agreed to settle this case and described the settlement terms. Petitioners allege that their son Joseph N. Lerro ("Joey") suffered injuries and death due to diphtheria-tetanus-acellular pertussis (DTaP), haemophilus influenza type B (HiB), inactivated polio (IPV), pneumococcal (Prevnar), and rotavirus vaccines which Joey received on January 23, 2012.

Respondent denies that Joey's injuries and death were caused by DTaP, HiB, IPV, Prevnar, and/or rotavirus vaccines.

Nonetheless, the parties agreed to resolve this matter informally. The court hereby adopts the parties' said stipulation, attached hereto, and awards compensation in the amount and on the terms set forth therein. Pursuant to the stipulation, the court awards petitioners a lump sum of $235,000.00 representing compensation for all damages that would be available under 42 U.S.C. § 300aa-15(a). The award shall be in the form of a check for $235,000.00 made payable to petitioners as administrators/executors of Joey's estate.

IT IS SO ORDERED.

Anthony Calise, personal representative of the estate of Lisa Calise, deceased, Petitioner v. Secretary of Health and Human Services, Respondent

Compensated Vaccine Injury: Death

Damages decision based on proffer; influenza vaccine; neuromyelitis optica (NMO); death.

Case No: 08-865V

Date Filed: July 3, 2013

Anthony Calise, personal representative of the estate of Lisa Calise, deceased, Petitioner v. Secretary of Health and Human Services, Respondent

DECISION AWARDING DAMAGES

Millman, Special Master

On July 3, 2013, respondent filed a Proffer on Award of Compensation. Based on the record as a whole, the special master finds that petitioner is entitled to the award as stated in the Proffer. Pursuant to the terms stated in the attached Proffer, the court awards petitioner a lump sum payment of $586,793.37 (representing $250,000.00 for pain and suffering, $86,793.37 for past unreimbursable expenses, and $250,000.00 for the statutory death award). The lump sum of $586,793.37 represents compensation for all damages that would be available under 42 U.S.C. § 300aa-15(a), and shall be made payable to petitioner.

IT IS SO ORDERED.

Margaret Rouse, Daughter and Executrix of the Estate of Henry Sundermeyer, Petitioner, v. Secretary of the Department of Health and Human Services, Respondent

Compensated Vaccine Injury: Death

Stipulation; Trivalent Influenza Vaccine; Significantly Aggravated COPD; Death

Case No: 12-439V

Date Filed: July 3, 2013

Margaret Rouse, Daughter and Executrix of the Estate of Henry Sundermeyer, Petitioner, v. Secretary of the Department of Health and Human Services, Respondent

DECISION ON JOINT STIPULATION

Vowell, Special Master

Margaret Rouse ["petitioner"] filed a petition for compensation under the National Vaccine Injury Compensation Program2 on behalf Henry Sundermyer ["vaccinee"] on July 9, 2012. Petitioner alleges that a flu vaccine administered on January 18, 2011, significantly aggravated the vaccinee's underlying COPD and other pulmonary conditions and that the vaccinee subsequently died as a result of this alleged vaccine related injury.

Respondent denies that influenza vaccine significantly aggravated any preexisting condition of the vaccinee and denies that the vaccination caused any other injury or is the cause of the vaccinee's death. Stipulation at ¶ 6. Nevertheless, the parties have agreed to settle the case. On July 2, 2013, the parties filed a joint stipulation agreeing to settle this case and describing the settlement terms. Respondent agrees to pay petitioner:

A lump sum of $60,000.00 in the form of a check payable to petitioner, as conservator/legal representative of Henry Sundermyer's estate. This amount represents compensation for all damages that would be available under § 300aa-15(a).

The special master adopts the parties' stipulation attached hereto, and awards compensation in the amount and on the terms set forth therein.

IT IS SO ORDERED.

Elisa Gould and Christopher Chupp, as co-personal representatives of the Estate of Joseph N. Chupp, Jr., deceased v. Secretary of Health and Human Services, Respondent

Compensated Vaccine Injury: Death

Damages decision based on stipulation; influenza vaccine; pneumonia; sepsis; systemic inflammatory response; death.

Case No: 12-775V

Date Filed: August 21, 2013

Elisa Gould and Christopher Chupp, as co-personal representatives of the Estate of Joseph N. Chupp, Jr., deceased v. Secretary of Health and Human Services, Respondent

DECISION AWARDING DAMAGES AND ATTORNEYS' FEES AND COSTS

Millman, Special Master

On August 21, 2013, the parties filed the attached stipulation in which they agreed to settle this case and described the settlement terms. Petitioners allege that Joseph N. Chupp, Jr. (J.N. Chupp) suffered pneumonia, sepsis, and/or a systemic inflammatory response as a result of his receipt of influenza vaccine on September 15, 2011. They further allege that J.N. Chupp's alleged reaction to the flu vaccine was a substantial factor in his death on September 23, 2011.

Respondent denies that flu vaccine caused J.N. Chupp's alleged injuries or was a substantial factor in his death.

Nonetheless, the parties agreed to resolve this matter informally. The court finds the terms to be reasonable, hereby adopts the parties' stipulation, and awards compensation in the amount and on the terms set forth therein. Pursuant to the stipulation, the court awards a lump sum of $225,000.00. The award shall be in the form of a check for $225,000.00 made payable to petitioners as Co-Personal Representatives of the Estate of Joseph N. Chupp, Jr.

IT IS SO ORDERED.

Sandra Steinberg, as the administrator of the Estate of, Isaiah, Petitioner v. Secretary of Health and Human Services, Respondent

Compensated Vaccine Injury: Death

Pediarix, Haemophilus Influenza Type B (Hib) Vaccine, Pneumococcal Conjugate Vaccine (PVC); Death; Decision; Stipulation.

Case No: 10-356V

Date Filed: November 13, 2013

Sandra Steinberg, as the administrator of the Estate of, Isaiah, Petitioner v. Secretary of Health and Human Services, Respondent

DECISION AWARDING DAMAGES

Special Master Hamilton-Fieldman

On June 9, 2010, Petitioner, Sandra Steinberg, filed a petition seeking compensation under the National Vaccine Injury Compensation Program (Athe Vaccine Program) on behalf of her son, Isaiah. Petitioner alleged that her son suffered a decrease in brain function and subsequent death, as a result of receiving the Pediarix vaccine, the Haemophilus influenza type B (Hib) vaccine, and the Pneumococcal Conjugate Vaccine (PVC).

Respondent denies that Isaiah's vaccinations caused his injury and resulting death. Nonetheless, both parties, while maintaining their above stated positions, agreed in a Stipulation, filed November 13, 2013, ("Stipulation") that the issues before them can be settled and that a decision should be entered awarding Petitioner compensation.

The undersigned finds said stipulation reasonable and adopts it as the decision of the Court in awarding damages, on the terms set forth therein.

The stipulation awards:

A lump sum of $40,000.00 in the form of a check payable to Petitioner, as legal representative of Isaiah Steinberg's estate. This amount represents compensation for all damages that would be available under 42 U.S.C. §300aa-15(a) to which Petitioner would be entitled.

IT IS SO ORDERED.

Sandra Myer, as next friend of Justin Myer, Petitioner v. Secretary of Health and Human Services, Respondent

Compensated Vaccine Injury: Death

Proffer; hepatitis B vaccine; autoimmune encephalitis; death

Case No: 06-148V

Date Filed: December 18, 2013

Sandra Myer, as next friend of Justin Myer, Petitioner v. Secretary of Health and Human Services, Respondent

DECISION AWARDING DAMAGES

Special Master Dorsey

On February 27, 2006, Justin Myer filed a petition for compensation under the National Vaccine Injury Compensation Program, 42 U.S.C. §§ 300aa-1 to -34 (2006), in which he alleged that he suffered autoimmune encephalitis as a result of a Hepatitis B vaccine he received on October 25, 2002. During the pendency of his claim, Justin died, and his mother, Sandra Myer ("petitioner"), was appointed guardian of Justin's estate.

The special master previously assigned to this case found that petitioner was entitled to compensation. Ruling on Entitlement, filed July 28, 2011, at 2.

On December 17, 2013, respondent filed a Proffer on Award of Compensation ("Proffer"). In that Proffer, respondent represented that petitioner agrees with the proffered award. Based on the record as a whole, the undersigned finds that petitioner is awarded is entitled to an award as stated in the Proffer.

Pursuant to the terms stated in the Proffer, attached to this decision as Appendix A, the undersigned awards petitioner:

A. A lump sum payment to petitioner, as Personal Representative of the Estate of Justin Myer, of $603,451.58, which amount includes the death benefit compensation ($250,000.00), past pain and suffering ($250,000.00), and past lost wages ($103,451.58). No payments shall be made until petitioner provides respondent with documentation establishing that she has been appointed as the Personal Representative of Justin Myer's estate;

B. A lump sum payment of $60,381.95, representing compensation for past unreimbursable expenses, payable to Sandra Myer, petitioner; and

C. A lump sum payment of $23,144.61, representing compensation for satisfaction of the State of Texas Medicaid lien, payable jointly to petitioner, Sandra Myer, as Personal Representative of Justin Myer's estate and petitioner agrees to endorse this payment to the State of Texas.

IT IS SO ORDERED.

Natalie S. Wait Hiebert, Petitioner v. Secretary of Health and Human Services, Respondent

Summary: In the following case, the special master accepts the parties' settlement and awards compensation for urticarial and angioedema injuries.

Compensated Vaccine Injury: Urticarial and Angioedema Injuries

Stipulation: DTap/Tdap Vaccine; Urticarial and Angioedema Injuries; Damages.

Case No: 11-251V

Date Filed: January 9, 2013

Natalie S. Wait Hiebert, Petitioner v. Secretary of Health and Human Services, Respondent

DECISION AWARDING DAMAGES

Chief Special Master Campbell-Smith

On April 22, 2011, petitioner, Natalie S. Wait Hiebert, filed a petition seeking compensation under the National Vaccine Injury Compensation Program alleging that she suffered certain injuries as a result of receiving a vaccination. Among the injuries petitioner alleged she suffered as a result of receiving a DTap/Tdap vaccine were urticarial (hives) and angioedema (swelling).

Respondent denies that Natalie's urticarial, angioedema, and/or any other injury was caused by her receipt of the DTaP/Tdap vaccine.

Nonetheless, both parties, while maintaining their above stated positions, agreed in a Stipulation filed January 7, 2013, that the issues before them can be settled and that a decision should be entered awarding petitioner compensation. The undersigned finds said stipulation reasonable and adopts it as the decision of the Court in awarding damages, on the terms set forth therein. Damages awarded in that stipulation include:

a. A lump sum of $650,000.00, which amount represents compensation for all damages that would be available under 42 U.S.C. §300aa-15(a), except as set forth in paragraph 8.b., in the form of a check payable to petitioner;

b. An amount sufficient to purchase the annuity contract described in paragraph 10 below, paid to the life insurance company from which the annuity will be purchased.

The undersigned approves the requested amount for petitioner's compensation.

IT IS SO ORDERED.

Laurie Roy, parent of Jamie Roy, a minor, Petitioner, v. Secretary of Health and Human Services, Respondent

Summary: In the following case, the special master accepts the parties' settlement and awards compensation for neurological injuries.

Compensated Vaccine Injury: Neurological Injury, Opsoclonus Myoclonus, and Ataxia

According to the National Institute of Neurological Disorders and Strokes, opsoclonus myoclonus is a rare neurological disorder characterized by an unsteady, trembling gait, myoclonus (brief, shock-like muscle spasms), and opsoclonus (irregular, rapid eye movements). Other symptoms may include difficulty speaking, poorly articulated speech, or an inability to speak. A decrease in muscle tone, lethargy, irritability, and malaise (a vague feeling of bodily discomfort) may also be present. Opsoclonus myoclonus may occur in association with tumors or viral infections. It is often seen in children with tumors.

Treatment for opsoclonus myoclonus may include corticosteroids or ACTH (adrenocorticotropic hormone). In cases where there is a tumor present, treatment such as chemotherapy, surgery, or radiation may be required.

The prognosis for opsoclonus myoclonus varies depending on the symptoms and the presence and treatment of tumors. With treatment of the underlying cause of the disorder, there may be an improvement of symptoms. The symptoms sometimes recur without warning. Generally the disorder is not fatal.

Decision by stipulation; HPV, TDaP and meningococcal conjugate vaccinations; neurological injury, opsoclonus myoclonus, and ataxia.

Case No: 10-0747V

Date Filed: January 11, 2013

Laurie Roy, parent of Jamie Roy, a minor, Petitioner, v. Secretary of Health and Human Services, Respondent

DECISION

Hastings, Special Master.

This is an action seeking an award under the National Vaccine Injury Compensation Program on account of an injury suffered by Jamie Roy. On January 9, 2013, counsel for both parties filed a Stipulation, stipulating that a decision should be entered granting compensation. The parties have stipulated that petitioner shall receive the following compensation:

A lump sum of $85,000.00, in the form of a check payable to petitioner, representing compensation for all damages that would be available under 42 U.S.C. §300aa-15(a).

I have reviewed the file, and based on that review, I conclude that the parties' stipulation appears to be an appropriate one. Accordingly, my decision is that a Program award shall be made to petitioner in the amount set forth above.

IT IS SO ORDERED.

Jesalee Parsons, Petitioner v. Secretary of Health and Human Services, Respondent

Summary: In this case the special master accepts the settlement between the parties and awards compensation for pancreatitis.

Compensated Vaccine Injury: Pancreatitis

Gardasil Vaccination; Pancreatitis; Decision; Stipulation.

Case No: 08-117V

Date Filed: April 16, 2013

Jesalee Parsons, Petitioner v. Secretary of Health and Human Services, Respondent

DECISION AWARDING DAMAGES

Special Master Hamilton-Fieldman

On June 17, 2008, Petitioner, Jesalee Parsons, filed a petition seeking compensation under the National Vaccine Injury Compensation Program. Petitioner alleged that she suffered pancreatitis, as a result of receiving a Gardasil Vaccination.

Respondent denies that Petitioner's Gardasil vaccination caused her pancreatitis, and/or any other injury.

Nonetheless, both parties, while maintaining their above stated positions, agreed in a Stipulation, filed April 15, 2013, ("Stipulation") that the issues before them can be settled and that a decision should be entered awarding Petitioner compensation. The undersigned finds said stipulation reasonable and adopts it as the decision of the Court in awarding damages, on the terms set forth therein. The stipulation awards:

A lump sum of $55,000.00 in the form of a check payable to Petitioner. This amount represents compensation for all damages that would be available under 42 U.S.C. §300aa-15(a) to which Petitioner would be entitled and a lump sum of $13,090.29, which represents reimbursement of a State of Oklahoma Medicaid lien (Oklahoma Health Care Authority, P.O. Drawer 18497) in the form of a check payable jointly to Petitioner. Petitioner agrees to endorse this payment to the State. The above amounts represent compensation for all damages that would be available under 42 U.S.C. 300aa-15(a).

IT IS SO ORDERED.

Erica Hill, Natural Mother and Guardian for E.J., a minor, Petitioner v. Secretary of Health and Human Services, Respondent

Summary: In this case the special master accepts the settlement between the parties and awards compensation for Bell's palsy.

Compensated Vaccine Injury: Bell's Palsy

According to the National Institute of Neurological Disorders and Strokes, Bell's palsy is a form of temporary facial paralysis resulting from damage or trauma to the facial nerves. The facial nerve—also called the 7th cranial nerve—travels through a narrow, bony canal (called the Fallopian canal) in the skull, beneath the ear, to the muscles on each side of the face. For most of its journey, the nerve is encased in this bony shell.

Each facial nerve directs the muscles on one side of the face, including those that control eye blinking and closing, and facial expressions such as smiling and frowning. Additionally, the facial nerve carries nerve impulses to the lacrimal or tear glands, the saliva glands, and the muscles of a small bone in the middle of the ear called the stapes. The facial nerve also transmits taste sensations from the tongue.

When Bell's palsy occurs, the function of the facial nerve is disrupted, causing an interruption in the messages the brain sends to the facial muscles. This interruption results in facial weakness or paralysis.

Bell's palsy is named for Sir Charles Bell, a 19th-century Scottish surgeon who was the first to describe the condition. The disorder, which is not related to stroke, is the most common cause of facial paralysis. Generally, Bell's palsy affects only one of the paired facial nerves and one side of the face; however, in rare cases, it can affect both sides.

Because the facial nerve has so many functions and is so complex, damage to the nerve or a disruption in its function can lead to many problems. Symptoms of Bell's palsy can vary from person to person and range in severity from mild weakness to total paralysis. These symptoms may include twitching, weakness, or paralysis on one or rarely both sides of the face. Other symptoms may include drooping of the eyelid and corner of the mouth, drooling, dryness of the eye or mouth, impairment of taste, and excessive tearing in one eye. Most often these symptoms, which usually begin suddenly and reach their peak within 48 hours, lead to significant facial distortion.

Other symptoms may include pain or discomfort around the jaw and behind the ear, ringing in one or both ears, headache, loss of taste, hypersensitivity to sound on the affected side, impaired speech, dizziness, and difficulty eating or drinking.

Bell's palsy occurs when the nerve that controls the facial muscles is swollen, inflamed, or compressed, resulting in facial weakness or paralysis. Exactly what causes this damage, however, is unknown.

Most scientists believe that a viral infection such as viral meningitis or the common cold sore virus—herpes simplex—causes the disorder. They believe that the facial nerve swells and becomes inflamed in reaction to the infection, causing pressure within the Fallopian canal and leading to ischemia (the restriction of blood and oxygen to the nerve cells). In some mild cases (where recovery is rapid), there is damage only to the myelin sheath of the nerve. The myelin sheath is the fatty covering—which acts as an insulator—on nerve fibers in the brain.

The disorder has also been associated with influenza or a flu-like illness, headaches, chronic middle ear infection, high blood pressure, diabetes, sarcoidosis, tumors, Lyme disease, and trauma such as skull fracture or facial injury.

Stipulation; meningococcal vaccine; Bell's palsy; joint stiffness; myalgia; sensory neuropathy; retinal vasculitis.

Case No: 12-411V

Date Filed: May 9, 2013

Erica Hill, Natural Mother and Guardian for E.J., a minor, Petitioner v. Secretary of Health and Human Services, Respondent

UNPUBLISHED DECISION

Special Master Zane

On May 8, 2013, the parties in the above-captioned case filed a Stipulation memorializing their agreement as to the appropriate amount of compensation in this case. Petitioner, Erica Hill, on behalf of E.J., alleged that E.J. suffered from jaw pain, bilateral Bell's palsy, joint stiffness, myalgia, sensory neuropathy, retinal vasculitis, and hypertension that were caused-in-fact by the receipt of the meningococcal vaccine on June 18, 2010, and which vaccine is contained in the Vaccine Injury Table, 42 C.F.R § 100.3(a). Ms. Hill also alleges that E.J. experienced the residual effects of this injury for more than six months and that neither Petitioner nor E.J. have otherwise received compensation for such injuries. Petitioner seeks compensation related to E.J.'s injuries pursuant to the National Vaccine Injury Compensation Program, 42 U.S.C. 300aa-10 to 34.

Respondent denies that the meningococcal vaccine caused E.J.'s claimed injuries or any other injury and denies that E.J.'s current disabilities are sequelae of the alleged vaccine-related injury.

Nonetheless, the parties have agreed informally to resolve this matter. Specifically, Petitioner is awarded: a lump sum of $90,000.00, in the form of a check payable to petitioner, as guardian of the Estate of E.J. This amount represents compensation for all damages that would be available under 42 U.S.C. § 300aa-15(a). The Court thanks the parties for their cooperative efforts in resolving this matter.

IT IS SO ORDERED.

Susan Williamsen, Petitioner v. Secretary of Health and Human Services, Respondent

Summary: In this case the special master accepts the settlement between the parties and awards compensation for systemic lupus erythematosus ("SLE").

Compensated Vaccine Injury: Systemic Lupus Erythematosus

Other common symptoms include:

- Chest pain when taking a deep breath
- Fatigue
- Fever with no other cause
- General discomfort, uneasiness, or ill feeling (malaise)
- Hair loss
- Mouth sores
- Sensitivity to sunlight
- Skin rash —a "butterfly" rash in about half people with SLE. The rash is most often seen over the cheeks and bridge of the nose, but can be wide-spread. It gets worse in sunlight.
- Swollen lymph nodes

Other symptoms depend on which part of the body is affected:
- Brain and nervous system: headaches, numbness, tingling, seizures, vision problems, personality changes
- Digestive tract: abdominal pain, nausea, and vomiting
- Heart: abnormal heart rhythms (arrhythmias)
- Lung: coughing up blood and difficulty breathing
- Skin: patchy skin color, fingers that change color when cold (Raynaud's phenomenon)

Some people have only skin symptoms. This is called discoid lupus.

Stipulation; tetanus-diptheria ("Td") vaccine; systemic lupus erythematosus ("SLE").

Case No: 10-223V

Date Filed: July 3, 2013

Susan Williamsen, Petitioner v. Secretary of Health and Human Services, Respondent

UNPUBLISHED DECISION

Special Master Daria J. Zane

On July 3, 2013, the parties in the above-captioned case filed a Stipulation memorializing their agreement as to the appropriate amount of compensation in this case. Petitioner alleged that she suffered from systemic lupus erythematosus ("SLE") as a consequence of her receipt of the tetanus-diptheria ("Td") vaccine, which is a vaccine contained in the Vaccine Injury Table, 42 C.F.R § 100.3(a), and which she received on or about April 21, 2009. Petitioner alleges that she experienced the residual effects of this injury for more than six months. Petitioner also represents that there have been no prior awards or settlement of a civil action for these damages. Petitioner seeks compensation related to her injuries pursuant to the National Vaccine Injury Compensation Program, 42 U.S.C. §300aa-10 to 34.

Respondent denies that the Td vaccine caused Petitioner's SLE or any other injury and denies that Petitioner's current disabilities are sequelae of her alleged vaccine-related injury.

Nonetheless, the parties have agreed informally to resolve this matter. The undersigned hereby ADOPTS the parties stipulation and awards compensation in the amount and on the terms set forth therein. Specifically, Petitioner is awarded:

a) a lump sum of $230,000.00, representing compensation for the reimbursement of a State of California Medicaid lien, payable jointly to petitioner and Department of Health Care Services, Personal Injury Unit, Sacramento, CA 95899-7421. Petitioner agrees to endorse this check.

b) a lump sum of $770,000.00 in the form of a check payable to Petitioner. This amount represents compensation for all damages that would be available under 42 U.S.C. § 300aa-15(a).

The Court thanks the parties for their cooperative efforts in resolving this matter.

IT IS SO ORDERED.

Deborah Grenon, Petitioner v. Secretary of Health and Human Services, Respondent

Summary: In this case the special master accepts the settlement between the parties and awards compensation for shoulder injury reactive to vaccine administration (SIRVA) and rheumatoid arthritis.

Compensated Vaccine Injury: SIRVA and Rheumatoid Arthritis

Damages decision based on stipulation; tetanus-diphtheria-acellular pertussis vaccine; Hepatitis B vaccine; injection-related shoulder injury; rheumatoid arthritis.

Case No: 12-528V

Date Filed: September 26, 2013

Deborah Grenon, Petitioner v. Secretary of Health and Human Services, Respondent

DECISION AWARDING DAMAGES

Millman, Special Master

On September 26, 2013, the parties filed the attached stipulation in which they agreed to settle this case and described the settlement terms. Petitioner alleges that she suffered an injection-related shoulder injury and rheumatoid arthritis that were caused by her August 25, 2009 receipt of tetanus-diphtheria-acellular pertussis ("Tdap") vaccine and her September 1, 2009 receipt of Hepatitis

B ("hep B") vaccine. Petitioner further alleges that she suffered the residual effects of these injuries for more than six months.

Respondent denies that petitioner suffered from an injection-related shoulder injury, rheumatoid arthritis, or any other injury that was caused by her Tdap or hep B vaccinations. Nonetheless, the parties agreed to resolve this matter informally.

The undersigned finds the terms of the stipulation to be reasonable. The court hereby adopts the parties' said stipulation, attached hereto, and awards compensation in the amount and on the terms set forth therein. Pursuant to the stipulation, the court awards a lump sum of $90,000.00, representing compensation for all damages that would be available under 42 U.S.C. § 300aa-15(a). The award shall be in the form of a check for $90,000.00 made payable to petitioner.

IT IS SO ORDERED.

Alyssa Vanscoy, a minor by her Parents and Natural Guardians, Scott Vanscoy and Caroline Vanscoy, Petitioners v. Secretary of Health and Human Services, Respondent

Summary: In this case the special master accepts the settlement between the parties and awards compensation for injuries suffered after fainting due to vaccine administration.

Compensated Vaccine Injury: Fainting Injuries

Damages; decision based on proffer; human papillomavirus (HPV) vaccine; Gardasil; fainting injuries.

Case No: 13-266V

Date Filed: October 2, 2013

Alyssa Vanscoy, a minor by her Parents and Natural Guardians, Scott Vanscoy and Caroline Vanscoy, Petitioners v. Secretary of Health and Human Services, Respondent

DECISION AWARDING DAMAGES

On April 15, 2013, Scott and Caroline Van Scoy filed a petition seeking compensation under the National Vaccine Injury Compensation Program alleging that the human papillomavirus vaccination (Gardasil) their daughter Alyssa received caused her to faint, resulting in multiple facial injuries. On July 3, 2013, the undersigned ruled, based upon respondent's concession, see Respondent's Report, filed July 1, 2013, that petitioners are entitled to compensation.

On September 30, 2013, respondent filed a Proffer on Award of Compensation. Based upon the record as a whole, the special master finds the Proffer reasonable and that petitioners are entitled to an award as stated in the Proffer. Pursuant to the attached Proffer (Appendix A), the court awards petitioners:

A. A lump sum payment of $32,205.00, representing compensation for actual and projected pain and suffering ($20,000.00) and projected unreimbursable expenses ($12,205.00) in the form of a check payable to petitioners.

B. A lump sum payment of $4,466.78, representing compensation for past unreimbursable expenses, payable to Scott Van Scoy and Caroline Van Scoy, petitioners.

IT IS SO ORDERED.

Marisol Ledesma Tirador, as the Parent and Natural Guardian of Paola Melissa Carbo Ledesma, an Infant, Petitioner v. Secretary of Health and Human Services, Respondent

Summary: In this case the special master accepts the settlement between the parties and awards compensation for idiopathic thrombocytopenic purpura (ITP).

Compensated Vaccine Injury: Idiopathic Thrombocytopenic Purpura (ITP)

Stipulation; varicella vaccine; hepatitis A vaccine; chronic idiopathic thrombocytopenic purpura; ITP

Case No: 12-192V

Date Filed: October 29, 2013

Marisol Ledesma Tirador, as the Parent and Natural Guardian of Paola Melissa Carbo Ledesma, an Infant, Petitioner v. Secretary of Health and Human Services, Respondent

DECISION

Special Master Christian J. Moran

On October 25, 2013, respondent filed a joint stipulation concerning the petition for compensation filed by Marisol Ledesma Tirador on March 26, 2012. In her petition, petitioner alleged that the varicella and hepatitis A vaccines, which are contained in the Vaccine Injury Table (the "Table"), 42 C.F.R. §100.3(a), and which her child, Paola, received on March 10, 2010, caused Paola to suffer chronic idiopathic thrombocytopenic purpura ("ITP"). Petitioner further alleges that Paola suffered the residual effects of this injury for more than six months. Petitioner represents that there has been no prior award or settlement of a civil action for damages on her behalf as a result of her condition.

Respondent denies that Paola's alleged injury and residual effects were caused-in-fact by either the varicella vaccine or the hepatitis A vaccine. Respondent further denies that either the varicella vaccine or the hepatitis A vaccine caused Paola any other injury or her current condition.

Nevertheless, the parties agree to the joint stipulation, attached hereto as Appendix A. The undersigned finds said stipulation reasonable and adopts it as the decision of the Court in awarding damages, on the terms set forth therein.

Damages awarded in that stipulation include:

A lump sum payment of $75,000.00 in the form of a check payable to petitioner as the Guardian/Conservator of the estate of Paola Melissa Carbo Ledesma, for the benefit of Paola Melissa Carbo Ledesma. This amount represents compensation for all damages that would be available under 42 U.S.C. § 300aa-15(a).

IT IS SO ORDERED.

Regan M. Colombatto, Petitioner v. Secretary of Health and Human Services, Respondent

Summary: In this case the special master accepts the settlement between the parties and awards compensation for focal lipodystrophy; paresthesias.

Compensated Vaccine Injury: Focal Lipodystrophy; Paresthesias

According to the National Institute of Neurological Disorders and Strokes, paresthesias refers to a burning or prickling sensation that is usually felt in the hands, arms, legs, or feet, but can also occur in other parts of the body. The sensation, which happens without warning, is usually painless and described as tingling or numbness, skin crawling, or itching.

Most people have experienced temporary paresthesia—a feeling of "pins and needles"—at some time in their lives when they have sat with legs crossed for too long, or fallen asleep with an arm crooked under their head. It happens when sustained pressure is placed on a nerve. The feeling quickly goes away once the pressure is relieved.

Chronic paresthesia is often a symptom of an underlying neurological disease or traumatic nerve damage. Paresthesia can be caused by disorders affecting the central nervous system, such as stroke and transient ischemic attacks (mini-strokes), multiple sclerosis, transverse myelitis, and encephalitis. A tumor or vascular lesion pressed up against the brain or spinal cord can also cause paresthesia. Nerve entrapment syndromes, such as carpal tunnel syndrome, can damage peripheral nerves and cause paresthesia accompanied by pain. Diagnostic evaluation is based on determining the underlying condition causing the paresthetic sensations. An individual's medical history, physical examination, and laboratory tests are essential for the diagnosis. Physicians may order additional tests depending on the suspected cause of the paresthesia.

Damages decision based on stipulation; Hepatitis B vaccine; focal lipodystrophy; paresthesias

Case No: 12-166V

Date Filed: November 8, 2013

Regan M. Colombatto, Petitioner v. Secretary of Health and Human Services, Respondent

DECISION AWARDING DAMAGES

Millman, Special Master

On November 8, 2013, the parties filed the attached stipulation in which they agreed to settle this case and described the settlement terms. Petitioner alleges her receipt of Hepatitis B vaccine on April 5, 2011, caused her to suffer from focal lipodystrophy and paresthesias. Respondent concedes that petitioner's focal lipodystrophy was caused-in-fact by her Hepatitis B vaccine, but denies that any other injuries were caused by the vaccine. Nonetheless, the parties agreed to resolve this matter informally.

The undersigned finds the terms of the stipulation to be reasonable. The court hereby adopts the parties' said stipulation, attached hereto, and awards compensation in the amount and on the terms set forth therein. Pursuant to the stipulation, the court awards a lump sum of $350,000.00, representing compensation for all damages that would be available under 42 U.S.C. § 300aa-15(a) (2012). The award shall be in the form of a check for $350,000.00 made payable to petitioner.

In the absence of a motion for review filed pursuant to RCFC Appendix B, the clerk of the court is directed to enter judgment herewith.

IT IS SO ORDERED.

James Melton, Petitioner v. Secretary of Health and Human Services, Respondent

Summary: In this case the special master accepts the settlement between the parties and awards compensation for neuro-ophthalmologic injury, including optic neuritis.

Compensated Vaccine Injury: Neuro-ophthalmologic Injury—Optic Nueritis

Stipulation; Influenza; Neuro-ophthalmologic Injury; Optic Neuritis

Case No: 11-589 V

Date Filed: December 2, 2013

James Melton, Petitioner v. Secretary of Health and Human Services, Respondent

DECISION ON JOINT STIPULATION

Vowell, Chief Special Master:

James Melton ["petitioner"] filed a petition for compensation under the National Vaccine Injury Compensation Program on September 14, 2011. Petitioner alleges that he suffered from a neuro-ophthalmologic injury, including optic neuritis, as a result of an influenza vaccination he received on September 30, 2008, and he further alleges that he experienced residual effects of this injury for more than six months.

Respondent denies that petitioner's influenza vaccine is the cause of his ophthalmologic injury, including optic neuritis, or any other injury or his current disabilities.

Nevertheless, the parties have agreed to settle the case. On December 2, 2013, the parties filed a joint stipulation agreeing to settle this case and describing the settlement terms.

Respondent agrees to pay petitioner:

A lump sum of $175,000.00 in the form of a check payable to petitioner, James Melton. This amount represents compensation for all damages that would be available under § 300aa-15(a).

IT IS SO ORDERED.

Angela Patten, Petitioner v. Secretary of Health and Human, Respondent

Summary: In this case the special master accepts the settlement between the parties and awards compensation for Gastroparesis.

Compensated Vaccine Injury: Gastroparesis

Damages decision based on stipulation; trivalent influenza vaccine; gastroparesis

Case No: 12-758V

Date Filed: December 11, 2013

Angela Patten, Petitioner v. Secretary of Health and Human, Respondent

DECISION AWARDING DAMAGES

Millman, Special Master

On December 9, 2013, the parties filed the attached stipulation in which they agreed to settle this case and described the settlement terms. Petitioner alleges that she suffered gastroparesis that was caused by her November 17, 2009 receipt of trivalent influenza ("flu") vaccine. Petitioner further alleges that she suffered the residual effects of this injury for more than six months. Respondent denies that petitioner suffered gastroparesis or any other injury that was caused by her flu vaccination. Nonetheless, the parties agreed to resolve this matter informally.

The undersigned finds the terms of the stipulation to be reasonable. The court hereby adopts the parties' said stipulation, attached hereto, and awards compensation in the amount and on the terms set forth therein. Pursuant to the stipulation, the court awards a lump sum of $60,000.00, representing compensation for all damages that would be available under 42 U.S.C. § 300aa-15(a). The award shall be in the form of a check for $60,000.00 made payable to petitioner.

IT IS SO ORDERED.

Minah Fowler, by her Mother and Next Friend, Hope Fowler, Petitioner v. Secretary of Health and Human Services, Respondent

Summary: The authors elected to end the listing of vaccine cases with this case in which the nature of the injury—despite a settlement of over $1,000,000.00—is not described.

The NVICP is supposed to provide information regarding vaccine injuries for the purpose of improving vaccine safety and encouraging public acceptance of vaccine. This was clearly stated in a ruling by Special Master Dee Lord on the February 2011 decision in the Langlord case. And yet here we have no information other than that a child was injured by a vaccine.

Compensated Vaccine Injury: Not Stated

Damages decision based on proffer—injury not stated.

Case No: 03-1974V

Date Filed: January 17, 2013

Minah Fowler, by her Mother and Next Friend, Hope Fowler, Petitioner v Secretary of Health and Human Services, Respondent

DECISION AWARDING DAMAGES

Millman, Special Master

On January 16, 2013, respondent filed a Proffer on Award of Compensation. Based on the record as a whole, the special master finds that petitioner is entitled to the award as stated in the Proffer. Pursuant to the terms stated in the attached Proffer, the court awards petitioner:

a. a lump sum payment of $1,061,756.00, representing compensation for lost future earnings ($705,856.00), pain and suffering ($205,000.00), and life care expenses for year one and a portion of years two through four ($150,900.00), in the form of a check payable to petitioner as guardian/conservator of Minah Fowler, for the benefit of Minah Fowler;

b. a lump sum payment of $26,491.09, representing compensation for past unreimbursable expenses, payable to Hope Fowler, petitioner;

c. a lump sum payment of $1,324.03, representing compensation for satisfaction of the Commonwealth of Pennsylvania Medicaid lien, payable jointly to petitioner, as guardian of the Estate of Minah Fowler, and Pennsylvania Department of Public Welfare, Bureau of Program Integrity, Division of Third Party Liability, Recovery Section, Harrisburg, PA 17105-8486; and

d. an amount sufficient to purchase an annuity contract subject to the conditions described in section II. D. of the attached Proffer.

IT IS SO ORDERED.

13

HISTORICAL DECISIONS REGARDING ENCEPHALOPATHY MANIFESTING AUTISM

What is autism?

Many people have come to believe that autism is a disease. We see autism represented in the media as a puzzle piece —a mystery, an enigma. We hear about research focused on finding "the autism gene." Yet the genetic research has yielded little progress.

And, while we hear about autism almost daily in the media, we are all reassured that autism is just believed to be more common because clinicians are better at diagnosing it now than they were in the past.

All of this thinking is flawed.

Children and young adults with autism are more common today than they were in the past because more individuals are suffering brain injuries than in the past. How much of the increase in autism is due to vaccine injury is not known. That question (and answer) is beyond the scope of this book. However, as the reader will soon realize, vaccine injury is one route—by no means the only route—to this behavioral disorder.

Autism is not defined in the medical literature as a disease. It is described by some in medicine as an indication of encephalopathy, a long acknowledged vaccine injury outcome.

Autism is defined in the *Diagnostic and Statistical Manual of Mental Disorders,* the *DSM*, as a behavioral disorder. In other words, if you have the behavior deficits described in the *DSM*—deficits in social-emotional reciprocity, deficits in nonverbal communicative behaviors, or deficits in developing, maintaining, and understanding relationships—it is quite possible that you are on the road to an autism diagnosis. If a person also exhibits "restricted, repetitive patterns of behavior, interests, or activities . . . stereotyped or repetitive motor movements, an insistence on sameness, inflexible adherence to routines, or ritualized patterns," a clinician is more likely to impart an autism diagnosis.

As the following publicly available case documents will show, the behavioral diagnosis of autism has long been known to occur in the presence of vaccine injuries that result in encephalopathy. While this claim is controversial, the cases speak for themselves.

Kienan Freeman, by his Mother, Rebekah Smothers, Petitioner v. Secretary of Health and Human Services, Respondent

Summary: In this MMR injury case, the special master finds that the child's seizure disorder and developmental delay ("retardation") likely were the result of his MMR vaccination. In a footnote it is reported that the child also developed an autism spectrum disorder.

Case No: 01-390V

Date Filed: September 25, 2003

Kienan Freeman, by his Mother, Rebekah Smothers, Petitioner v. Secretary of Health and Human Services, Respondent

Hastings, Special Master

This is an action in which the petitioner seeks an award under the National Vaccine Injury Compensation Program on account of an injury to her son, Kienan Freeman. For the reasons stated below, I conclude that petitioner is entitled to such an award, in an amount yet to be determined.

Kienan Freeman was born on March 21, 1998. For the first 16 months of life, although he experienced a number of ear infections, Kienan seemed to develop normally and experience generally good health.

On July 30, 1999, at the age of 16 months, Kienan received a measles-mumps-rubella ("MMR") inoculation. Eight days later, on August 7, 1999, Kienan was taken to a hospital emergency room, after he was found to be exhibiting seemingly involuntary movements described as "twitching" and eye deviations. He was then observed to suffer an extended seizure in the emergency room, which finally subsided after he was administered anti-seizure medications. While some hospital records indicate that the duration of Kienan's seizure episode was about 45 minutes, careful analysis of those records indicates that more likely his seizure episode lasted 60 to 75 minutes, or more.

During the next several weeks, Kienan did not experience any seizures. However, on October 30, 1999, Kienan suffered another prolonged seizure, again prompting a two-day hospitalization. Thereafter, Kienan began to suffer increasingly frequent seizures of short duration, without fever. By early February, he was experiencing several seizures per week.

In the weeks after Kienan's first seizure episode on August 7, 1999, according to his mother, his ability to speak seemed to regress. By early 2000, as his seizures became frequent, concern about Kienan's development increased. In March of that year, Kienan was assessed by a multi-disciplinary team, and found to be significantly delayed in his development. Since that time, Kienan has continued to suffer from seizures, and has proven to be significantly delayed in mental and other developmental abilities. No cause for his seizures and retardation has ever been definitively diagnosed.

EVIDENCE SUPPORTS AN ASSOCIATION BETWEEN MEASLES VACCINATION AND NEUROLOGICAL DISORDERS

The record in this case contains strong evidence indicating that neurologic disorders, in the form of both encephalopathy (brain disorder) and seizure disorder, have been found to be associated with both the measles virus in its natural, "*wild*" form, and with the measles *vaccine*. One item of evidence is an article authored by certain officials of the Department of Health and Human Services, in fact the very officials who administer the Program for the Secretary of Health and Human Services. The article notes that encephalopathy serious enough to cause death or permanent nervous system impairment is known to be associated with infection by the *wild* measles virus. The article's authors then examined cases in which persons suffered encephalopathies without determined cause within 15 days after a measles *vaccination*. Observing that such encephalopathies most often occurred on the eighth or ninth day after vaccination, the authors concluded that this result "suggests that a causal relationship between measles vaccine and encephalopathy exists as a rare complication of measles immunization."

In addition, Dr. Kinsbourne stated that his review of the medical literature indicates that the literature supports the view that both the *wild* measles virus and the measles *vaccine* can cause encephalopathies, resulting in both seizures and retardation. And Dr. Snyder also acknowledged both that the *wild* measles virus "has been known to cause encephalitis and seizure disorders," and that medical literature "has associated MMR *vaccination* with seizure disorders."

OVERALL CONCLUSION CONCERNING "CAUSATION-IN-FACT" ISSUE

In . . . this Section . . . I concluded that Kienan's seizure of August 7, 1999, likely was caused by his MMR vaccination of July 30, 1999. I then concluded that the seizure of August 7, in turn, was likely the cause of Kienan's subsequent seizure disorder and retardation. Putting those two factual conclusions together, I find as fact that Kienan's seizure disorder and retardation likely were the result of his MMR vaccination of July 30, 1999.

For the reasons stated above, I find that petitioner is entitled to a Program award on Kienan's behalf.

ALTERNATIVE STORY—AUTISM

It was noted at the hearing that Kienan's neurologic disorder has features that might cause it to be labeled as "atypical autism," a condition within the category of "autistic spectrum disorder." (Tr. 103-108.) I note, however, that even assuming that Kienan's disorder is correctly classified within the "atypical autism" category, that is essentially irrelevant to my ruling concerning the entitlement issue in this case. As Dr. Kinsbourne explained, Kienan's autistic-type features seem to be a result of the brain damage that caused his severe mental retardation. (Tr. 9, 21-22.) As Dr. Kinsbourne further explained, brain damage is one of the many possible causes of autism. (Tr. 108.) Thus, I cannot see why the fact that Kienan's disorder may fall within the autism spectrum has any substantial relevance to the question of what caused Kienan's seizure disorder and mental retardation.

Accordingly, I also note that, as far as I can see, the outcome of this case has no significant relevance to the many pending cases before me in which it is asserted that a MMR vaccination caused the vaccinee's autism disorder. As far as I am aware, none of those cases involves a prolonged seizure happening a week or so after vaccination. Therefore, I do not perceive that the petitioner's theory of causation in this case would be of relevance to those cases.

Further, I note that my conclusion that Kienan's neurologic disorder probably was caused by his MMR inoculation should not be interpreted as a conclusion that the MMR inoculation is a particularly dangerous vaccination. To the contrary, given the huge number of MMR inoculations that have been administered world-wide and the very small number of seizures or neurologic disorders reported after such inoculations, it is clear that any risk of neurologic injury from such inoculations is an extremely small one, confined to very rare instances. It remains clear that MMR vaccination is generally a very safe procedure, and that the risks resulting from *failure to run the such vaccinations* far exceed any very slight risk involved in *receiving* them.

Bailey Banks, by his father Kenneth Banks, Petitioner v. Secretary of the Department of Health and Human Services, Respondent

Summary: In this MMR injury case, the special master finds that the MMR vaccine injury resulted in the child developing ADEM which "was severe enough to cause lasting, residual damage, and retarded his developmental progress, which fits under the generalized heading of Pervasive Developmental Delay, or PDD (an Autism Spectrum Disorder). Additionally, this chain of causation was not too remote, but was rather a proximate sequence of cause and effect leading inexorably from vaccination to Pervasive Developmental Delay."

Case No: 02-0738V

Date Filed: July 20, 2007

Bailey Banks, by his father Kenneth Banks, Petitioner v. Secretary of the Department of Health and Human Services, Respondent

Abell, Special Master

On 26 June 2002, the Petitioner filed a petition for compensation under the National Childhood Vaccine Injury Act alleging that, as a result of the MMR vaccination received on 14 March 2000, his child, Bailey, suffered a seizure and Acute Disseminated Encephalomyelitis ("ADEM"), which led to Pervasive Developmental Delay ("PDD"), a condition from which he continues to suffer.

FACTS

Bailey Banks was born 26 October 1998. Bailey's development before his vaccination (both before and after birth) was normal and healthy.

At Bailey's fifteenth month check-up on 14 March 2000, no health concerns were noted, and he received the MMR vaccination at issue, his first.

Bailey then experienced a seizure 16 days later, on 30 March 2000, during which Bailey's mother witnessed his eyes rolling back and him choking, and he was taken to the Emergency Room. At the Emergency Room, Bailey was found to be afebrile and irritable and to have vomited three times. The treating doctor at the time characterized Bailey's condition as "new onset seizure" and Bailey was admitted to the hospital for observation, where he remained apparently healthy for the remainder of his stay there.

The following day, on 31 March 2007, an MRI scan was taken of Bailey's brain, which was interpreted by the treating radiologist, Bret Sleight, M.D., as "most consistent with a demyelinating process of immune etiology such as may be seen with ADEM or perhaps post-vaccination."

Bailey then underwent, on 10 April 2000, a full neurological examination, administered by another neurologist, Bryan Philbrook, M.D. Dr. Philbrook concluded that Bailey suffered from "mild gross motor developmental delay." Dr. Philbrook also noted his medical opinion that "[w]e reviewed the patient's MRI and felt that moderate hypomyelination was more likely than a demyelinating process like ADEM, but cannot rule out the latter with certainty."

An EEG performed while Bailey slept on 5 May 2000 was unremarkable. Also, a brain MRI performed on 5 January 2001 evidenced in the same results as the MRI performed on 31 March 2000, with no significant changes since then.

On 22 January 2001 Bailey was examined by another neurologist, Frank Berenson, M.D., who noted that Bailey was suffering from global developmental delays, which included features associated with pervasive developmental delay. However, he added that "[s]ocially there continues to be difficulty. His eye contact is variable. He has limited to no imaginary pretend play. He continues to bite excessively. . . ." Furthermore, even though Bailey remained alert during the visit, his speech development was found to be delayed. Lastly,

Bailey continued to walk with a "somewhat toddling gait" that Dr. Berenson described as "somewhat puppet-like" in appearance.

Beyond the medical records mentioned above, Petitioner's brief references several others, engendered between 2001 and the present, that support the claim that Bailey continued to display neurological developmental delays requiring therapeutic services.

Among the physicians treating Bailey, a neurologist named Dr. Ivan Lopez personally examined Bailey and diagnosed Bailey as follows:

This patient has developmental delay probably secondary to an episode of acute demyelinating encephalomyelitis that he had at 18 months of age after the vaccine. He certainly does not ___[sic] for autism because over here we can find a specific reason for his condition and this is not just coming up with no reason.

Dr. Lopez's diagnosis appears to conflict with the diagnosis given by Bailey's pediatrician on 20 May 2004, who saddled Bailey's condition with the generalized term "autism"; however, that pediatrician later acknowledged that use of the term autism was used merely as a simplification for non-medical school personnel, and that pervasive developmental delay "is the correct [i.e., technical] diagnosis." Another pediatrician's diagnosis noted that Bailey's condition "seems to be a global developmental delay with autistic features as opposed to an actual autistic spectrum disorder."

EXPERT TESTIMONY AT THE ENTITLEMENT HEARING

Moving on to the alternative hypothesis/diagnosis of autism, Dr. Lopez distinguishes autism as a more generalized condition without a known etiology, and contrasted it to Bailey's condition, which he says is clearly attributable to demyelination based on neuroimaging evidence. Dr. Lopez also differentiated Bailey's condition from autism, because Bailey has been affected in more than one developmental skill area; he clarified by stating that Bailey has "induced pervasive developmental delay . . . due to ADEM." He noted that the conflation of designations resulted from a medical convention created for the sake of explanation to laymen, but that the two are not properly interchangeable, but actually quite distinct. Speaking more directly, Dr. Lopez stated that "Bailey does not have autism because he has a reason for his deficits."

Regarding the medical records that indicated that Bailey was or is autistic, Dr. MacDonald said, "I think he falls into that autistic spectrum pervasive developmental disorder category, and that seems to be fairly consistent." He noted, however, that a majority of people "use these terms somewhat interchangeably."

When questioned about the existence of medical literature which establishes a "relationship between MMR and autism or PDD," Dr. MacDonald indicated his thought that "all the medical literature is negative in that regard." Also, he referenced a dearth of known literature to explain why he sees no connection between ADEM and PDD:

I can find no literature relating ADEM to autism or pervasive developmental disorder, and by its nature ADEM is a primary demyelinating disorder of the nervous system. . . . PDD is a problem with the neurons, not the white matter of the brain, so it doesn't make sense that autistic children would have had a demyelinating disorder before. In fact, MRI scans [that] have been done repeatedly in children with PDD/autism don't show demyelination, so there is no connection. Even if one believes the child has ADEM, there is no connection to the diagnosis of PDD.

When questioned by the Court . . . Dr. MacDonald . . . ultimately concluded that "Bailey falls into the large group of children with autism/PDD in which by our current evidence-based medicine we rarely can make a specific diagnosis."

The Court specifically asked Dr. Lopez to explain the causative, logical link between the disputed occurrence ADEM and the undisputed PDD from which Bailey now suffers. Dr. Lopez conceded that "the majority of patients with ADEM improve significantly," but added that "the exception to this rule is when patients have been exposed to measles, just like in the case of MMR vaccine," in which case "sequela may occur in up to 50 percent of patients." He elaborated that such sequela potentially include "mental syndromes such as PDD and others" and opined that "up to 50 percent of patients . . . who have had ADEM will show[,] as a consequence of this monophasic condition[,] PDD."

THE COURT'S CONCLUSIONS

On its face, Petitioner has proffered a credible theory that, if the Court accepts its component parts, evidences a chain of logical and biological connection. It seems that Respondent's challenge in disputing and denying Petitioner's case in chief is a question of degree not kind: whether Bailey's lack of balance amounts to ataxia, whether Bailey's PDD constitutes a mental handicap, etc. Respondent acknowledges that Bailey currently suffers from PDD, and that the MMR vaccine can cause ADEM. The only link on the logical "chain" of Petitioner's theory that Respondent really disputes, as it relates to the question of "can it?" (i.e., biologic plausibility), is whether ADEM can lead to PDD. Most of Respondent's contentions focus more narrowly on the issue of "did it?": i.e., was the mechanism proffered by Petitioner's expert really at work in this individual in this set of facts?

Respondent seems to have abandoned the earlier argument that Bailey suffered from autism, instead of PDD. The Court notes the various similarities between Bailey's condition and autism as defined above, but nonetheless rules that PDD better and more precisely describes Bailey's condition and symptoms than does autism. Respondent's acknowledgment serves to reaffirm the Court's conclusion on this point.

This series of circumstances, corroborated by the medical records prepared by treating doctors, fits much more closely with the monophasic illness of ADEM than it does with any other etiology proffered by either party. Combined with the radiologists' analysis of the MRI scans, and the Court's finding of ataxia, the Court accepts that Petitioner has met the burden of proof in showing the fact that Bailey more likely than not suffered from ADEM.

Having suffered from ADEM, it remains to be discussed if and how the ADEM led directly to PDD as a sequela. In sum, the Court's factual findings are fourfold:

1. Bailey did show evidence of ataxia in the period surrounding his seizure, following his vaccination;
2. Such ataxia, when considered in conjunction with the radiological results and some other "soft indicia", together support the Court's finding that Bailey did, in fact, suffer from ADEM.
3. Bailey's ADEM was caused-in-fact and proximately caused by his vaccination. It is well-understood that the vaccination at issue *can* cause ADEM, and the Court finds, on the record filed herein, that it *did* actually cause the ADEM.

4.   Bailey's ADEM was severe enough to cause lasting, residual damage, and retarded his developmental progress, which fits under the generalized heading of Pervasive Developmental Delay, or PDD. Additionally, this chain of causation was not too remote, but was rather a proximate sequence of cause and effect leading inexorably from vaccination to Pervasive Developmental Delay.

Therefore, in light of the foregoing, the Court rules in favor of entitlement in this matter.

DEFINITIONS

Acute disseminated encephalomyelitis (ADEM) is "an acute or subacute encephalomyelitis or infiltration and demyelination; it occurs most commonly following an acute viral infection, especially measles, but may occur without a recognizable antecedent. . . . It is believed to be a manifestation of an autoimmune attack on the myelin of the central nervous system. Clinical manifestations include fever, headache, vomiting, and drowsiness progressing to lethargy and coma; tremor, seizures, and paralysis may also occur; mortality ranges from 5 to 20 per cent; many survivors have residual neurological deficits." *Dorland's Illustrated Medical Dictionary* (30th ed. 2003) (Saunders) at 610.

Pervasive Developmental Delay describes a class of conditions, and it is apparent from the record that the parties and the medical records are referring to Pervasive Developmental Disorder Not Otherwise Specified ("PDD-NOS"):

Pervasive Developmental Disorder, Not Otherwise Specified (PDD-NOS) is a 'subthreshold' condition in which some—but not all—features of autism or another explicitly identified Pervasive Developmental Disorder are identified. PDD-NOS is often incorrectly referred to as simply "PDD." The term PDD refers to the class of conditions to which autism belongs. PDD is NOT itself a diagnosis, while PDD-NOS IS a diagnosis. The term Pervasive Developmental Disorder—Not Otherwise Specified (PDD-NOS; also referred to as "atypical personality development," "atypical PDD," or "atypical autism") is included in *DSM-IV* to encompass cases where there is marked impairment of social interaction, communication, and/or stereotyped behavior patterns or interest, but when full features for autism or another explicitly defined PDD are not met.

It should be emphasized that this "subthreshold" category is thus defined implicitly, that is, no specific guidelines for diagnosis are provided. While deficits in peer relations and unusual sensitivities are typically noted, social skills are less impaired than in classical autism. The lack of definition(s) for this relatively heterogeneous group of children presents problems for research on this condition. The limited available evidence suggest that children with PDD-NOS probably come to professional attention rather later than is the case with autistic children, and that intellectual deficits are less common. The Yale Child Study Center's Developmental Disabilities Clinic Webpage, article on PDD-NOS, available at http://www.med.yale.edu/chldstdy/autism/pddnos. html. See also *Diagnostic and Statistical Manual of Mental Disorders* (4th ed., 2000) at 69 *et seq.* In the interest of consistency, the Court will follow the convention adhered to by the medical records and by the parties in this case, and this condition will be referred to herein as "PDD."

"An autism spectrum disorder is a brain disorder affecting a person's ability to communicate, form relationships, and/or respond appropriately to the environment. Such disorders sometimes result in death. The 'spectrum' of such disorders includes relatively high-functioning persons with speech and language intact, as well as persons who are mentally retarded, mute, or with serious language delays. Symptoms may include, but are not limited to, avoidance of eye contact, seeming 'deafness,' abrupt loss of language, unawareness of environment, physical abusiveness, inaccessibility, fixation, bizarre behavior, 'flapping,' repetitive and/or obsessive behavior, insensitivity to pain, social withdrawal, and extreme sensitivity to sounds, textures, tastes, smells, and light." *Autism General Order # 1* (Fed. Cl. Spec. Mstr. Jul. 3, 2002), quoting National Institute of Mental Health, Publication 97-4023.

David and Sandra Bastian, Legal Representatives of Kyle Bastian, v. Secretary of the Department of Health and Human Services.

Summary: In this DPT injury case, the special master rules that the child suffered a Table encephalopathy with sequelae, including autism.

Case No: 90-1161V

Date Filed: September 22, 1994

David and Sandra Bastian, Legal Representatives of Kyle Bastian, v. Secretary of the Department of Health and Human Services.

Abell, Special Master

Petitioners alleged that as a direct result of a 28 September 1984 diphtheria-pertussis-tetanus (DPT) vaccination, Kyle suffered a Table encephalopathy with sequelae.

Kyle M. Bastian was born on 5 March 1983 at Holy Cross Hospital, Silver Spring, Maryland. Prior to his fourth DPT vaccination, Kyle suffered from a series of colds, ear and throat infections, and fevers. On 28 September 1984, at approximately 10:00 a.m., Kyle received his fourth DPT vaccination at the offices of Dr. Richard J. Hollander, Silver Spring, Maryland. Kyle had received a well baby checkup that morning by Dr. Hollander and according to Mrs. Bastian, Dr. Hollander thought Kyle had "excellent hand skills" and was "impressed with [Kyle's] intelligence and curiosity." Mrs. Bastian was instructed to give Kyle Tylenol when she got home.

Upon arriving home, Mrs. Bastian put Kyle down for a nap. On this day, Kyle awoke from his nap with a "screeching sound," as though he was in pain and a temperature of 103 degrees F. Mrs. Bastian called her physician's office and as a consequence thereto administered Tylenol to Kyle and sponged him down every half hour. Kyle's screeching continued off and on for most of the afternoon of the 28th. By 7:30 p.m. Kyle's temperature was 104.5 degrees. After speaking to Dr. Hollander again, Mrs. Bastian continued with the Tylenol and sponging until around 11:00 p.m. Mrs. Bastian put Kyle to bed with her. At about 1:30 a.m. on 29 September 1984 she found Kyle cyanotic, his whole body rigid, and his eyes "up in his head." She immediately called the paramedics and Kyle was rushed to Holy Cross Hospital. In the hospital emergency room, Kyle continued "screeching" on and off. Kyle was kept at the hospital less than an hour and then returned home.

At approximately 9:30 a.m. on 29 September 1984 Mrs. Bastian took Kyle to Dr. Hollander's office for a recheck. When they returned home an hour or two later, Kyle began developing hives all over his body. When Mrs. Bastian put Kyle down, "he just toppled over." He had a fever of 105 degrees and he "started shaking all over." Accordingly, Mrs. Bastian took Kyle to the emergency room for a second time on the 29th. The contemporaneous medical records clearly indicate Kyle had a febrile seizure and hives within 72 hours of the inoculation

and, in fact, was seen at the Holy Cross Hospital Emergency Room for his seizure. Kyle returned home from the emergency room, apparently upon Mrs. Bastian's request.

Mrs. Bastian noted that on 30 September 1984 Kyle was "totally out of it," he could
not sit up, had a fixed stare, and made no eye contact. This condition continues to
this day. Mrs. Bastian testified that after the DPT vaccination Kyle's eating habits
"completely changed." Immediately following the vaccination he had "no appetite
for a couple of days" and would only consume liquids, not solid foods. Kyle's parents subsequently expressed concern regarding possible hearing loss.

To Mrs. Bastian, Kyle never seemed to come back—he was never the same
child he had been prior to the immunization.

EXPERT TESTIMONY

Dr. Quinn unequivocally stated that Kyle suffers today from an encephalopathy. She testified he manifested the following signs and symptoms of an
encephalopathy within 72 hours of the injection in question: screaming, loss of
muscle tone or hypotonia, lethargy, irritability, a 10 minute seizure, cyanosis,
listlessness, and inconsolable crying.

Dr. Quinn opined that Kyle suffers from pervasive developmental disorder
(PDD). Dr. Spiro, however, opined that Kyle is autistic.

Dr. Quinn explicated on the differences between autism and PDD. Dr. Quinn
pointed out that PDD and autism are sometimes incorrectly used interchangeably. She stated that autism may be one of a spectrum of disorders under PDD
but that it is a separate classifiable disorder. She concluded that Kyle does not
have autism, but has PDD. Dr. Quinn explained that PDD is caused by a brain
insult. Dr. Quinn indicated Kyle's post-vaccinal encephalopathy was the brain
insult which in turn resulted in his PDD. Dr. Quinn opined, to a reasonable
degree of medical certainty, that Kyle's condition is permanent.

Dr. Ira Lourie, treating child psychiatrist, also testified. Kyle was first referred
to Dr. Lourie's practice in 1990. Dr. Lourie indicated that Kyle is not autistic,
and, in fact, he is not certain that he even has PDD—although he has characteristics of PDD. Kyle has never actually been diagnosed with autism according
to Dr. Lourie's analysis of the medical records. Nor is he mentally retarded.

Dr. Spiro opined that Kyle suffers from "autistic spectrum disorder" which is the cause of his developmental problems. Nevertheless, he admitted that no one else has ever diagnosed Kyle as autistic. Further, he testified that to his knowledge, there is no medically recognized evidence that PDD can be a sequel to some sort of brain trauma.

In sum, Dr. Spiro recognized that there are other pediatric neurologists who acknowledge brain trauma as a cause of autism encompassed within PDD, but he is in disagreement with them.

Regarding sequelae herein, petitioners have met their burden by proving by a preponderance of the evidence that Kyle suffers from PDD and that the on-Table encephalopathy medically could have caused the PDD. In addition, respondent has failed to prove by a preponderance of the evidence that Kyle's injury was caused by any factor unrelated to the administration of the vaccine.

When the undersigned weighs the totality of the medical records and the credible fact testimony, the following neurological signs and symptoms are found to have occurred by a preponderance of the evidence on Table: (a) a ten minute grand mal or generalized seizure, (b) high-pitched screaming, (c) hypotonia, (d) lethargy and/or listlessness, (e) cyanosis, and (f) the beginning of a loss of language/speech development and eye contact. Subsequent to the Table period there was an evident loss of milestones. The sum of the evidence establishes that Kyle presented as a normal child antecedent to the fourth DPT inoculation of 28 September 1984, within three days manifested numerous ominous indicia, as indicated *supra,* and thereafter, "he just never seemed to come back. He was not the same child he was before the shot."

Based upon the facts presented herein, this court is reluctant to find by a preponderance of the evidence that Kyle is autistic when no examining physician has ever diagnosed him as such.

Dr. Quinn, who has conscientiously diagnosed Kyle over time, linked Kyle's current condition to his DPT vaccination. Both Drs. Quinn and Lourie testified that Kyle exhibits some autistic symptomatology but is not autistic. Dr. Quinn opined that Kyle suffers from PDD, a disorder exhibited by autistic-like qualities, but lacking a sufficient number of autistic-like qualities to be labeled autism. Dr. Quinn opined that post-natal static encephalopathy is a cause of PDD. In reaching her conclusion she referenced Dr. Rapin's article.[**] Dr. Rapin's article recognizes there are some children with autistic symptomatology that follows an acute encephalopathy. Dr. Quinn's reasoning is logical and convincing and is accepted by this court.

The undersigned finds, after a review of the entire record, that petitioners are entitled to compensation under the Act.

[**] Isabelle Rapin, *Autistic Children: Diagnosis and Clinical Features,* Pediatrics 751 (1991).

CONCLUSION: WHY RECOGNIZING VACCINE INJURY IS IMPORTANT

The public health establishment constantly reminds us to vaccinate our children and keep our own vaccinations up-to-date. Every "flu season" features waves of advertisements to get a flu shot. One can now receive the yearly flu vaccine in a local pharmacy. Every school year begins with notifications to American families to vaccinate their children as the mandated by the various states.

Vaccines are the only drugs that people are compelled to give to their children. The government agency that compels the use of these drugs—the Department of Health and Human Services—also runs the National Vaccine Injury Compensation Program (NVICP). While millions are spent on pro-vaccination messages, few dollars are spent notifying the public about the NVICP. The NVICP may be the most secret public program in federal government. Hardly anyone knows of its existence. The people who work in the program rarely speak out (although some have after leaving) and seem driven to say as little about the reality of vaccine injury as possible.

When Congressman Darrell Issa, chairman of the House Oversight and Government Reform Committee, sought to hold hearings on the NVICP in the fall of 2013, pro-vaccine advocates exerted political pressure to shut the congressional investigation down. Once again, the program avoided the spotlight, and the reality of vaccine injury was kept away from the public.

In writing this book, we have sought to pull the cover off of the program and let the public see actual cases of vaccine injury. We believe that doing so is a public service because the public ought to be clearly informed about adverse reactions to the only drugs that they are required to give their children. Vaccine injuries happen, and not knowing about them helps no one.

Further, the past public disclosures on vaccine injuries have led to real and significant improvements in vaccine safety and effectiveness. Raising public awareness and encouraging discourse on vaccine injury is critical to increasing understanding of the value and limitations of these drugs.

It is critical to study vaccine injuries in the same way that it is critical to study aviation accidents. The National Transportation Safety Board investigates and analyzes all air travel crashes and issues aviation accident reports, which are open and available to the public. We need the same for vaccine injuries.

It is important that people learn to recognize and respond to vaccine injuries. That is why we have included information about the vaccines covered by the NVICP, how to file a claim with the program, and how to utilize the Vaccine Adverse Event Reporting System. As of this writing, the NVICP is the only legal venue for filing a claim for vaccine injury. The interpretation of the 1986 Act by the United States Supreme Court in the *Brusewitz* case all but excluded other civil remedies.

The National Vaccine Injury Compensation Program is the only redress for people who feel that they have been injured by a vaccine to receive compensation.

The venue for such people to receive justice has not yet been realized.

APPENDIX

VAERS : THE VACCINE ADVERSE EVENT REPORTING SYSTEM

From vaers.hhs.gov

What is VAERS?

The Vaccine Adverse Event Reporting System (VAERS) is a national vaccine safety surveillance program co-sponsored by the Centers for Disease Control and Prevention (CDC) and the Food and Drug Administration (FDA). VAERS collects and analyzes information from reports of adverse events (possible side effects) following vaccination. Since 1990, VAERS has received more than two hundred thousand reports, most of which describe mild side effects such as fever. Very rarely, people experience serious adverse events. By monitoring these events, VAERS helps identify new safety concerns, and helps make sure the benefits of vaccines continue to be far greater than the risks. VAERS data are monitored to

- Detect new, unusual, or rare vaccine adverse events
- Monitor increases in known adverse events
- Identify potential patient risk factors for particular types of adverse events
- Identify vaccine lots with increased numbers or types of reported adverse events
- Assess the safety of newly licensed vaccines

Who reports to VAERS?

Anyone can file a VAERS report, including health-care providers, manufacturers, and vaccine recipients. The majority of VAERS reports are sent in by vaccine manufacturers (37 percent) and health care providers (36 percent). The remaining reports are obtained from state immunization programs (10 percent), vaccine recipients (or their parents/guardians, 7 percent) and other sources (10 percent). Vaccine recipients or their parents or guardians are encouraged to seek the help of their health-care professional in filling out the VAERS form. Each report provides valuable information that is added to the VAERS database. Accurate and complete reporting of post-vaccination events supplies the information needed for evaluation of vaccine safety. The CDC and FDA use VAERS information to ensure the safest strategies of vaccine use and to further reduce the rare risks associated with vaccines.

What can be reported to VAERS?

VAERS seeks reports of any clinically significant medical event that occurs after vaccination, even if the reporter cannot be certain that the event was caused by the vaccine. CDC/ISO and FDA review adverse reports; VAERS has identified important signals that after further research resulted in changes to vaccine recommendations. VAERS encourages the reporting of any clinically significant adverse event that occurs after the administration of any vaccine licensed in the United States. You should report adverse events even if you are unsure whether a vaccine caused the event. Knowingly filing a false VAERS report with the intent to mislead the Department of Health and Human Services is a violation of federal law (18 U.S. Code § 1001) punishable by fine and imprisonment.

Why should I report to VAERS?

Each report provides valuable information that is added to the VAERS database. Accurate and complete reporting of post-vaccination adverse events supplies the information needed for evaluation of vaccine safety. CDC and FDA use VAERS information to ensure the safest strategies of vaccine use, and to further reduce the rare risks associated with vaccines.

Are VAERS reports kept confidential?

VAERS is required to meet the highest government security standards for using confidential patient medical records. Individual identifiers are removed from all data posted on our website.

How do I report to VAERS?

You can submit reports online through our Web reporting system or on a paper VAERS report form. You may use photocopies of the form to submit reports.

You can obtain pre-addressed postage-paid report forms via fax, mail, or e-mail by calling the VAERS Information Line at (800) 822-7967.

Completed paper VAERS forms may be sent via fax to (877) 721-0366 or by mail to:

VAERS
PO Box 1100
Rockville, MD 20849

Which adverse events should I report to VAERS?

We encourage you to report any adverse event that occurs after the administration of any vaccine licensed in the United States. You should report adverse events even if you are unsure whether a vaccine caused them. The National Childhood Vaccine Injury Act (NCVIA) requires health-care providers to report:

- Any adverse event listed by the vaccine manufacturer as a contraindication to further doses of the vaccine.

- Any adverse event listed in the VAERS Table of Reportable Events Following Vaccination that occurs within the specified time period after vaccination.

Will I receive confirmation that the report I filed was received?

Yes. If you file a report online, you will receive a confirmation number, called an "E-number," automatically. If you file a paper report, you will receive your case number and VAERS identification number by mail within a few days.

How can I get a copy of my report?

You can get a copy of a report you filed by calling the VAERS Information Line at (800) 822-7967.

If you would like a copy of a report filed by someone else, you may ask the person who filed the report to give you a copy, or contact FDA's Freedom of Information Office, which charges a fee for copying the report. All identifying information is removed from the report. For more information, contact the Freedom of Information Office at the following address:

Food and Drug Administration
Office of Shared Services
Division of Freedom of Information
Office of Public Information and Library Services
12420 Parklawn Drive ELEM-1029
Rockville, MD 20857
Phone: 301-796-3900
Fax: 301-827-9267

How do I provide follow-up information for a case?

You may provide additional information about a report you filed via fax, mail, or telephone (by calling our Information Line at (800) 822-7967). Be sure to include your E-number or VAERS identification number. We do not recommend you send e-mail, as the confidentiality of your information can not be assured.

You may also provide follow-up information in response to a VAERS acknowledgment or follow-up letter you may receive. If you have questions about how the Health Insurance Portability and Accountability Act of 1996 (HIPAA) applies to VAERS, please visit our VAERS Privacy Policies and Disclaimers section.

How are VAERS reports analyzed?

Data collected on the VAERS form includes information about the patient, the vaccination(s) given, the reported adverse event, and the person reporting the event.

The CDC and FDA require additional information on selected VAERS reports for the public health purpose of helping ensure the safety of US-licensed vaccines. You or your health-care provider may be contacted for follow-up information by VAERS staff after your report is received. These selected reports are followed up by a team of health-care professionals to obtain additional information (such as medical records and autopsy reports) to provide as complete a picture of the case as possible. All records sent to VAERS are kept confidential as required by law. The patient's consent is not required to release the medical records to VAERS. If you have questions about how the Health Insurance Portability and Accountability Act of 1996 (HIPAA) applies to VAERS, please visit our VAERS Privacy Policies and Disclaimers section.

The signs, symptoms, and diagnoses provided are assigned codes and affixed to the case for indexing purposes. Information obtained from the original VAERS report, follow-up inquiries, and coding activities are stored in a secure computerized database for analysis. Scanned facsimiles of the original reports are also maintained in a computerized image-base for FDA and CDC vaccine surveillance activities. VAERS data stripped of personal identifiers are available for download and review on the Public Access Data page.

How are VAERS reports followed up?

The CDC and FDA require additional information on selected VAERS reports for the public health purpose of helping to ensure the safety of US-licensed vaccines. You or your health-care provider may be contacted for follow-up information by VAERS staff after your report is received. These selected reports are followed up by a team of health-care professionals to obtain additional information (such as medical records and autopsy reports) to provide as complete a picture of the case as possible. All records sent to VAERS are kept confidential as required by law. The patient's consent is not required to release the medical records to VAERS. If you have questions about how the Health Insurance Portability and Accountability Act of 1996 (HIPAA) applies to VAERS, please visit our VAERS Privacy Policies and Disclaimers section.

Are all adverse events reported to VAERS caused by vaccines?

No. VAERS receives reports of many adverse events that occur after vaccination. Some occur coincidentally following vaccination, while others may be caused by vaccination. Studies help determine if a vaccine really caused an adverse event. Just because an adverse event happened after a person received a vaccine does not mean the vaccine caused the adverse event. Other factors, such as the person's medical history and other medicines the person took near the time of the vaccination, may have caused the adverse event. It is important to remember that many adverse events reported to VAERS may not be caused by vaccines. Although VAERS can rarely provide definitive evidence of causal associations between vaccines and particular risks, its unique role as a national spontaneous reporting system enables the early detection of signals that can then be more rigorously investigated.

How Do I find out what adverse events have been reported to VAERS?

The adverse events reported to VAERS are included in the public data sets. After accepting the terms of use, you can follow the instructions to sort the records by vaccine type, or search for a specific adverse event.

Which government agencies manage VAERS?

VAERS is a national passive reporting system co-managed by the Centers for Disease Control and Prevention (CDC) and the Food and Drug Administration (FDA) agencies of the US Department of Health and Human Services.

Does VAERS provide medical advice?

No. Please contact a health-care provider to discuss the specifics of your case.

Is VAERS involved in the Vaccine Injury Compensation Program?

No. The Vaccine Injury Compensation Program (VICP), which compensates people whose injuries may have been caused by vaccines recommended by CDC for routine use in children, is administered by the Health Resources and Services Administration. The VICP is separate from the VAERS program, and reporting an event to VAERS does not file a claim for compensation to the VICP.

For more information about the VICP, call (800) 338-2382 or visit the VICP website.

Is there a compensation program for individuals who are injured by the H1N1 vaccine?

Yes, the Countermeasures Injury Compensation Program (CICP) is a separate federal government program directed to compensate certain individuals seriously injured by countermeasures covered, such as the pandemic 2009 H1N1 influenza, smallpox, and anthrax vaccines, under declarations issued by the Secretary of the US Department of Health and Human Services. Information on the CICP can be obtained by visiting their website at http://www.hrsa.gov/cicp/ or calling (855) 266-2427 (855-266-CICP). Please be aware that reporting an event to VAERS does not constitute filing for compensation with the CICP.

Does VAERS provide general vaccine information?

No. VAERS only collects and analyzes adverse event reports. For general information about vaccine safety, visit CDC's Vaccine Safety website. For information about specific vaccines, immunization schedules, publications on vaccine-preventable diseases, and more, visit CDC's Vaccines and Immunizations website or call the CDC INFO Contact Center Information Line at (800) 232-4636.

Where can more information about VAERS be found?

You can get more information about VAERS by:
- Sending e-mail to info@vaers.org
- Calling the toll-free VAERS Information Line at (800) 822 7967
- Faxing inquiries to the toll-free fax line at (877) 721-0366
- Visiting the Food and Drug Administration
- Visiting the Centers for Disease Control and Prevention

HOW TO FILE A CLAIM WITH THE NATIONAL VACCINE INJURY COMPENSATION PROGRAM

From www.hrsa.gov

You may file a claim if you believe you were injured by a vaccine, if you are the parent or legal guardian of a child or disabled adult believed to have been injured by a vaccine, or if you are the legal representative of the estate of a deceased individual whose death you believe was caused by a vaccine. An injury must have lasted for more than six months after the vaccine was given or resulted in a hospital stay and surgery.

All claims must be filed with the US Court of Federal Claims and must include the claim (or petition) and two copies, a Court of Federal Claims cover sheet, medical records and/or other documentation, and a $350 filing fee.

Compensation varies, depending on the injury, and can include as much as $250,000 for pain and suffering, lost earnings, legal fees, and/or a reasonable amount for past and future care. For a death, you may receive as much as $250,000 for the estate and legal fees.

You must file your claim within three years after the first symptom of the vaccine injury or within two years of a death and four years after the start of the first symptom of the vaccine injury that resulted in the death.

1. *Understand the process.* Vaccine compensation claims are managed and adjudicated by the Office of Special Masters, within the US Court of Federal Claims. You do not need a lawyer to file a claim; however, since this is a legal process, most people use a lawyer.

2. *Who may file.* You may file a claim if you received a vaccine covered by the VICP and believe that you have been injured by this vaccine. You may file if you are the parent or legal guardian of a child or disabled adult who received and who you believe was injured by a covered vaccine, or if you are the legal representative of the estate of a deceased person who received

a covered vaccine and whose death you believe resulted from that vaccina-tion. You may file a claim if you are not a US citizen.

- Some people who receive vaccines outside of the U.S. may be eligible for compensation. The vaccines must have been covered by the VICP and given in the following circumstances:
  - o the injured person must have received a vaccine in the US trust ter-ritories; or
  - o if the vaccine was administered outside of the United States or its trust territories:
    1. the injured person must have been a US citizen serving in the mili-tary or a US government employee, or have been a dependent of such a citizen; or
    2. the injured person must have received a vaccine manufactured by a vaccine company located in the United States and returned to the United States within six months after the date of vaccination.
- In addition, to be eligible to file a claim, the effects of the person's injury must have:
  1. lasted for more than six months after the vaccine was given; or
  2. resulted in a hospital stay and surgery; or
  3. resulted in death.

3. *Filing information and deadlines.* To be eligible to file a claim, the effects of the person's injury must have:
   1. lasted for more than six months after the vaccine was given; or
   2. resulted in a hospital stay and surgery; or
   3. resulted in death.

You must file your claim within three years after the first symptom of the vac-cine injury or within two years of a death and four years after the start of the first symptom of the vaccine injury that resulted in the death.

When a *new vaccine* is covered by the VICP or when a *new injury/condition* is added to the vaccine injury table (Table), claims that do not meet the general filing deadlines must be filed within two years from the date the vaccine or injury/condition is added to the table for injuries or deaths that occurred up to eight years before the table change. The table lists and explains injuries that are presumed to be caused by vaccines.

For example, the hepatitis A vaccine was covered by the VICP as of December 1, 2004. Under the general filing deadline for an injury, the claim must be filed within three years after the first symptom of the vaccine injury. However, claims that do not meet the general filing deadlines must be filed by December 1, 2006, for injuries or deaths that occurred on or after December 1, 1996.

As a general filing rule, for individuals who are filing a claim, the appropriate filing deadline is the one above that provides the most time to file an injury or a death claim.

First, a claim must be filed by or on the behalf of the individual thought to be injured by a vaccine covered by the VICP. A claim is started by filing a legal document called a petition that is prepared by you or your lawyer to request compensation under the VICP. Anyone who files a claim is called a petitioner. The only form required is the court's cover sheet for the claim. You may obtain a copy of the cover sheet and a sample claim by calling 202-357-6400. Your claim should address the following information:

- who was injured by the vaccine;
- which vaccine caused the injury;
- when the vaccine was given;
- the city and state or country where the vaccine was given;
- the type of injury;
- when the first symptom of the injury appeared; and
- how long the effects of the injury lasted.

Your claim should also include your medical records and/or other appropriate documents, the court's cover sheet, and the $400 filing fee. If you are unable to pay this fee, call 202-357-6400 for assistance. The original claim and two copies plus a $400 filing fee should be sent to:

> Clerk
> US Court of Federal Claims
> 717 Madison Place, NW
> Washington, DC 20439

Medical Records and Other Documentation

You must include certain medical records and/or other appropriate documents with the claim. If some medical records are unavailable, you must identify those records and explain why they are unavailable. The medical review and processing of the claim may be delayed if you do not include the appropriate medical records and other documents with the claim.

In order to ensure that your claim is processed in a timely manner, the VICP suggests that you include the following medical records and other documents when filing your claim with the Court and the Secretary of Health and Human Services, c/o Director, Division of Vaccine Injury Compensation.

Types of Medical Records
1. Prenatal and Birth Records*
   - Mother's prenatal record
   - Delivery record
   - Birth certificate
   - Newborn hospital record, including providers' notes, and radiology/lab results
   - Any hospitalization face sheet with final diagnosis
2. Medical Records Prior to Vaccination
   - Clinic notes (such as well-baby visits)
   - Private doctor visits
   - Growth charts/lab/radiology results
   - Consultation reports and evaluations
   - Developmental charts
3. Vaccination Record (if available)
   - Lot number
   - Manufacturer
4. Post-Injury Hospital/Emergency Treatment Records
   - Admission/discharge summaries
   - History and physical records
   - Progress notes (including doctors'/nurses' notes)
   - Medication records
   - Lab/radiology/EEG results
   - Flow sheets (respiratory care/treatment)
   - Consultation reports and evaluations
5. Post-Injury Outpatient Records
   - History and physical records
   - Progress notes (including doctors'/nurses' notes)
   - Medication records
   - Lab/radiology/EEG results
   - Clinic notes
   - All evaluations
6. Vaccine Adverse Event Reporting System (VAERS) Form (if submitted)

7. Long-Term Records (that apply to your injury)
   - School records
   - Consultation reports and evaluations
   - Educational testing records
   - Psychological testing records
   - Police/ambulance records
8. Death Records (if applicable)
   - Death certificate
   - Autopsy report (if done)
   - Autopsy slides

*Note: Number 1 may be omitted if the injured person is an adult.

Filing a Claim with or without a Lawyer

You do not need a lawyer to file a claim. However, since this is a legal process, most people use a lawyer. If certain minimal requirements are met, the VICP will pay your lawyer's fees and other legal costs related to your claim, whether or not you are paid for a vaccine injury or death. The VICP will not pay the fees of petitioners representing themselves, but will pay their legal costs, whether or not the claim is paid, as long as certain minimal requirements are met.

Filing a Claim Outside the VICP

Most of the time, you must *first* file and have your claim processed with the VICP before a civil lawsuit can be filed against the vaccine company or the person who gave the vaccine. If you would like to file a civil lawsuit outside of the VICP, contact a lawyer for advice.

Obtaining a List of Lawyers Who File VICP Claims

Vaccine Attorneys lists attorneys who have agreed, upon request, to accept referrals in certain vaccine injury cases and is compiled by the US Court of Federal Claims. The link to the list is provided for informational purposes only and does not constitute an endorsement or recommendation by HHS or HRSA. HHS and HRSA do not endorse or recommend representation by attorneys on the list or discourage representation by attorneys not on the list.

Contact:

Clerk
U.S. Court of Federal Claims
717 Madison Place, N.W.
Washington, DC 20439

202-357-6400 or your state or local bar association

A Summary of the Claims Process

The court has documents that explain the process in more detail. To obtain these documents, you may visit the US Court of Federal Claims website or call 202-357-6400. Most petitioners use a lawyer, since this is a legal process and the rules of the court are very specific and must be followed. The process for filing a claim is:

1. the petitioner or petitioner's lawyer sends one original and two copies of the claim along with the medical records, other appropriate documents, and a $400 filing fee to the court;
2. the petitioner or petitioner's lawyer sends one copy of the claim, including the medical records and other appropriate documents, to the Secretary of Health and Human Services, c/o Director, Division of Vaccine Injury Compensation;
3. the court sends one copy of the claim and medical records to the DOJ;
4. HHS reviews the medical information in the claim, and this review is sent to the DOJ lawyer who represents the Secretary of Health and Human Services;
5. the DOJ lawyer reviews the legal aspects of the claim and writes a report;
6. the HHS and DOJ reviews are combined into one report that is sent to the court and the petitioner or the petitioner's lawyer;
7. the DOJ and the petitioner or the petitioner's lawyer take legal action to resolve the claim;
8. a "special master" (a lawyer appointed by the judges of the Court) decides whether the claim will be paid and how much will be paid for the claim;
9. if the special master decides to pay the claim, the petitioner must make a decision to accept or reject the special master's decision in writing; and
10. the special master's decision may be appealed to a judge of the court by the petitioner or HHS, then to the US Court of Appeals for the Federal Circuit, and, finally, to the US Supreme Court.

Reasons for Compensation

To be paid, you must prove that:

- the injured person received a vaccine listed on the vaccine injury table (table); and
- the first symptom of the injury/condition on the table as defined in the Qualifications and Aids to Interpretation (Aids) occurred within the time period listed on the table; or

- the vaccine caused the injury; or
- the vaccine caused an existing illness to get worse (significantly aggravated). In addition, the court must determine that the injury or death did not result from any other possible causes.

Types of Payments Awarded

For an *injury*, you may be paid:

- a reasonable amount for past and future nonreimbursable medical, custodial care, and rehabilitation costs, and related expenses (there is no limit on the amount a person with an injury may be paid for these types of expenses; payments are based on your vaccine injury needs);
- up to $250,000 for actual and projected pain and suffering;
- lost earnings; and/or
- reasonable lawyers' fees and other legal costs or *legal costs, not fees, of petitioners representing themselves*, if your claim was filed on a reasonable basis and in good faith.

For a *death,* you may be paid:

- up to $250,000 as a death benefit for the estate of the deceased; and
- reasonable lawyers' fees and other legal costs or *legal costs, not fees, of petitioners representing themselves*, if your claim was filed on a reasonable basis and in good faith.

4. File a claim with the US Court of Federal Claims. The claim for compensation is a legal document, called a petition, that you or your lawyer prepares and files by sending it to the US Court of Federal Claims.

Who determines compensation:

The U.S. Court of Federal Claims makes the final decision regarding petitions, compensation and the amount of the award.

Vaccines covered by the NVICP:

Diphtheria, tetanus, pertussis (DTP, DTaP, Tdap, DT, Td, or TT)

Haemophilus influenzae type b (Hib)

Hepatitis A (HAV)

Hepatitis B (HBV)

Human papillomavirus (HPV)

Influenza (TIV, LAIV) [given each year during the flu season]

Measles, mumps, rubella (MMR, MR, M, R)

Meningococcal (MCV4, MPSV4)

Polio (OPV or IPV)

Pneumococcal conjugate (PCV)

Rotavirus (RV)

Varicella (VZV)

Vaccine injury table:

The vaccine injury table (table) makes it easier for some people to get compensation. The table lists and explains injuries/conditions that are presumed to be caused by vaccines. It also lists time periods in which the first symptom of these injuries/conditions must occur after receiving the vaccine. If the first symptom of these injuries/conditions occurs within the listed time periods, it is presumed that the vaccine was the cause of the injury or condition unless another cause is found. For example, if you received the tetanus vaccines and had a severe allergic reaction (anaphylaxis) within four hours after receiving the vaccine, it is presumed that the tetanus vaccine caused the injury if no other cause is found.

If your injury/condition is not on the table or if your injury/condition did not occur within the time period on the table, you must prove that the vaccine caused the injury/condition. Such proof must be based on medical records or opinion, which may include expert witness testimony.

Due to a technical error, the table posted on the VICP website from October 25, 2013, to November 4, 2013, should not be referenced or used. The table that is currently posted is correct.

§100.3 Vaccine injury table.

(a) In accordance with section 312(b) of the National Childhood Vaccine Injury Act of 1986, title III of Pub. L. 99-660, 100 Stat. 3779 (42 U.S.C. 300aa-1 note) and section 2114(c) of the Public Health Service Act (42 U.S.C. 300aa-14(c)), the following is a table of vaccines, the injuries, disabilities, illnesses, conditions, and deaths resulting from the administration of such vaccines, and the time period in which the first symptom or manifestation of onset or of the significant aggravation of such injuries, disabilities, illnesses, conditions, and deaths is to occur after vaccine administration for purposes of receiving compensation under the program:

Vaccine Injury Table

Vaccine	Illness, disability, injury or condition covered	Time period for first symptom or manifestation of onset or of significant aggravation after vaccine administration
I. Vaccines containing tetanus toxoid (e.g., DTaP, DTP, DT, Td, or TT)	A. Anaphylaxis or anaphylactic shock	4 hours.
	B. Brachial Neuritis	2-28 days.
	C. Any acute complication or sequela (including death) of an illness, disability, injury, or condition referred to above which illness, disability, injury, or condition arose within the time period prescribed	Not applicable.
II. Vaccines containing whole cell pertussis bacteria, extracted or partial cell pertussis bacteria, or specific pertussis antigen(s) (e.g., DTP, DTaP, P, DTP-Hib)	A. Anaphylaxis or anaphylactic shock	4 hours.
	B. Encephalopathy (or encephalitis)	72 hours.
	C. Any acute complication or sequela (including death) of an illness, disability, injury, or condition referred to above which illness, disability, injury, or condition arose within the time period prescribed	Not applicable.

Vaccine	Illness, disability, injury or condition covered	Time period for first symptom or manifestation of onset or of significant aggravation after vaccine administration
III. Measles, mumps, and rubella vaccine or any of its components (e.g., MMR, MR, M, R)	A. Anaphylaxis or anaphylactic shock	4 hours.
	B. Encephalopathy (or encephalitis)	5–15 days (not less than 5 days and not more than 15 days).
	C. Any acute complication or sequela (including death) of an illness, disability, injury, or condition referred to above which illness, disability, injury, or condition arose within the time period prescribed	No applicable.
IV. Vaccines containing rubella virus (e.g., MMR, MR, R)	A. Chronic arthritis	7–42 days.
	B. Any acute complication or sequela (including death) of an illness, disability, injury, or condition referred to above which illness, disability, injury, or condition arose within the time period prescribed	Not applicable.
V. Vaccines containing measles virus (e.g., MMR, MR, M)	A. Thrombocytopenic purpura	7–30 days.
	B. Vaccine-Strain Measles Viral Infection in an immunodeficient recipient	6 months.

Table (*Continued*)

Vaccine Injury Table (*Continued*)

Vaccine	Illness, disability, injury or condition covered	Time period for first symptom or manifestation of onset or of significant aggravation after vaccine administration
	C. Any acute complication or sequela (including death) of an illness, disability, injury, or condition referred to above which illness, disability, injury, or condition arose within the time period prescribed	Not applicable.
VI. Vaccines containing polio live virus (OPV)	A. Paralytic Polio	
	—in a non-immunodeficient recipient	30 days.
	—in an immunodeficient recipient	6 months.
	—in a vaccine associated community case	Not applicable.
	B. Vaccine-Strain Polio Viral Infection	
	—in a non-immunodeficient recipient	30 days.
	—in an immunodeficient recipient	6 months.
	—in a vaccine associated community case	Not applicable.
	C. Any acute complication or sequela (including death) of an illness, disability, injury, or condition referred to above which illness, disability, injury, or condition arose within the time period prescribed	Not applicable.
VII. Vaccines containing polio inactivated virus (e.g., IPV)	A. Anaphylaxis or anaphylactic shock	4 hours

Vaccine	Illness, disability, injury or condition covered	Time period for first symptom or manifestation of onset or of significant aggravation after vaccine administration
	B. Any acute complication or sequela (including death of an illness, disability, injury, or condition referred to above which illness, disability, injury, or condition arose within the time period prescribed.	Not applicable.
VIII. Hepatitis B vaccines	A. Anaphylaxis or anaphylactic shock	4 hours.
	B. Any acute complication or sequela (including death) of an illness, disability, injury, or condition referred to above which illness, disability, injury, or condition arose within the time period prescribed	Not applicable.
IX. Hemophilus influenzae type b polysaccharide conjugate vaccines	No Condition Specified	Not applicable.
X. Varicella vaccine	No Condition Specified	Not applicable.
XI. Rotavirus vaccine	No Condition Specified	Not applicable.
XII. Pneumococcal conjugate vaccines	No Condition Specified	Not applicable.
XIII. Hepatitis A vaccines	No Condition Specified	Not applicable.

Table (*Continued*)

Vaccine Injury Table (*Continued*)

Vaccine	Illness, disability, injury or condition covered	Time period for first symptom or manifestation of onset or of significant aggravation after vaccine administration
XIV. Trivalent influenza vaccines	No Condition Specified	Not applicable.
XV. Meningococcal vaccines	No Condition Specified	Not applicable.
XVI. Human papillomavirus (HPV) vaccines	No Condition Specified	Not applicable.
XVII. Any new vaccine recommended by the Centers for Disease Control and Prevention for routine administration to children, after publication by the Secretary of a notice of coverage*	No Condition Specified	Not applicable.

*Now includes all vaccines against seasonal influenza (except trivalent influenza vaccines, which are already covered), effective November 12, 2013.

(b) *Qualifications and aids to interpretation.* The following qualifications and aids to interpretation shall apply to the vaccine injury table to paragraph (a) of this section:

(1) *Anaphylaxis and anaphylactic shock.* For purposes of paragraph (a) of this section, anaphylaxis and anaphylactic shock mean an acute, severe, and potentially lethal systemic allergic reaction. Most cases resolve without sequelae. Signs and symptoms begin minutes to a few hours after exposure. Death, if it occurs, usually results from airway obstruction caused by laryngeal edema or bronchospasm and may be associated with cardiovascular collapse. Other significant clinical signs and symptoms may include the following: cyanosis, hypotension, bradycardia, tachycardia, arrhythmia, edema of the pharynx and/or trachea and/or larynx with stridor and dyspnea. Autopsy findings may include acute emphysema which results from lower respiratory tract obstruction, edema of the hypopharynx, epiglottis, larynx, or trachea and minimal findings of eosinophilia in the liver, spleen, and lungs. When death occurs within minutes of exposure and without signs of respiratory distress, there may not be significant pathologic findings.

(2) *Encephalopathy.* For purposes of paragraph (a) of this section, a vaccine recipient shall be considered to have suffered an encephalopathy only if such recipient manifests, within the applicable period, an injury meeting the description below of an acute encephalopathy, and then a chronic encephalopathy persists in such person for more than six months beyond the date of vaccination.

(i) An acute encephalopathy is one that is sufficiently severe so as to require hospitalization (whether or not hospitalization occurred).

(A) *For children less than eighteen months of age* who present without an associated seizure event, an acute encephalopathy is indicated by a significantly decreased level of consciousness lasting for at least twenty-four hours. Those children less than eighteen months of age who present following a seizure shall be viewed as having an acute encephalopathy if their significantly decreased level of consciousness persists beyond twenty-four hours and cannot be attributed to a postictal state (seizure) or medication.

(B) *For adults and children eighteen months of age or older,* an acute encephalopathy is one that persists for at least twenty-four hours and characterized by at least two of the following:

(*1*) A significant change in mental status that is not medication related; specifically, a confusional state, or a delirium, or a psychosis;

(2) A significantly decreased level of consciousness, which is independent of a seizure and cannot be attributed to the effects of medication; and

(3) A seizure associated with loss of consciousness.

(C) Increased intracranial pressure may be a clinical feature of acute encephalopathy in any age group.

(D) A "significantly decreased level of consciousness" is indicated by the presence of at least one of the following clinical signs for at least twenty-four hours or greater (see paragraphs (b)(2)(i)(A) and (b)(2)(i)(B) of this section for applicable timeframes):

(1) Decreased or absent response to environment (responds, if at all, only to loud voice or painful stimuli);

(2) Decreased or absent eye contact (does not fix gaze upon family members or other individuals); or

(3) Inconsistent or absent responses to external stimuli (does not recognize familiar people or things).

(E) The following clinical features alone, or in combination, do not demonstrate an acute encephalopathy or a significant change in either mental status or level of consciousness as described above: sleepiness; irritability (fussiness); high-pitched and unusual screaming; persistent, inconsolable crying; and bulging fontanelle. Seizures in themselves are not sufficient to constitute a diagnosis of encephalopathy. In the absence of other evidence of an acute encephalopathy, seizures shall not be viewed as the first symptom or manifestation of the onset of an acute encephalopathy.

(ii) *Chronic encephalopathy* occurs when a change in mental or neurologic status, first manifested during the applicable time period, persists for a period of at least six months from the date of vaccination. Individuals who return to a normal neurologic state after the acute encephalopathy shall not be presumed to have suffered residual neurologic damage from that event; any subsequent chronic encephalopathy shall not be presumed to be a sequela of the acute encephalopathy. If a preponderance of the evidence indicates that a child's chronic encephalopathy is secondary to genetic, prenatal, or perinatal factors, that chronic encephalopathy shall not be considered to be a condition set forth in the table.

(iii) An encephalopathy shall not be considered to be a condition set forth in the table if in a proceeding on a petition, it is shown by a preponderance of the evidence that the encephalopathy was caused by an infection, a toxin, a metabolic disturbance, a structural lesion, a genetic disorder or trauma (without regard to whether the cause of the infection, toxin, trauma, metabolic disturbance, structural lesion, or genetic disorder is known). If at the time a decision is made on a petition filed under section 2111(b) of the act for a vaccine-related injury or death, it is not possible to determine the cause by a preponderance of the evidence of an encephalopathy, the encephalopathy shall be considered to be a condition set forth in the table.

(iv) In determining whether or not an encephalopathy is a condition set forth in the table, the court shall consider the entire medical record.

(3) [Reserved]

(4) *Seizure and convulsion.* For purposes of paragraphs (b) (2) of this section, the terms, "seizure" and "convulsion" include myoclonic, generalized tonic-clonic (grand mal), and simple and complex partial seizures. Absence (petit mal) seizures shall not be considered to be a condition set forth in the table. Jerking movements or staring episodes alone are not necessarily an indication of seizure activity.

(5) *Sequela.* The term "sequela" means a condition or event which was actually caused by a condition listed in the vaccine injury table.

(6) *Chronic arthritis.* (i) For purposes of paragraph (a) of this section, chronic arthritis may be found in a person with no history in the three years prior to vaccination of arthropathy (joint disease) on the basis of:

(A) Medical documentation, recorded within thirty days after the onset, of objective signs of acute arthritis (joint swelling) that occurred between seven and forty-two days after a rubella vaccination;

(B) Medical documentation (recorded within three years after the onset of acute arthritis) of the persistence of objective signs of intermittent or continuous arthritis for more than six months following vaccination; and

(C) Medical documentation of an antibody response to the rubella virus.

(ii) For purposes of paragraph (a) of this section, the following shall not be considered as chronic arthritis: musculoskeletal disorders such as diffuse connective tissue diseases (including but not limited to rheumatoid arthritis, juvenile rheumatoid arthritis, systemic lupus erythematosus, systemic sclerosis, mixed connective tissue disease, polymyositis/determatomyositis, fibromyalgia, necrotizing vascultitis and vasculopathies and Sjögren's Syndrome), degenerative joint disease, infectious agents other than rubella (whether by direct invasion or as an immune reaction), metabolic and endocrine diseases, trauma, neoplasms, neuropathic disorders, bone and cartilage disorders and arthritis associated with ankylosing spondylitis, psoriasis, inflammatory bowel disease, Reiter's syndrome, or blood disorders.

(iii) Arthralgia (joint pain) or stiffness without joint swelling shall not be viewed as chronic arthritis for purposes of paragraph (a) of this section.

(7) *Brachial neuritis.* (i) This term is defined as dysfunction limited to the upper extremity nerve plexus (i.e., its trunks, divisions, or cords) without involvement of other peripheral (e.g., nerve roots or a single peripheral nerve) or central (e.g., spinal cord) nervous system structures. A deep, steady, often severe aching pain in the shoulder and upper arm usually heralds onset of the condition. The pain is followed in days or weeks by weakness and atrophy in upper extremity muscle groups. Sensory loss may accompany the motor deficits, but is generally a less notable clinical feature. The neuritis, or plexopathy, may be present on the same side as or the opposite side of the injection; it is sometimes bilateral, affecting both upper extremities.

(ii) Weakness is required before the diagnosis can be made. Motor, sensory, and reflex findings on physical examination and the results of nerve conduction and electromyographic studies must be consistent in confirming that dysfunction is attributable to the brachial plexus. The condition should thereby be distinguishable from conditions that may give rise to dysfunction of nerve roots (i.e., radiculopathies) and peripheral nerves (i.e., including multiple monoeuropathies), as well as other peripheral and central nervous system structures (e.g., cranial neuropathies and myelopathies).

(8) *Thrombocytopenic purpura.* This term is defined by a serum platelet count less than 50,000/mm^3. Thrombocytopenic purpura does not include cases of thrombocytopenia associated with other causes such as hypersplenism, autoimmune disorders (including alloantibodies from previous transfusions), myelodysplasias, lymphoproliferative disorders, congenital thrombocytopenia, or hemolytic uremic syndrome. This does not include cases of immune (formerly called idiopathic) thrombocytopenic purpura (ITP) that are mediated,

for example, by viral or fungal infections, toxins, or drugs. Thrombocytopenic purpura does not include cases of thrombocytopenia associated with disseminated intravascular coagulation, as observed with bacterial and viral infections. Viral infections include, for example, those infections secondary to Epstein-Barr virus, cytomegalovirus, hepatitis A and B, rhinovirus, human immunodeficiency virus (HIV), adenovirus, and dengue virus. An antecedent viral infection may be demonstrated by clinical signs and symptoms and need not be confirmed by culture or serologic testing. Bone marrow examination, if performed, must reveal a normal or an increased number of megakaryocytes in an otherwise normal marrow.

(9) *Vaccine-strain measles viral infection.* This term is defined as a disease caused by the vaccine-strain that should be determined by vaccine-specific monoclonal antibody or polymerase chain reaction tests.

(10) *Vaccine-strain polio viral infection.* This term is defined as a disease caused by poliovirus that is isolated from the affected tissue and should be determined to be the vaccine-strain by oligonucleotide or polymerase chain reaction. Isolation of poliovirus from the stool is not sufficient to establish a tissue specific infection or disease caused by vaccine-strain poliovirus.

(c) *Coverage provisions.* (1) Except as provided in paragraph (c)(2), (3), (4), (5), (6), or (7) of this section, the revised table of injuries set forth in paragraph (a) of this section and the qualifications and aids to interpretation set forth in paragraph (b) of this section apply to petitions for compensation under the program filed with the US Court of Federal Claims on or after March 24, 1997. Petitions for compensation filed before such date shall be governed by section 2114(a) and (b) of the Public Health Service Act as in effect on January 1, 1995, or by §100.3 as in effect on March 10, 1995 (see 60 FR 7678, *et seq.,* February 8, 1995), as applicable.

(2) Hepatitis B, Hib, and varicella vaccines (items VIII, IX, and X of the table) are included in the table as of August 6, 1997.

(3) Rotavirus vaccines (item XI of the table) are included in the table as of October 22, 1998.

(4) Pneumococcal conjugate vaccines (item XII of the table) are included in the table as of December 18, 1999.

(5) Hepatitis A vaccines (item XIII of the table) are included on the table as of December 1, 2004.

(6) Trivalent influenza vaccines (item XIV of the table) are included on the table as of July 1, 2005.

(7) Meningococcal vaccines and human papillomavirus vaccines (items XV and XVI of the table) are included on the table as of February 1, 2007.

(8) Other new vaccines (item XVII of the table) will be included in the table as of the effective date of a tax enacted to provide funds for compensation paid with respect to such vaccines. An amendment to this section will be published in the Federal Register to announce the effective date of such a tax.

THE NATIONAL CHILDHOOD VACCINE SAFETY ACT

42 USC CHAPTER 6A - PUBLIC HEALTH SERVICE
TITLE 42 - THE PUBLIC HEALTH AND WELFARE
CHAPTER 6A - PUBLIC HEALTH SERVICE
SUBCHAPTER XIX - VACCINES

PART 2 - NATIONAL VACCINE INJURY COMPENSATION PROGRAM

Table of Contents

SUBPART A - PROGRAM REQUIREMENTS

-HEAD-
    Sec. 300aa-10. Establishment of program

-STATUTE-
    (a) Program established
    There is established the National Vaccine Injury Compensation
Program to be administered by the Secretary under which
compensation may be paid for a vaccine-related injury or death.
    (b) Attorney's obligation
    It shall be the ethical obligation of any attorney who is
consulted by an individual with respect to a vaccine-related injury
or death to advise such individual that compensation may be
available under the program (!1) for such injury or death.

    (c) Publicity

The Secretary shall undertake reasonable efforts to inform the public of the availability of the Program.

-SOURCE-
(July 1, 1944, ch. 373, title XXI, Sec. 2110, as added Pub. L. 99-660, title III, Sec. 311(a), Nov. 14, 1986, 100 Stat. 3758; amended Pub. L. 101-239, title VI, Sec. 6601(b), Dec. 19, 1989, 103 Stat. 2285.)

-MISC1-
PRIOR PROVISIONS
A prior section 300aa-10, act July 1, 1944, Sec. 2111, was successively renumbered by subsequent acts and transferred, see section 238h of this title.
A prior section 2110 of act July 1, 1944, was successively renumbered by subsequent acts and transferred, see section 238g of this title.

AMENDMENTS
1989 - Subsec. (c). Pub. L. 101-239 added subsec. (c).

EFFECTIVE DATE OF 1989 AMENDMENT
Section 6601(s) of Pub. L. 101-239, as amended by Pub. L. 102-572, title IX, Sec. 902(b)(1), Oct. 29, 1992, 106 Stat. 4516, provided that:
"(1) Except as provided in paragraph (2), the amendments made by this section [amending this section and sections 300aa-11 to 300aa-17, 300aa-21, 300aa-23, 300aa-26, and 300aa-27 of this title] shall apply as follows:
"(A) Petitions filed after the date of enactment of this section [Dec. 19, 1989] shall proceed under the National Vaccine Injury Compensation Program under title XXI of the Public Health Service Act [this subchapter] as amended by this section.
"(B) Petitions currently pending in which the evidentiary record is closed shall continue to proceed under the Program in accordance with the law in effect before the date of the enactment of this section, except that if the United States Court of Federal Claims is to review the findings of fact and conclusions of law of a special master on such a petition, the court may receive further evidence in conducting such review.
"(C) Petitions currently pending in which the evidentiary record is not closed shall proceed under the Program in accordance with the law as amended by this section.
All pending cases which will proceed under the Program as amended by this section shall be immediately suspended for 30 days to enable the special masters and parties to prepare for proceeding under the Program as amended by this section. In determining the 240-day period prescribed by section 2112(d) of the Public Health Service Act [42 U.S.C. 300aa-12(d)], as amended by this section, or the 420-day period prescribed by section 2121(b) of such Act [42 U.S.C. 300aa-21(b)], as so amended, any period of suspension under the preceding sentence shall be excluded.
"(2) The amendments to section 2115 of the Public Health Service Act [42 U.S.C. 300aa-15] shall apply to all pending and subsequently filed petitions."

EFFECTIVE DATE

Subpart effective Oct. 1, 1988, see section 323 of Pub. L. 99-660, as amended, set out as a note under section 300aa-1 of this title.

-FOOTNOTE-
(!1) So in original. Probably should be capitalized.

-End-

-CITE-
42 USC Sec. 300aa-11
01/08/2008

-EXPCITE-
TITLE 42 - THE PUBLIC HEALTH AND WELFARE
CHAPTER 6A - PUBLIC HEALTH SERVICE
SUBCHAPTER XIX - VACCINES
Part 2 - National Vaccine Injury Compensation Program
subpart a - program requirements

-HEAD-
Sec. 300aa-11. Petitions for compensation

-STATUTE-
(a) General rule

(1) A proceeding for compensation under the Program for a vaccine-related injury or death shall be initiated by service upon the Secretary and the filing of a petition containing the matter prescribed by subsection (c) of this section with the United States Court of Federal Claims. The clerk of the United States Court of Federal Claims shall immediately forward the filed petition to the chief special master for assignment to a special master under section 300aa-12(d)(1) of this title.

(2)(A) No person may bring a civil action for damages in an amount greater than $1,000 or in an unspecified amount against a vaccine administrator or manufacturer in a State or Federal court for damages arising from a vaccine-related injury or death associated with the administration of a vaccine after October 1, 1988, and no such court may award damages in an amount greater than $1,000 in a civil action for damages for such a vaccine-related injury or death, unless a petition has been filed, in accordance with section 300aa-16 of this title, for compensation under the Program for such injury or death and -

(i)(I) the United States Court of Federal Claims has issued a judgment under section 300aa-12 of this title on such petition, and

(II) such person elects under section 300aa-21(a) of this title to file such an action, or

(ii) such person elects to withdraw such petition under section 300aa-21(b) of this title or such petition is considered withdrawn under such section.

(B) If a civil action which is barred under subparagraph (A) is filed in a State or Federal court, the court shall dismiss the action. If a petition is filed under this section with respect to the injury or death for which such civil action was brought, the date such dismissed action was filed shall, for purposes of the limitations of actions prescribed by section 300aa-16 of this title, be considered the date the petition was filed if the petition was filed within one year of the date of the dismissal of the civil action.

(3) No vaccine administrator or manufacturer may be made a party to a civil action (other than a civil action which may be brought under paragraph (2)) for damages for a vaccine-related injury or death associated with the administration of a vaccine after October 1, 1988.

(4) If in a civil action brought against a vaccine administrator or manufacturer before October 1, 1988, damages were denied for a vaccine-related injury or death or if such civil action was dismissed with prejudice, the person who brought such action may file a petition under subsection (b) of this section for such injury or death.

(5)(A) A plaintiff who on October 1, 1988, has pending a civil action for damages for a vaccine-related injury or death may, at any time within 2 years after October 1, 1988, or before judgment, whichever occurs first, petition to have such action dismissed without prejudice or costs and file a petition under subsection (b) of this section for such injury or death.

(B) If a plaintiff has pending a civil action for damages for a vaccine-related injury or death, such person may not file a petition under subsection (b) of this section for such injury or death.

(6) If a person brings a civil action after November 15, 1988 (!1) for damages for a vaccine-related injury or death associated with the administration of a vaccine before November 15, 1988, such person may not file a petition under subsection (b) of this section for such injury or death.

(7) If in a civil action brought against a vaccine administrator or manufacturer for a vaccine-related injury or death damages are awarded under a judgment of a court or a settlement of such action, the person who brought such action may not file a petition under subsection (b) of this section for such injury or death.

(8) If on October 1, 1988, there was pending an appeal or rehearing with respect to a civil action brought against a vaccine administrator or manufacturer and if the outcome of the last appellate review of such action or the last rehearing of such action is the denial of damages for a vaccine-related injury or death, the person who brought such action may file a petition under subsection (b) of this section for such injury or death.

(9) This subsection applies only to a person who has sustained a vaccine-related injury or death and who is qualified to file a petition for compensation under the Program.

(10) The Clerk of the United States Claims Court (!2) is authorized to continue to receive, and forward, petitions for compensation for a vaccine-related injury or death associated with the administration of a vaccine on or after October 1, 1992.

(b) Petitioners

(1)(A) Except as provided in subparagraph (B), any person who has sustained a vaccine-related injury, the legal representative of such person if such person is a minor or is disabled, or the legal representative of any person who died as the result of the administration of a vaccine set forth in the Vaccine Injury Table may, if the person meets the requirements of subsection (c)(1) of this section, file a petition for compensation under the Program.

(B) No person may file a petition for a vaccine-related injury or death associated with a vaccine administered before October 1, 1988, if compensation has been paid under this part for 3500 petitions for such injuries or deaths.

(2) Only one petition may be filed with respect to each administration of a vaccine.

(c) Petition content

A petition for compensation under the Program for a vaccine-related injury or death shall contain -

(1) except as provided in paragraph (3), an affidavit, and supporting documentation, demonstrating that the person who suffered such injury or who died -

(A) received a vaccine set forth in the Vaccine Injury Table or, if such person did not receive such a vaccine, contracted polio, directly or indirectly, from another person who received an oral polio vaccine,

(B)(i) if such person received a vaccine set forth in the Vaccine Injury Table -

(I) received the vaccine in the United States or in its trust territories,

(II) received the vaccine outside the United States or a trust territory and at the time of the vaccination such person was a citizen of the United States serving abroad as a member of the Armed Forces or otherwise as an employee of the United States or a dependent of such a citizen, or

(III) received the vaccine outside the United States or a trust territory and the vaccine was manufactured by a vaccine manufacturer located in the United States and such person returned to the United States not later than 6 months after the date of the vaccination,

(ii) if such person did not receive such a vaccine but contracted polio from another person who received an oral polio vaccine, was a citizen of the United States or a dependent of such a citizen,

(C)(i) sustained, or had significantly aggravated, any illness, disability, injury, or condition set forth in the Vaccine Injury Table in association with the vaccine referred to in subparagraph (A) or died from the administration of such vaccine, and the first symptom or manifestation of the onset or of the significant aggravation of any such illness, disability, injury, or condition or the death occurred within the time period after vaccine administration set forth in the Vaccine Injury Table, or

(ii)(I) sustained, or had significantly aggravated, any illness, disability, injury, or condition not set forth in the Vaccine Injury Table but which was caused by a vaccine referred to in subparagraph (A), or

(II) sustained, or had significantly aggravated, any illness, disability, injury, or condition set forth in the Vaccine

Injury Table the first symptom or manifestation of the onset or significant aggravation of which did not occur within the time period set forth in the Table but which was caused by a vaccine referred to in subparagraph (A),

(D)(i) suffered the residual effects or complications of such illness, disability, injury, or condition for more than 6 months after the administration of the vaccine, or (ii) died from the administration of the vaccine, or (iii) suffered such illness, disability, injury, or condition from the vaccine which resulted in inpatient hospitalization and surgical intervention, and

(E) has not previously collected an award or settlement of a civil action for damages for such vaccine-related injury or death,

(2) except as provided in paragraph (3), maternal prenatal and delivery records, newborn hospital records (including all physicians' and nurses' notes and test results), vaccination records associated with the vaccine allegedly causing the injury, pre- and post-injury physician or clinic records (including all relevant growth charts and test results), all post-injury inpatient and outpatient records (including all provider notes, test results, and medication records), if applicable, a death certificate, and if applicable, autopsy results, and

(3) an identification of any records of the type described in paragraph (1) or (2) which are unavailable to the petitioner and the reasons for their unavailability.

(d) Additional information

A petition may also include other available relevant medical records relating to the person who suffered such injury or who died from the administration of the vaccine.

(e) Schedule

The petitioner shall submit in accordance with a schedule set by the special master assigned to the petition assessments, evaluations, and prognoses and such other records and documents as are reasonably necessary for the determination of the amount of compensation to be paid to, or on behalf of, the person who suffered such injury or who died from the administration of the vaccine.

-SOURCE-

(July 1, 1944, ch. 373, title XXI, Sec. 2111, as added Pub. L. 99-660, title III, Sec. 311(a), Nov. 14, 1986, 100 Stat. 3758; amended Pub. L. 100-203, title IV, Secs. 4302(b), 4304(a), (b), 4306, 4307(1), (2), Dec. 22, 1987, 101 Stat. 1330-221, 1330-223, 1330-224; Pub. L. 101-239, title VI, Sec. 6601(c)(1)-(7), Dec. 19, 1989, 103 Stat. 2285, 2286; Pub. L. 101-502, Sec. 5(a), Nov. 3, 1990, 104 Stat. 1286; Pub. L. 102-168, title II, Sec. 201(h)(1), Nov. 26, 1991, 105 Stat. 1104; Pub. L. 102-572, title IX, Sec. 902(b)(1), Oct. 29, 1992, 106 Stat. 4516; Pub. L. 103-43, title XX, Sec. 2012, June 10, 1993, 107 Stat. 214; Pub. L. 105-277, div. C, title XV, Sec. 1502, Oct. 21, 1998, 112 Stat. 2681-741; Pub. L. 106-310, div. A, title XVII, Sec. 1701(a), Oct. 17, 2000, 114 Stat. 1151.)

-COD-

CODIFICATION

In subsecs. (a)(2)(A), (3), (4), (5)(A), (8), and (b)(1)(B), "October 1, 1988" substituted for "the effective date of this subpart" on authority of section 323 of Pub. L. 99-660, as amended, set out as an Effective Date note under section 300aa-1 of this title.

-MISC1-

PRIOR PROVISIONS

A prior section 300aa-11, act July 1, 1944, Sec. 2112, was successively renumbered by subsequent acts and transferred, see section 238i of this title.

A prior section 2111 of act July 1, 1944, was successively renumbered by subsequent acts and transferred, see section 238h of this title.

AMENDMENTS

2000 - Subsec. (c)(1)(D)(iii). Pub. L. 106-310 added cl. (iii).

1998 - Subsec. (c)(1)(D)(i). Pub. L. 105-277 struck out "and incurred unreimbursable expenses due in whole or in part to such illness, disability, injury, or condition in an amount greater than $1,000" before ", or (ii) died".

1993 - Subsec. (a)(10). Pub. L. 103-43 added par. (10).

1992 - Subsec. (a)(1), (2)(A)(i)(T). Pub. L. 102-572 substituted "United States Court of Federal Claims" for "United States Claims Court" wherever appearing.

1991 - Subsec. (a)(2)(A)(i), (ii). Pub. L. 102-168 realigned margins of cls. (i) and (ii).

1990 - Subsec. (a)(2)(A). Pub. L. 101-502, Sec. 5(a)(1), substituted "unless a petition has been filed, in accordance with section 300aa-16 of this title, for compensation under the Program for such injury or death and - " and cls. (i) and (ii) for "unless

"(i) a petition has been filed, in accordance with section 300aa-16 of this title, for compensation under the Program for such injury or death,

"(ii) the United States Claims Court has issued a judgment under section 300aa-12 of this title on such petition, and

"(iii) such person elects under section 300aa-21(a) of this title to file such an action."

Subsec. (a)(5)(A). Pub. L. 101-502, Sec. 5(a)(2), struck out "without prejudice" after "without prejudice or costs".

Subsec. (a)(5)(B). Pub. L. 101-502, Sec. 5(a)(3), substituted "plaintiff" for "plaintiff who".

Subsec. (d). Pub. L. 101-502, Sec. 5(a)(4), struck out "(d) except as provided in paragraph (3)," before "(d) Additional information".

Subsec. (e). Pub. L. 101-502, Sec. 5(a)(5), substituted "(e) Schedule" for "(e)(e) Schedule".

1989 - Subsec. (a)(1). Pub. L. 101-239, Sec. 6601(c)(1), substituted "filing of a petition containing the matter prescribed in subsection (c) of this section" for "filing of a petition" and inserted at end "The clerk of the United States Claims Court shall immediately forward the filed petition to the chief special master for assignment to a special master under section 300aa-12(d)(1) of this title."

Subsec. (a)(2)(A)(i). Pub. L. 101-239, Sec. 6601(c)(2), struck out "under subsection (b) of this section" after "section 300aa-16 of this title,".

Subsec. (a)(5)(A). Pub. L. 101-239, Sec. 6601(c)(3)(A), substituted "petition to have such action dismissed without prejudice or costs" for "elect to withdraw such action".

Subsec. (a)(5)(B). Pub. L. 101-239, Sec. 6601(c)(3)(B), substituted "has pending" for "on October 1, 1988, had pending" and struck out "does not withdraw the action under subparagraph (A)" after "vaccine-related injury or death".

Subsec. (a)(6). Pub. L. 101-239, Sec. 6601(c)(4), substituted "November 15, 1988" for "the effective date of this subpart" in two places.

Subsec. (a)(8). Pub. L. 101-239, Sec. 6601(c)(5), added par. (8). Former par. (8) redesignated (9).

Subsec. (a)(9). Pub. L. 101-239, Sec. 6601(c)(5), (7), redesignated par. (8) as (9) and realigned margin.

Subsec. (c)(1). Pub. L. 101-239, Sec. 6601(c)(6)(A), inserted "except as provided in paragraph (3)," after "(1)" in introductory provisions.

Subsec. (c)(2). Pub. L. 101-239, Sec. 6601(c)(6)(B), (C), added par. (2) and redesignated former par. (2) as subsec. (d).

Pub. L. 101-239, Sec. 6601(c)(6)(A), inserted "except as provided in paragraph (3)," after "(2)".

Subsec. (c)(3). Pub. L. 101-239, Sec. 6601(c)(6)(C), (D), added par. (3). Former par. (3) redesignated subsec. (e).

Subsec. (d). Pub. L. 101-239, Sec. 6601(c)(6)(B), redesignated former subsec. (c)(2) as subsec. (d), expanded margin to full measure, inserted subsec. designation and heading, substituted "A petition may also include other available" for "all available", struck out "(including autopsy reports, if any)" after "relevant medical records", and substituted "administration of the vaccine." for "administration of the vaccine and an identification of any unavailable records known to the petitioner and the reasons for their unavailability, and".

Subsec. (e). Pub. L. 101-239, Sec. 6601(c)(6)(D), redesignated former subsec. (c)(3) as subsec. (e), expanded margin to full measure, inserted subsec. designation and heading, and substituted "The petitioner shall submit in accordance with a schedule set by the special master assigned to the petition" for "appropriate".

1987 - Subsec. (a)(1). Pub. L. 100-203, Sec. 4307(1), which directed that par. (1) be amended by substituting "with the United States Claims Court" for "with the United States district court for the district in which the petitioner resides or the injury or death occurred", was executed making the substitution for "with the United States district court for the district in which the petitioner resides or in which the injury or death occurred", as the probable intent of Congress.

Subsec. (a)(2)(A). Pub. L. 100-203, Sec. 4306, substituted "vaccine administrator or manufacturer" for "vaccine manufacturer".

Pub. L. 100-203, Sec. 4302(b)(1), substituted "effective date of this subpart" for "effective date of this part".

Subsec. (a)(2)(A)(ii). Pub. L. 100-203, Sec. 4307(2), substituted "the United States Claims Court" for "a district court of the United States".

Subsec. (a)(3). Pub. L. 100-203, Sec. 4306, substituted "vaccine administrator or manufacturer" for "vaccine manufacturer".

Pub. L. 100-203, Sec. 4302(b)(1), substituted "effective date of this subpart" for "effective date of this part".

Subsec. (a)(4). Pub. L. 100-203, Sec. 4306, substituted "vaccine administrator or manufacturer" for "vaccine manufacturer".

Pub. L. 100-203, Sec. 4302(b)(1), substituted "effective date of this subpart" for "effective date of this part".

Subsec. (a)(5)(A). Pub. L. 100-203, Sec. 4302(b)(2), substituted "after the effective date of this subpart" for "after the effective date of this subchapter".

Pub. L. 100-203, Sec. 4302(b)(1), substituted "who on the effective date of this subpart" for "who on the effective date of this part".

Subsec. (a)(5)(B). Pub. L. 100-203, Sec. 4302(b)(1), substituted "effective date of this subpart" for "effective date of this part".

Subsec. (a)(6). Pub. L. 100-203, Sec. 4302(b)(1), substituted "effective date of this subpart" for "effective date of this part" in two places.

Subsec. (a)(7). Pub. L. 100-203, Sec. 4306, substituted "vaccine administrator or manufacturer" for "vaccine manufacturer".

Subsec. (a)(8). Pub. L. 100-203, Sec. 4304(a), added par. (8).

Subsec. (b)(1)(A). Pub. L. 100-203, Sec. 4304(b)(1), substituted "may, if the person meets the requirements of subsection (c)(1) of this section, file" for "may file".

Subsec. (b)(1)(B). Pub. L. 100-203, Sec. 4302(b)(1), substituted "effective date of this subpart" for "effective date of this part".

Subsec. (c)(1)(D). Pub. L. 100-203, Sec. 4304(b)(2), substituted "for more than 6 months" for "for more than 1 year", "and incurred" for ", (ii) incurred", and "(ii)" for "(iii)".

-CHANGE-

CHANGE OF NAME

References to United States Claims Court deemed to refer to United States Court of Federal Claims, see section 902(b) of Pub. L. 102-572, set out as a note under section 171 of Title 28, Judiciary and Judicial Procedure.

-MISC2-

EFFECTIVE DATE OF 2000 AMENDMENT

Pub. L. 106-310, div. A, title XVII, Sec. 1701(b), Oct. 17, 2000, 114 Stat. 1151, provided that: "The amendment made by subsection (a) [amending this section] takes effect upon the date of the enactment of this Act [Oct. 17, 2000], including with respect to petitions under section 2111 of the Public Health Service Act [this section] that are pending on such date."

EFFECTIVE DATE OF 1992 AMENDMENT

Amendment by Pub. L. 102-572 effective Oct. 29, 1992, see section 911 of Pub. L. 102-572, set out as a note under section 171 of Title 28, Judiciary and Judicial Procedure.

EFFECTIVE DATE OF 1991 AMENDMENT

Section 201(i) of Pub. L. 102-168 provided that:

"(1) Except as provided in paragraph (2), the amendments made by this section [amending this section and sections 300aa-12, 300aa-15, 300aa-16, 300aa-19, and 300aa-21 of this title and provisions

set out as a note under section 300aa-1 of this title] shall take
effect on the date of the enactment of this Act [Nov. 26, 1991].
  "(2) The amendments made by subsections (d) and (f) [amending
sections 300aa-12, 300aa-15, 300aa-16, and 300aa-21 of this title]
shall take effect as if the amendments had been in effect on and
after October 1, 1988."

EFFECTIVE DATE OF 1990 AMENDMENT
  Section 5(h) of Pub. L. 101-502 provided that: "The amendments
made by subsections (f)(1) and (g) [amending section 300aa-21 of
this title and provisions set out as a note under section 300aa-1
of this title and enacting provisions set out as a note under
section 300aa-12 of this title] shall take effect as of November
14, 1986, and the amendments made by subsections (a) through (e)
and subsection (f)(2) [amending this section and sections 300aa-12,
300aa-13, 300aa-15, 300aa-16, and 300aa-21 of this title] shall
take effect as of September 30, 1990."

EFFECTIVE DATE OF 1989 AMENDMENT
  For applicability of amendments by Pub. L. 101-239 to petitions
filed after Dec. 19, 1989, petitions currently pending in which the
evidentiary record is closed, and petitions currently pending in
which the evidentiary record is not closed, with provision for an
immediate suspension for 30 days of all pending cases, see section
6601(s)(1) of Pub. L. 101-239, set out as a note under section
300aa-10 of this title.

-FOOTNOTE-
  (!1) So in original. Probably should be followed by a comma.

  (!2) See Change of Name note below.

-End-

-CITE-
  42 USC Sec. 300aa-12
01/08/2008

-EXPCITE-
  TITLE 42 - THE PUBLIC HEALTH AND WELFARE
  CHAPTER 6A - PUBLIC HEALTH SERVICE
  SUBCHAPTER XIX - VACCINES
  Part 2 - National Vaccine Injury Compensation Program
  subpart a - program requirements

-HEAD-
  Sec. 300aa-12. Court jurisdiction

-STATUTE-
  (a) General rule
    The United States Court of Federal Claims and the United States
  Court of Federal Claims special masters shall, in accordance with
  this section, have jurisdiction over proceedings to determine if a
  petitioner under section 300aa-11 of this title is entitled to

compensation under the Program and the amount of such compensation. The United States Court of Federal Claims may issue and enforce such orders as the court deems necessary to assure the prompt payment of any compensation awarded.

(b) Parties

(1) In all proceedings brought by the filing of a petition under section 300aa-11(b) of this title, the Secretary shall be named as the respondent, shall participate, and shall be represented in accordance with section 518(a) of title 28.

(2) Within 30 days after the Secretary receives service of any petition filed under section 300aa-11 of this title, the Secretary shall publish notice of such petition in the Federal Register. The special master designated with respect to such petition under subsection (c) of this section shall afford all interested persons an opportunity to submit relevant, written information –

(A) relating to the existence of the evidence described in section 300aa-13(a)(1)(B) of this title, or

(B) relating to any allegation in a petition with respect to the matters described in section 300aa-11(c)(1)(C)(ii) of this title.

(c) United States Court of Federal Claims special masters

(1) There is established within the United States Court of Federal Claims an office of special masters which shall consist of not more than 8 special masters. The judges of the United States Court of Federal Claims shall appoint the special masters, 1 of whom, by designation of the judges of the United States Court of Federal Claims, shall serve as chief special master. The appointment and reappointment of the special masters shall be by the concurrence of a majority of the judges of the court.

(2) The chief special master and other special masters shall be subject to removal by the judges of the United States Court of Federal Claims for incompetency, misconduct, or neglect of duty or for physical or mental disability or for other good cause shown.

(3) A special master's office shall be terminated if the judges of the United States Court of Federal Claims determine, upon advice of the chief special master, that the services performed by that office are no longer needed.

(4) The appointment of any individual as a special master shall be for a term of 4 years, subject to termination under paragraphs (2) and (3). Individuals serving as special masters on December 19, 1989, shall serve for 4 years from the date of their original appointment, subject to termination under paragraphs (2) and (3). The chief special master in office on December 19, 1989, shall continue to serve as chief special master for the balance of the master's term, subject to termination under paragraphs (2) and (3).

(5) The compensation of the special masters shall be determined by the judges of the United States Court of Federal Claims, upon advice of the chief special master. The salary of the chief special master shall be the annual rate of basic pay for level IV of the Executive Schedule, as prescribed by section 5315, title 5. The salaries of the other special masters shall not exceed the annual rate of basic pay of level V of the Executive Schedule, as prescribed by section 5316, title 5.

(6) The chief special master shall be responsible for the following:

(A) Administering the office of special masters and their staff, providing for the efficient, expeditious, and effective handling of petitions, and performing such other duties related to the Program as may be assigned to the chief special master by a concurrence of a majority of the United States Claims Courts (!1) judges.

(B) Appointing and fixing the salary and duties of such administrative staff as are necessary. Such staff shall be subject to removal for good cause by the chief special master.

(C) Managing and executing all aspects of budgetary and administrative affairs affecting the special masters and their staff, subject to the rules and regulations of the Judicial Conference of the United States. The Conference rules and regulations pertaining to United States magistrate judges shall be applied to the special masters.

(D) Coordinating with the United States Court of Federal Claims the use of services, equipment, personnel, information, and facilities of the United States Court of Federal Claims without reimbursement.

(E) Reporting annually to the Congress and the judges of the United States Court of Federal Claims on the number of petitions filed under section 300aa-11 of this title and their disposition, the dates on which the vaccine-related injuries and deaths for which the petitions were filed occurred, the types and amounts of awards, the length of time for the disposition of petitions, the cost of administering the Program, and recommendations for changes in the Program.

(d) Special masters

(1) Following the receipt and filing of a petition under section 300aa-11 of this title, the clerk of the United States Court of Federal Claims shall forward the petition to the chief special master who shall designate a special master to carry out the functions authorized by paragraph (3).

(2) The special masters shall recommend rules to the Court of Federal Claims and, taking into account such recommended rules, the Court of Federal Claims shall promulgate rules pursuant to section 2071 of title 28. Such rules shall -

(A) provide for a less-adversarial, expeditious, and informal proceeding for the resolution of petitions,

(B) include flexible and informal standards of admissibility of evidence,

(C) include the opportunity for summary judgment,

(D) include the opportunity for parties to submit arguments and evidence on the record without requiring routine use of oral presentations, cross examinations, or hearings, and

(E) provide for limitations on discovery and allow the special masters to replace the usual rules of discovery in civil actions in the United States Court of Federal Claims.

(3)(A) A special master to whom a petition has been assigned shall issue a decision on such petition with respect to whether compensation is to be provided under the Program and the amount of such compensation. The decision of the special master shall -

(i) include findings of fact and conclusions of law, and

(ii) be issued as expeditiously as practicable but not later than 240 days, exclusive of suspended time under subparagraph (C), after the date the petition was filed.

The decision of the special master may be reviewed by the United States Court of Federal Claims in accordance with subsection (e) of this section.

(B) In conducting a proceeding on a petition a special master -

(i) may require such evidence as may be reasonable and necessary,

(ii) may require the submission of such information as may be reasonable and necessary,

(iii) may require the testimony of any person and the production of any documents as may be reasonable and necessary,

(iv) shall afford all interested persons an opportunity to submit relevant written information -

(I) relating to the existence of the evidence described in section 300aa-13(a)(1)(B) of this title, or

(II) relating to any allegation in a petition with respect to the matters described in section 300aa-11(c)(1)(C)(ii) of this title, and

(v) may conduct such hearings as may be reasonable and necessary.

There may be no discovery in a proceeding on a petition other than the discovery required by the special master.

(C) In conducting a proceeding on a petition a special master shall suspend the proceedings one time for 30 days on the motion of either party. After a motion for suspension is granted, further motions for suspension by either party may be granted by the special master, if the special master determines the suspension is reasonable and necessary, for an aggregate period not to exceed 150 days.

(D) If, in reviewing proceedings on petitions for vaccine-related injuries or deaths associated with the administration of vaccines before October 1, 1988, the chief special master determines that the number of filings and resultant workload place an undue burden on the parties or the special master involved in such proceedings, the chief special master may, in the interest of justice, suspend proceedings on any petition for up to 30 months (but for not more than 6 months at a time) in addition to the suspension time under subparagraph (C).

(4)(A) Except as provided in subparagraph (B), information submitted to a special master or the court in a proceeding on a petition may not be disclosed to a person who is not a party to the proceeding without the express written consent of the person who submitted the information.

(B) A decision of a special master or the court in a proceeding shall be disclosed, except that if the decision is to include information -

(i) which is trade secret or commercial or financial information which is privileged and confidential, or

(ii) which are medical files and similar files the disclosure of which would constitute a clearly unwarranted invasion of privacy,

and if the person who submitted such information objects to the inclusion of such information in the decision, the decision shall be disclosed without such information.

(e) Action by United States Court of Federal Claims

(1) Upon issuance of the special master's decision, the parties shall have 30 days to file with the clerk of the United States Court of Federal Claims a motion to have the court review the decision. If such a motion is filed, the other party shall file a response with the clerk of the United States Court of Federal Claims no later than 30 days after the filing of such motion.

(2) Upon the filing of a motion under paragraph (1) with respect to a petition, the United States Court of Federal Claims shall have jurisdiction to undertake a review of the record of the proceedings and may thereafter –

(A) uphold the findings of fact and conclusions of law of the special master and sustain the special master's decision,

(B) set aside any findings of fact or conclusion of law of the special master found to be arbitrary, capricious, an abuse of discretion, or otherwise not in accordance with law and issue its own findings of fact and conclusions of law, or

(C) remand the petition to the special master for further action in accordance with the court's direction.

The court shall complete its action on a petition within 120 days of the filing of a response under paragraph (1) excluding any days the petition is before a special master as a result of a remand under subparagraph (C). The court may allow not more than 90 days for remands under subparagraph (C).

(3) In the absence of a motion under paragraph (1) respecting the special master's decision or if the United States Court of Federal Claims takes the action described in paragraph (2)(A) with respect to the special master's decision, the clerk of the United States Court of Federal Claims shall immediately enter judgment in accordance with the special master's decision.

(f) Appeals

The findings of fact and conclusions of law of the United States Court of Federal Claims on a petition shall be final determinations of the matters involved, except that the Secretary or any petitioner aggrieved by the findings or conclusions of the court may obtain review of the judgment of the court in the United States court of appeals for the Federal Circuit upon petition filed within 60 days of the date of the judgment with such court of appeals within 60 days of the date of entry of the United States Claims Court's (!2) judgment with such court of appeals.

(g) Notice

If –

(1) a special master fails to make a decision on a petition within the 240 days prescribed by subsection (d)(3)(A)(ii) of this section (excluding (A) any period of suspension under subsection (d)(3)(C) or (d)(3)(D) of this section, and (B) any days the petition is before a special master as a result of a remand under subsection (e)(2)(C) of this section), or

(2) the United States Court of Federal Claims fails to enter a judgment under this section on a petition within 420 days (excluding (A) any period of suspension under subsection (d)(3)(C) or (d)(3)(D) of this section, and (B) any days the petition is before a special master as a result of a remand under subsection (e)(2)(C) of this section) after the date on which the petition was filed,

the special master or court shall notify the petitioner under such petition that the petitioner may withdraw the petition under section 300aa-21(b) of this title or the petitioner may choose under section 300aa-21(b) of this title to have the petition remain before the special master or court, as the case may be.

-SOURCE-

(July 1, 1944, ch. 373, title XXI, Sec. 2112, as added Pub. L. 99-660, title III, Sec. 311(a), Nov. 14, 1986, 100 Stat. 3761; amended Pub. L. 100-203, title IV, Secs. 4303(d)(2)(A), 4307(3), 4308(a), (b), Dec. 22, 1987, 101 Stat. 1330-222, 1330-224; Pub. L. 100-360, title IV, Sec. 411(o)(2), (3)(A), July 1, 1988, 102 Stat. 808; Pub. L. 101-239, title VI, Sec. 6601(d)-(i), Dec. 19, 1989, 103 Stat. 2286-2290; Pub. L. 101-502, Sec. 5(b), Nov. 3, 1990, 104 Stat. 1286; Pub. L. 101-650, title III, Sec. 321, Dec. 1, 1990, 104 Stat. 5117; Pub. L. 102-168, title II, Sec. 201(c), (d)(1), (h)(2), (3), Nov. 26, 1991, 105 Stat. 1103, 1104; Pub. L. 102-572, title IX, Sec. 902(b), Oct. 29, 1992, 106 Stat. 4516; Pub. L. 103-66, title XIII, Sec. 13632(c), Aug. 10, 1993, 107 Stat. 646.)

-COD-

CODIFICATION

In subsec. (c)(4), "on December 19, 1989," substituted for "upon the date of the enactment of this subsection" and "on the date of the enactment of this subsection".

In subsec. (d)(3)(D), "October 1, 1988," substituted for "the effective date of this part".

MISC1

PRIOR PROVISIONS

A prior section 300aa-12, act July 1, 1944, Sec. 2113, was successively renumbered by subsequent acts and transferred, see section 238j of this title.

A prior section 2112 of act July 1, 1944, was successively renumbered by subsequent acts and transferred, see section 238i of this title.

AMENDMENTS

1993 - Subsec. (d)(3)(D). Pub. L. 103-66 substituted "30 months (but for not more than 6 months at a time)" for "540 days".

1992 - Subsecs. (a), (c) to (g). Pub. L. 102-572 substituted "United States Court of Federal Claims" for "United States Claims Court" and "Court of Federal Claims" for "Claims Court", wherever appearing.

1991 - Subsec. (d)(3)(D). Pub. L. 102-168, Sec. 201(c), (h)(2), realigned margin and substituted "540 days" for "180 days".

Subsec. (g). Pub. L. 102-168, Sec. 201(h)(3), made technical amendment to underlying provisions of original Act.

Pub. L. 102-168, Sec. 201(d)(1), substituted "or the petitioner may choose under section 300aa-21(b) of this title to have the petition remain before the special master or court, as the case may be" for "and the petition will be considered withdrawn under such section if the petitioner, the special master, or the court do not take certain actions" before period at end.

1990 - Subsec. (d)(3)(D). Pub. L. 101-502, Sec. 5(b)(1), added subpar. (D).

Subsec. (g). Pub. L. 101-502, Sec. 5(b)(2), added subsec. (g).

1989 - Subsec. (a). Pub. L. 101-239, Sec. 6601(d), substituted "and the United States Claims Court special masters shall, in accordance with this section, have jurisdiction" for "shall have jurisdiction (1)", ". The United States Claims Court may issue" for ", and (2) to issue", and "deems" for "deem".

Subsec. (b)(1). Pub. L. 101-239, Sec. 6601(f), substituted "In all proceedings brought by the filing of a petition under section 300aa-11(b) of this title, the Secretary shall be named as the respondent, shall participate, and shall be represented in accordance with section 518(a) of title 28." for "The Secretary shall be named as the respondent in all proceedings brought by the filing of a petition under section 300aa-11(b) of this title. Except as provided in paragraph (2), no other person may intervene in any such proceeding."

Subsec. (c). Pub. L. 101-239, Sec. 6601(e)(2), added subsec. (c). Former subsec. (c) redesignated (d).

Subsec. (d). Pub. L. 101-239, Sec. 6601(e)(1), redesignated subsec. (c) as (d). Former subsec. (d) redesignated (e).

Subsec. (d)(1). Pub. L. 101-239, Sec. 6601(g)(1), amended par. (1) generally. Prior to amendment, par. (1) read as follows: "Following receipt of a petition under subsection (a) of this section, the United States Claims Court shall designate a special master to carry out the functions authorized by paragraph (2)."

Subsec. (d)(2) to (4). Pub. L. 101-239, Sec. 6601(g)(2), added pars. (2) to (4) and struck out former par. (2) which prescribed functions of special masters.

Subsec. (e). Pub. L. 101-239, Sec. 6601(h), substituted "Action by United States Claims Court" for "Action by court" as heading and amended text generally. Prior to amendment, text read as follows:

"(1) Upon objection by the petitioner or respondent to the proposed findings of fact or conclusions of law prepared by the special master or upon the court's own motion, the court shall undertake a review of the record of the proceedings and may thereafter make a de novo determination of any matter and issue its judgment accordingly, including findings of fact and conclusions of law, or remand for further proceedings.

"(2) If no objection is filed under paragraph (1) or if the court does not choose to review the proceeding, the court shall adopt the proposed findings of fact and conclusions of law of the special master as its own and render judgment thereon.

"(3) The court shall render its judgment on any petition filed under the Program as expeditiously as practicable but not later than 365 days after the date on which the petition was filed."

Pub. L. 101-239, Sec. 6601(e)(1), redesignated subsec. (d) as (e). Former subsec. (e) redesignated (f).

Subsec. (f). Pub. L. 101-239, Sec. 6601(i), inserted "within 60 days of the date of entry of the United States Claims Court's judgment with such court of appeals" after "with such court of appeals".

Pub. L. 101-239, Sec. 6601(e)(1), redesignated subsec. (e) as (f).

1988 - Subsec. (c)(2). Pub. L. 100-360, Sec. 411(o)(3)(A), added Pub. L. 100-203, Sec. 4308(a), see 1987 Amendment note below.

Subsec. (e). Pub. L. 100-360, Sec. 411(o)(2), made technical amendment to directory language of Pub. L. 100-203, Sec. 4307(3)(C), see 1987 Amendment note below.

Pub. L. 100-360, Sec. 411(o)(3)(A), added Pub. L. 100-203, Sec. 4308(b), see 1987 Amendment note below.

1987 - Subsec. (a). Pub. L. 100-203, Sec. 4307(3)(A), substituted "United States Claims Court" for "district courts of the United States" and "the court" for "the courts".

Subsec. (c)(1). Pub. L. 100-203, Sec. 4307(3)(B), substituted "the United States Claims Court" for "the district court of the United States in which the petition is filed".

Subsec. (c)(2), Pub. L. 100-203, Sec. 4308(a), as added by Pub. L. 100-360, Sec. 411(o)(3)(A), inserted ", shall perform, and submit to the court proposed findings of fact and conclusions of law," in introductory provisions and struck out subpar. (E) which read as follows: "prepare and submit to the court proposed findings of fact and conclusions of law."

Subsec. (e). Pub. L. 100-203, Sec. 4308(b), as added by Pub. L. 100-360, Sec. 411(o)(3)(A), inserted "within 60 days of the date of the judgment" after "petition filed".

Pub. L. 100-203, Sec. 4307(3)(C), as amended by Pub. L. 100-360, Sec. 411(o)(2), substituted "the United States Claims Court" for "a district court of the United States" and "for the Federal Circuit" for "for the circuit in which the court is located".

Pub. L. 100-203, Sec. 4303(d)(2)(A), redesignated subsec. (g) as (e) and struck out former subsec. (e) relating to administration of an award.

Subsec. (f). Pub. L. 100-203, Sec. 4303(d)(2)(A), struck out subsec. (f) which related to revision of an award.

Subsec. (g). Pub. L. 100-203, Sec. 4303(d)(2)(A), redesignated subsec. (g) as (e).

-CHANGE-
CHANGE OF NAME
"United States magistrate judges" substituted for "United States magistrates" in subsec. (c)(6)(C) pursuant to section 321 of Pub. L. 101-650, set out as a note under section 631 of Title 28, Judiciary and Judicial Procedure.

-MISC2-
EFFECTIVE DATE OF 1992 AMENDMENT
Amendment by Pub. L. 102-572 effective Oct. 29, 1992, see section 911 of Pub. L. 102-572, set out as a note under section 171 of Title 28, Judiciary and Judicial Procedure.

EFFECTIVE DATE OF 1991 AMENDMENT
Amendment by section 201(d)(1) of Pub. L. 102-168 effective as if in effect on and after Oct. 1, 1988, see section 201(i)(2) of Pub. L. 102-168, set out as a note under section 300aa-11 of this title.

EFFECTIVE DATE OF 1990 AMENDMENT
Amendment by Pub. L. 101-502 effective Sept. 30, 1990, see section 5(h) of Pub. L. 101-502, set out as a note under section 300aa-11 of this title.

EFFECTIVE DATE OF 1989 AMENDMENT
For applicability of amendments by Pub. L. 101-239 to petitions filed after Dec. 19, 1989, petitions currently pending in which the evidentiary record is closed, and petitions currently pending in

which the evidentiary record is not closed, with provision for an immediate suspension for 30 days of all pending cases, except that such suspension be excluded in determining the 240-day period prescribed in subsec. (d) of this section, see section 6601(s)(1) of Pub. L. 101-239, set out as a note under section 300aa-10 of this title.

EFFECTIVE DATE OF 1988 AMENDMENT

Except as specifically provided in section 411 of Pub. L. 100-360, amendment by Pub. L. 100-360, as it relates to a provision in the Omnibus Budget Reconciliation Act of 1987, Pub. L. 100-203, effective as if included in the enactment of that provision in Pub. L. 100-203, see section 411(a) of Pub. L. 100-360, set out as a Reference to OBRA; Effective Date note under section 106 of Title 1, General Provisions.

TERMINATION OF REPORTING REQUIREMENTS

For termination, effective May 15, 2000, of provisions in subsec. (c)(6)(E) of this section relating to reporting annually to the Congress, see section 3003 of Pub. L. 104-66, as amended, set out as a note under section 1113 of Title 31, Money and Finance, and page 13 of House Document No. 103-7.

REVIEW BY 3-JUDGE PANEL

Section 322(c) of Pub. L. 99-660, as added by Pub. L. 101-502, Sec. 5(g)(2), Nov. 3, 1990, 104 Stat. 1288, and amended by Pub. L. 102-572, title IX, Sec. 902(b)(1), Oct. 29, 1992, 106 Stat. 4516, provided that: "If the review authorized by section 2112(f) [subsec. (f) of this section] is held invalid because the judgment of the United States Court of Federal Claims being reviewed did not arise from a case or controversy under Article III of the Constitution, such judgment shall be reviewed by a 3-judge panel of the United States Court of Federal Claims. Such panel shall not include the judge who participated in such judgment."

[Enactment of section 322(c) of Pub. L. 99-660 by section 5(g)(2) of Pub. L. 101-502, set out above, effective Nov. 14, 1986, see section 5(h) of Pub. L. 101-502, set out as an Effective Date of 1990 Amendment note under section 300aa-11 of this title.]

-FOOTNOTE-
(!1) So in original. Probably should be a reference to the United States Court of Federal Claims.

(!2) So in original. Probably should be a reference to the United States Court of Federal Claims.

-End-

-CITE-
42 USC Sec. 300aa-13
01/08/2008

-EXPCITE-
TITLE 42 - THE PUBLIC HEALTH AND WELFARE

CHAPTER 6A - PUBLIC HEALTH SERVICE
SUBCHAPTER XIX - VACCINES
Part 2 - National Vaccine Injury Compensation Program
subpart a - program requirements

-HEAD-
Sec. 300aa-13. Determination of eligibility and compensation

-STATUTE-
(a) General rule
(1) Compensation shall be awarded under the Program to a
petitioner if the special master or court finds on the record as a
whole -
(A) that the petitioner has demonstrated by a preponderance of
the evidence the matters required in the petition by section
300aa-11(c)(1) of this title, and
(B) that there is not a preponderance of the evidence that the
illness, disability, injury, condition, or death described in the
petition is due to factors unrelated to the administration of the
vaccine described in the petition.

The special master or court may not make such a finding based on
the claims of a petitioner alone, unsubstantiated by medical
records or by medical opinion.
(2) For purposes of paragraph (1), the term "factors unrelated to
the administration of the vaccine" -
(A) does not include any idiopathic, unexplained, unknown,
hypothetical, or undocumentable cause, factor, injury, illness,
or condition, and
(B) may, as documented by the petitioner's evidence or other
material in the record, include infection, toxins, trauma
(including birth trauma and related anoxia), or metabolic
disturbances which have no known relation to the vaccine
involved, but which in the particular case are shown to have been
the agent or agents principally responsible for causing the
petitioner's illness, disability, injury, condition, or death.
(b) Matters to be considered
(1) In determining whether to award compensation to a petitioner
under the Program, the special master or court shall consider, in
addition to all other relevant medical and scientific evidence
contained in the record -
(A) any diagnosis, conclusion, medical judgment, or autopsy or
coroner's report which is contained in the record regarding the
nature, causation, and aggravation of the petitioner's illness,
disability, injury, condition, or death, and
(B) the results of any diagnostic or evaluative test which are
contained in the record and the summaries and conclusions.

Any such diagnosis, conclusion, judgment, test result, report, or
summary shall not be binding on the special master or court. In
evaluating the weight to be afforded to any such diagnosis,
conclusion, judgment, test result, report, or summary, the special
master or court shall consider the entire record and the course of
the injury, disability, illness, or condition until the date of the
judgment of the special master or court.
(2) The special master or court may find the first symptom or
manifestation of onset or significant aggravation of an injury,

disability, illness, condition, or death described in a petition occurred within the time period described in the Vaccine Injury Table even though the occurrence of such symptom or manifestation was not recorded or was incorrectly recorded as having occurred outside such period. Such a finding may be made only upon demonstration by a preponderance of the evidence that the onset or significant aggravation of the injury, disability, illness, condition, or death described in the petition did in fact occur within the time period described in the Vaccine Injury Table.
(c) "Record" defined
  For purposes of this section, the term "record" means the record established by the special masters of the United States Court of Federal Claims in a proceeding on a petition filed under section 300aa-11 of this title.

-SOURCE-
  (July 1, 1944, ch. 373, title XXI, Sec. 2113, as added Pub. L. 99-660, title III, Sec. 311(a), Nov. 14, 1986, 100 Stat. 3763; amended Pub. L. 100-203, title IV, Sec. 4307(4), Dec. 22, 1987, 101 Stat. 1330-224; Pub. L. 101-239, title VI, Sec. 6601(j), Dec. 19, 1989, 103 Stat. 2290; Pub. L. 101-502, Sec. 5(c), Nov. 3, 1990, 104 Stat. 1287; Pub. L. 102-572, title IX, Sec. 902(b)(1), Oct. 29, 1992, 106 Stat. 4516.)

-MISC1-
PRIOR PROVISIONS
  A prior section 300aa-13, act July 1, 1944, Sec. 2114, was successively renumbered by subsequent acts and transferred, see section 238k of this title.
  A prior section 2113 of act July 1, 1944, was successively renumbered by subsequent acts and transferred, see section 238j of this title.

AMENDMENTS
  1992 - Subsec. (c). Pub. L. 102-572 substituted "United States Court of Federal Claims" for "United States Claims Court".
  1990 - Subsec. (c). Pub. L. 101-502 inserted "the" after "special masters of".
  1989 - Subsecs. (a)(1), (b). Pub. L. 101-239, Sec. 6601(j)(1), substituted "special master or court" for "court" wherever appearing.
  Subsec. (c). Pub. L. 101-239, Sec. 6601(j)(2), inserted "special masters of" after "established by the".
  1987 - Subsec. (c). Pub. L. 100-203 substituted "the United States Claims Court" for "a district court of the United States".

EFFECTIVE DATE OF 1992 AMENDMENT
  Amendment by Pub. L. 102-572 effective Oct. 29, 1992, see section 911 of Pub. L. 102-572, set out as a note under section 171 of Title 28, Judiciary and Judicial Procedure.

EFFECTIVE DATE OF 1990 AMENDMENT
  Amendment by Pub. L. 101-502 effective Sept. 30, 1990, see section 5(h) of Pub. L. 101-502, set out as a note under section 300aa-11 of this title.

EFFECTIVE DATE OF 1989 AMENDMENT

For applicability of amendments by Pub. L. 101-239 to petitions filed after Dec. 19, 1989, petitions currently pending in which the evidentiary record is closed, and petitions currently pending in which the evidentiary record is not closed, with provision for an immediate suspension for 30 days of all pending cases, see section 6601(s)(1) of Pub. L. 101-239, set out as a note under section 300aa-10 of this title.

-End-

-CITE-
42 USC Sec. 300aa-14
01/08/2008

-EXPCITE-
TITLE 42 - THE PUBLIC HEALTH AND WELFARE
CHAPTER 6A - PUBLIC HEALTH SERVICE
SUBCHAPTER XIX - VACCINES
Part 2 - National Vaccine Injury Compensation Program
subpart a - program requirements

-HEAD-
Sec. 300aa-14. Vaccine Injury Table

-STATUTE-
(a) Initial table
The following is a table of vaccines, the injuries, disabilities, illnesses, conditions, and deaths resulting from the administration of such vaccines, and the time period in which the first symptom or manifestation of onset or of the significant aggravation of such injuries, disabilities, illnesses, conditions, and deaths is to occur after vaccine administration for purposes of receiving compensation under the Program:

NOTE: This Table is no longer in effect. See the <u>Vaccine Injury Table</u> for vaccines and injuries covered under claims currently being filed.

```
                      VACCINE INJURY TABLE
--------------------------------------------------------------------
```

I.   DTP; P; DTP/Polio
                   Combination; or Any
                   Other Vaccine
                   Containing Whole Cell
                   Pertussis Bacteria,
                   Extracted or Partial
                   Cell Bacteria, or
                   Specific Pertussis
                   Antigen(s).

Illness, disability, injury, or condition covered:	Time period for first symptom or manifestation of onset or of significant aggravation after vaccine administration:
A. Anaphylaxis or anaphylactic shock	24 hours
B. Encephalopathy (or encephalitis)	3 days
C. Shock-collapse or hypotonic-hyporesponsive collapse	3 days
D. Residual seizure disorder in accordance with subsection (b)(2)	3 days
E. Any acute complication or sequela (including death) of an illness, disability, injury, or condition referred to above which illness, disability, injury, or condition arose within the time period prescribed	Not applicable

II.   Measles, mumps,
                   rubella, or any vaccine
                   containing any of the
                   foregoing as a
                   component; DT; Td; or
                   Tetanus Toxoid.

A. Anaphylaxis or anaphylactic shock	24 hours
B. Encephalopathy (or encephalitis)	15 days (for mumps, rubella, measles, or any vaccine containing any of the foregoing as a component). 3 days (for DT, Td, or tetanus toxoid).
C. Residual seizure disorder in accordance with subsection (b)(2)	15 days (for mumps, rubella, measles, or any vaccine containing any of the foregoing as a component). 3 days (for DT, Td, or tetanus toxoid).

D. Any acute complication or sequela (including death) of an illness, disability, injury, or condition referred to above which illness, disability, injury, or condition arose within the time period prescribed	Not applicable	
III.	Polio Vaccines (other than Inactivated Polio Vaccine).	
	A. Paralytic polio	
	- in a non-immunodeficient recipient	30 days
	- in an immunodeficient recipient	6 months
	- in a vaccine-associated community case	Not applicable
	B. Any acute complication or sequela (including death) of an illness, disability, injury, or condition referred to above which illness, disability, injury, or condition arose within the time period prescribed	Not applicable
IV.	Inactivated Polio Vaccine.	
	A. Anaphylaxis or anaphylactic shock	24 hours
	B. Any acute complication or sequela (including death) of an illness, disability, injury, or condition referred to above which illness, disability, injury, or condition arose within the time period prescribed	Not applicable

----

(b) Qualifications and aids to interpretation

The following qualifications and aids to interpretation shall apply to the Vaccine Injury Table in subsection (a) of this section:

(1) A shock-collapse or a hypotonic-hyporesponsive collapse may be evidenced by indicia or symptoms such as decrease or loss of muscle tone, paralysis (partial or complete), hemiplegia or hemiparesis, loss of color or turning pale white or blue, unresponsiveness to environmental stimuli, depression of consciousness, loss of consciousness, prolonged sleeping with difficulty arousing, or cardiovascular or respiratory arrest.

(2) A petitioner may be considered to have suffered a residual seizure disorder if the petitioner did not suffer a seizure or

convulsion unaccompanied by fever or accompanied by a fever of less than 102 degrees Fahrenheit before the first seizure or convulsion after the administration of the vaccine involved and if -

    (A) in the case of a measles, mumps, or rubella vaccine or any combination of such vaccines, the first seizure or convulsion occurred within 15 days after administration of the vaccine and 2 or more seizures or convulsions occurred within 1 year after the administration of the vaccine which were unaccompanied by fever or accompanied by a fever of less than 102 degrees Fahrenheit, and

    (B) in the case of any other vaccine, the first seizure or convulsion occurred within 3 days after administration of the vaccine and 2 or more seizures or convulsions occurred within 1 year after the administration of the vaccine which were unaccompanied by fever or accompanied by a fever of less than 102 degrees Fahrenheit.

    (3)(A) The term "encephalopathy" means any significant acquired abnormality of, or injury to, or impairment of function of the brain. Among the frequent manifestations of encephalopathy are focal and diffuse neurologic signs, increased intracranial pressure, or changes lasting at least 6 hours in level of consciousness, with or without convulsions. The neurological signs and symptoms of encephalopathy may be temporary with complete recovery, or may result in various degrees of permanent impairment. Signs and symptoms such as high pitched and unusual screaming, persistent unconsolable crying, and bulging fontanel are compatible with an encephalopathy, but in and of themselves are not conclusive evidence of encephalopathy. Encephalopathy usually can be documented by slow wave activity on an electroencephalogram.

    (B) If in a proceeding on a petition it is shown by a preponderance of the evidence that an encephalopathy was caused by infection, toxins, trauma, or metabolic disturbances the encephalopathy shall not be considered to be a condition set forth in the table. If at the time a judgment is entered on a petition filed under section 300aa-11 of this title for a vaccine-related injury or death it is not possible to determine the cause, by a preponderance of the evidence, of an encephalopathy, the encephalopathy shall be considered to be a condition set forth in the table. In determining whether or not an encephalopathy is a condition set forth in the table, the court shall consider the entire medical record.

    (4) For purposes of paragraphs (2) and (3), the terms "seizure" and "convulsion" include grand mal, petit mal, absence, myoclonic, tonic-clonic, and focal motor seizures and signs. If a provision of the table to which paragraph (1), (2), (3), or (4) applies is revised under subsection (c) or (d) of this section, such paragraph shall not apply to such provision after the effective date of the revision unless the revision specifies that such paragraph is to continue to apply.

(c) Administrative revision of table

    (1) The Secretary may promulgate regulations to modify in accordance with paragraph (3) the Vaccine Injury Table. In promulgating such regulations, the Secretary shall provide for

notice and opportunity for a public hearing and at least 180 days of public comment.

(2) Any person (including the Advisory Commission on Childhood Vaccines) may petition the Secretary to propose regulations to amend the Vaccine Injury Table. Unless clearly frivolous, or initiated by the Commission, any such petition shall be referred to the Commission for its recommendations. Following -

(A) receipt of any recommendation of the Commission, or

(B) 180 days after the date of the referral to the Commission,

whichever occurs first, the Secretary shall conduct a rulemaking proceeding on the matters proposed in the petition or publish in the Federal Register a statement of reasons for not conducting such proceeding.

(3) A modification of the Vaccine Injury Table under paragraph (1) may add to, or delete from, the list of injuries, disabilities, illnesses, conditions, and deaths for which compensation may be provided or may change the time periods for the first symptom or manifestation of the onset or the significant aggravation of any such injury, disability, illness, condition, or death.

(4) Any modification under paragraph (1) of the Vaccine Injury Table shall apply only with respect to petitions for compensation under the Program which are filed after the effective date of such regulation.

(d) Role of Commission

Except with respect to a regulation recommended by the Advisory Commission on Childhood Vaccines, the Secretary may not propose a regulation under subsection (c) of this section or any revision thereof, unless the Secretary has first provided to the Commission a copy of the proposed regulation or revision, requested recommendations and comments by the Commission, and afforded the Commission at least 90 days to make such recommendations.

(e) Additional vaccines

(1) Vaccines recommended before August 1, 1993

By August 1, 1995, the Secretary shall revise the Vaccine Injury Table included in subsection (a) of this section to include -

(A) vaccines which are recommended to the Secretary by the Centers for Disease Control and Prevention before August 1, 1993, for routine administration to children,

(B) the injuries, disabilities, illnesses, conditions, and deaths associated with such vaccines, and

(C) the time period in which the first symptoms or manifestations of onset or other significant aggravation of such injuries, disabilities, illnesses, conditions, and deaths associated with such vaccines may occur.

(2) Vaccines recommended after August 1, 1993

When after August 1, 1993, the Centers for Disease Control and Prevention recommends a vaccine to the Secretary for routine administration to children, the Secretary shall, within 2 years of such recommendation, amend the Vaccine Injury Table included in subsection (a) of this section to include -

(A) vaccines which were recommended for routine administration to children,

(B) the injuries, disabilities, illnesses, conditions, and deaths associated with such vaccines, and

(C) the time period in which the first symptoms or

manifestations of onset or other significant aggravation of such injuries, disabilities, illnesses, conditions, and deaths associated with such vaccines may occur.

-SOURCE-

(July 1, 1944, ch. 373, title XXI, Sec. 2114, as added Pub. L. 99-660, title III, Sec. 311(a), Nov. 14, 1986, 100 Stat. 3764; amended Pub. L. 101-239, title VI, Sec. 6601(k), Dec. 19, 1989, 103 Stat. 2290; Pub. L. 103-66, title XIII, Sec. 13632(a)(2), Aug. 10, 1993, 107 Stat. 645.)

-MISC1-

PRIOR PROVISIONS

A prior section 300aa-14, act July 1, 1944, Sec. 2115, was successively renumbered by subsequent acts and transferred, see section 238l of this title.

A prior section 2114 of act July 1, 1944, was successively renumbered by subsequent acts and transferred, see section 238k of this title.

AMENDMENTS

1993 - Subsec. (e). Pub. L. 103-66 amended heading and text of subsec. (e) generally. Prior to amendment, text read as follows: "The Secretary may recommend to Congress revisions of the table to change the vaccines covered by the table."

1989 - Subsec. (a). Pub. L. 101-239, Sec. 6601(k)(1), substituted "(b)(2)" for "(c)(2)" in items I.D. and II.C. in table.

Subsec. (b)(3)(B). Pub. L. 101-239, Sec. 6601(k)(2), substituted "300aa-11 of this title" for "300aa-11(b) of this title".

EFFECTIVE DATE OF 1989 AMENDMENT

For applicability of amendments by Pub. L. 101-239 to petitions filed after Dec. 19, 1989, petitions currently pending in which the evidentiary record is closed, and petitions currently pending in which the evidentiary record is not closed, with provision for an immediate suspension for 30 days of all pending cases, see section 6601(s)(1) of Pub. L. 101-239, set out as a note under section 300aa-10 of this title.

REVISIONS OF VACCINE INJURY TABLE

The Vaccine Injury Table as modified by regulations promulgated by the Secretary of Health and Human Services is set out at 42 CFR 100.3.

Section 13632(a)(3) of Pub. L. 103-66 provided that: "A revision by the Secretary under section 2114(e) of the Public Health Service Act (42 U.S.C. 300aa-14(e)) (as amended by paragraph (2)) shall take effect upon the effective date of a tax enacted to provide funds for compensation paid with respect to the vaccine to be added to the vaccine injury table in section 2114(a) of the Public Health Service Act (42 U.S.C. 300aa-14(a))."

-End-

-CITE-

42 USC Sec. 300aa-15
01/08/2008

-EXPCITE-
    TITLE 42 - THE PUBLIC HEALTH AND WELFARE
    CHAPTER 6A - PUBLIC HEALTH SERVICE
    SUBCHAPTER XIX - VACCINES
    Part 2 - National Vaccine Injury Compensation Program
    subpart a - program requirements

-HEAD-
    Sec. 300aa-15. Compensation

-STATUTE-
    (a) General rule
        Compensation awarded under the Program to a petitioner under
    section 300aa-11 of this title for a vaccine-related injury or
    death associated with the administration of a vaccine after October
    1, 1988, shall include the following:
        (1)(A) Actual unreimbursable expenses incurred from the date of
    the judgment awarding such expenses and reasonable projected
    unreimbursable expenses which -
            (i) result from the vaccine-related injury for which the
        petitioner seeks compensation,
            (ii) have been or will be incurred by or on behalf of the
        person who suffered such injury, and
            (iii)(I) have been or will be for diagnosis and medical or
        other remedial care determined to be reasonably necessary, or
            (II) have been or will be for rehabilitation, developmental
        evaluation, special education, vocational training and
        placement, case management services, counseling, emotional or
        behavioral therapy, residential and custodial care and service
        expenses, special equipment, related travel expenses, and
        facilities determined to be reasonably necessary.

        (B) Subject to section 300aa-16(a)(2) of this title, actual
    unreimbursable expenses incurred before the date of the judgment
    awarding such expenses which -
            (i) resulted from the vaccine-related injury for which the
        petitioner seeks compensation,
            (ii) were incurred by or on behalf of the person who suffered
        such injury, and
            (iii) were for diagnosis, medical or other remedial care,
        rehabilitation, developmental evaluation, special education,
        vocational training and placement, case management services,
        counseling, emotional or behavioral therapy, residential and
        custodial care and service expenses, special equipment, related
        travel expenses, and facilities determined to be reasonably
        necessary.

        (2) In the event of a vaccine-related death, an award of
    $250,000 for the estate of the deceased.
        (3)(A) In the case of any person who has sustained a vaccine-
    related injury after attaining the age of 18 and whose earning
    capacity is or has been impaired by reason of such person's
    vaccine-related injury for which compensation is to be awarded,
    compensation for actual and anticipated loss of earnings

determined in accordance with generally recognized actuarial principles and projections.

(B) In the case of any person who has sustained a vaccine-related injury before attaining the age of 18 and whose earning capacity is or has been impaired by reason of such person's vaccine-related injury for which compensation is to be awarded and whose vaccine-related injury is of sufficient severity to permit reasonable anticipation that such person is likely to suffer impaired earning capacity at age 18 and beyond, compensation after attaining the age of 18 for loss of earnings determined on the basis of the average gross weekly earnings of workers in the private, non-farm sector, less appropriate taxes and the average cost of a health insurance policy, as determined by the Secretary.

(4) For actual and projected pain and suffering and emotional distress from the vaccine-related injury, an award not to exceed $250,000.

(b) Vaccines administered before effective date

Compensation awarded under the Program to a petitioner under section 300aa-11 of this title for a vaccine-related injury or death associated with the administration of a vaccine before October 1, 1988, may include the compensation described in paragraphs (1)(A) and (2) of subsection (a) of this section and may also include an amount, not to exceed a combined total of $30,000, for -

(1) lost earnings (as provided in paragraph (3) of subsection (a) of this section),

(2) pain and suffering (as provided in paragraph (4) of subsection (a) of this section), and

(3) reasonable attorneys' fees and costs (as provided in subsection (e) of this section.(!1)

(c) Residential and custodial care and service

The amount of any compensation for residential and custodial care and service expenses under subsection (a)(1) of this section shall be sufficient to enable the compensated person to remain living at home.

(d) Types of compensation prohibited

Compensation awarded under the Program may not include the following:

(1) Punitive or exemplary damages.

(2) Except with respect to compensation payments under paragraphs (2) and (3) of subsection (a) of this section, compensation for other than the health, education, or welfare of the person who suffered the vaccine-related injury with respect to which the compensation is paid.

(e) Attorneys' fees

(1) In awarding compensation on a petition filed under section 300aa-11 of this title the special master or court shall also award as part of such compensation an amount to cover -

(A) reasonable attorneys' fees, and

(B) other costs,

incurred in any proceeding on such petition. If the judgment of the United States Court of Federal Claims on such a petition does not award compensation, the special master or court may award an amount of compensation to cover petitioner's reasonable attorneys' fees and other costs incurred in any proceeding on such petition if the special master or court determines that the petition was brought in good faith and there was a reasonable basis for the claim for which the petition was brought.

(2) If the petitioner, before October 1, 1988, filed a civil action for damages for any vaccine-related injury or death for which compensation may be awarded under the Program, and petitioned under section 300aa-11(a)(5) of this title to have such action dismissed and to file a petition for compensation under the Program, in awarding compensation on such petition the special master or court may include an amount of compensation limited to the costs and expenses incurred by the petitioner and the attorney of the petitioner before October 1, 1988, in preparing, filing, and prosecuting such civil action (including the reasonable value of the attorney's time if the civil action was filed under contingent fee arrangements).

(3) No attorney may charge any fee for services in connection with a petition filed under section 300aa-11 of this title which is in addition to any amount awarded as compensation by the special master or court under paragraph (1).

(f) Payment of compensation

(1) Except as provided in paragraph (2), no compensation may be paid until an election has been made, or has been deemed to have been made, under section 300aa-21(a) of this title to receive compensation.

(2) Compensation described in subsection (a)(1)(A)(iii) of this section shall be paid from the date of the judgment of the United States Court of Federal Claims under section 300aa-12 of this title awarding the compensation. Such compensation may not be paid after an election under section 300aa-21(a) of this title to file a civil action for damages for the vaccine-related injury or death for which such compensation was awarded.

(3) Payments of compensation under the Program and the costs of carrying out the Program shall be exempt from reduction under any order issued under part C of the Balanced Budget and Emergency Deficit Control Act of 1985 [2 U.S.C. 900 et seq.].

(4)(A) Except as provided in subparagraph (B), payment of compensation under the Program shall be determined on the basis of the net present value of the elements of the compensation and shall be paid from the Vaccine Injury Compensation Trust Fund established under section 9510 of title 26 in a lump sum of which all or a portion may be used as ordered by the special master to purchase an annuity or otherwise be used, with the consent of the petitioner, in a manner determined by the special master to be in the best interests of the petitioner.

(B) In the case of a payment of compensation under the Program to a petitioner for a vaccine-related injury or death associated with the administration of a vaccine before October 1, 1988, the compensation shall be determined on the basis of the net present value of the elements of compensation and shall be paid from appropriations made available under subsection (j) of this section in a lump sum of which all or a portion may be used as ordered by the special master to purchase an annuity or otherwise be used, with the consent of the petitioner, in a manner determined by the special master to be in the best interests of the petitioner. Any reasonable attorneys' fees and costs shall be paid in a lump sum. If the appropriations under subsection (j) of this section are

insufficient to make a payment of an annual installment, the
limitation on civil actions prescribed by section 300aa-21(a) of
this title shall not apply to a civil action for damages brought by
the petitioner entitled to the payment.

(C) In purchasing an annuity under subparagraph (A) or (B), the
Secretary may purchase a guarantee for the annuity, may enter into
agreements regarding the purchase price for and rate of return of
the annuity, and may take such other actions as may be necessary to
safeguard the financial interests of the United States regarding
the annuity. Any payment received by the Secretary pursuant to the
preceding sentence shall be paid to the Vaccine Injury Compensation
Trust Fund established under section 9510 of title 26, or to the
appropriations account from which the funds were derived to
purchase the annuity, whichever is appropriate.

(g) Program not primarily liable

Payment of compensation under the Program shall not be made for
any item or service to the extent that payment has been made, or
can reasonably be expected to be made, with respect to such item or
service (1) under any State compensation program, under an
insurance policy, or under any Federal or State health benefits
program (other than under title XIX of the Social Security Act [42
U.S.C. 1396 et seq.]), or (2) by an entity which provides health
services on a prepaid basis.

(h) Liability of health insurance carriers, prepaid health plans,
   and benefit providers

No policy of health insurance may make payment of benefits under
the policy secondary to the payment of compensation under the
Program and -

   (1) no State, and

   (2) no entity which provides health services on a prepaid basis
   or provides health benefits,

may make the provision of health services or health benefits
secondary to the payment of compensation under the Program, except
that this subsection shall not apply to the provision of services
or benefits under title XIX of the Social Security Act [42 U.S.C.
1396 et seq.].

(i) Source of compensation

   (1) Payment of compensation under the Program to a petitioner for
a vaccine-related injury or death associated with the
administration of a vaccine before October 1, 1988, shall be made
by the Secretary from appropriations under subsection (j) of this
section.

   (2) Payment of compensation under the Program to a petitioner for
a vaccine-related injury or death associated with the
administration of a vaccine on or after October 1, 1988, shall be
made from the Vaccine Injury Compensation Trust Fund established
under section 9510 of title 26.

(j) Authorization

For the payment of compensation under the Program to a petitioner
for a vaccine-related injury or death associated with the
administration of a vaccine before October 1, 1988, there are
authorized to be appropriated to the Department of Health and Human
Services $80,000,000 for fiscal year 1989, $80,000,000 for fiscal
year 1990, $80,000,000 for fiscal year 1991, $80,000,000 for fiscal
year 1992, $110,000,000 for fiscal year 1993, and $110,000,000 for
each succeeding fiscal year in which a payment of compensation is

required under subsection (f)(4)(B) of this section. Amounts appropriated under this subsection shall remain available until expended.

-SOURCE-
(July 1, 1944, ch. 373, title XXI, Sec. 2115, as added Pub. L. 99-660, title III, Sec. 311(a), Nov. 14, 1986, 100 Stat. 3767; amended Pub. L. 100-203, title IV, Secs. 4302(b), 4303(a)-(d)(1), (e), (g), 4307(5), (6), Dec. 22, 1987, 101 Stat. 1330-221 to 1330-223, 1330-225; Pub. L. 100-360, title IV, Sec, 411(o)(1), July 1, 1988, 102 Stat, 808· Pub. L. 101-239, title VI, Sec. 6601(c)(8), (f), Dec. 19, 1989, 103 Stat. 2286, 2290; Pub. L. 101-502, Sec. 5(d), Nov. 3, 1990, 104 Stat. 1287; Pub. L. 102-168, title II, Sec. 201(e), (f), Nov. 26, 1991, 105 Stat. 1103; Pub. L. 102-531, title III, Sec. 314, Oct. 27, 1992, 106 Stat. 3508; Pub. L. 102-572, title IX, Sec. 902(b)(1), Oct. 29, 1992, 106 Stat. 4516; Pub. L. 103-66, title XIII, Sec. 13632(b), Aug. 10, 1993, 107 Stat. 646.)

-REFTEXT-
REFERENCES IN TEXT
The Balanced Budget and Emergency Deficit Control Act of 1985, referred to in subsec. (f)(3), is title II of Pub. L. 99-177, Dec. 12, 1985, 99 Stat. 1038. Part C of the Act is classified generally to subchapter I (Sec. 900 et seq.) of chapter 20 of Title 2, The Congress. For complete classification of this Act to the Code, see Short Title note set out under section 900 of Title 2 and Tables.

The Social Security Act, referred to in subsecs. (g) and (h), is act Aug. 14, 1935, ch. 531, 49 Stat. 620, as amended. Title XIX of the Social Security Act is classified generally to subchapter XIX (Sec. 1396 et seq.) of chapter 7 of this title. For complete classification of this Act to the Code, see section 1305 of this title and Tables.

-COD-
CODIFICATION
In subsecs. (a), (b), (e)(2), (f)(4)(B), (i), and (j), "October 1, 1988" substituted for "the effective date of this subpart" on authority of section 323 of Pub. L. 99-660, as amended, set out as an Effective Date note under section 300aa-1 of this title.

-MISC1-
PRIOR PROVISIONS
A prior section 300aa-15, act July 1, 1944, Sec. 2116, was successively renumbered by subsequent acts and transferred, see section 238m of this title.

A prior section 2115 of act July 1, 1944, was successively renumbered by subsequent acts and transferred, see section 2381 of this title.

AMENDMENTS
1993 - Subsec. (j). Pub. L. 103-66 substituted "$110,000,000 for each succeeding fiscal year" for "$80,000,000 for each succeeding fiscal year".

1992 - Subsecs. (e)(1), (f)(2). Pub. L. 102-572 substituted "United States Court of Federal Claims" for "United States Claims Court".

Subsec. (j). Pub. L. 102-531 increased authorization for fiscal year 1993 from $80,000,000 to $110,000,000.

1991 - Subsec. (f)(4)(A). Pub. L. 102-168, Sec. 201(e)(1)(A), (2), struck out "of the proceeds" after "portion" and substituted "Vaccine Injury Compensation Trust Fund established under section 9510 of title 26" for "trust fund".

Subsec. (f)(4)(B). Pub. L. 102-168, Sec. 201(e)(1)(B), which directed substitution of "shall be paid from appropriations made available under subsection (j) of this section in a lump sum of which all or a portion" for "paid in 4 equal installments of which all or portion of the proceeds" was executed by making the substitution for "paid in 4 equal annual installments of which all or a portion of the proceeds" to reflect the probable intent of Congress.

Subsec. (f)(4)(C). Pub. L. 102-168, Sec. 201(f), added subpar. (C).

1990 - Subsec. (e)(2). Pub. L. 101-502, Sec. 5(d)(1), inserted "of compensation" before "limited to the costs".

Subsec. (f)(2). Pub. L. 101-502, Sec. 5(d)(2)(A), substituted "section 300aa-21(a)" for "section 300aa-21(b)".

Subsec. (f)(4)(B). Pub. L. 101-502, Sec. 5(d)(2)(B), substituted "subsection (j)" for "subsection (i)" and "the limitation on civil actions prescribed by section 300aa-21(a) of this title" for "section 300aa-11(a) of this title".

Subsec. (j). Pub. L. 101-502, Sec. 5(d)(3), inserted before period at end of first sentence ", and $80,000,000 for each succeeding fiscal year in which a payment of compensation is required under subsection (f)(4)(B) of this section".

1989 - Subsec. (b). Pub. L. 101-239, Sec. 6601(l)(1), substituted "may include the compensation described in paragraphs (1)(A) and (2) of subsection (a) of this section and may also include an amount, not to exceed a combined total of $30,000, for - " and cls. (1) to (3) for "may not include the compensation described in paragraph (1)(B) of subsection (a) of this section and may include attorneys' fees and other costs included in a judgment under subsection (e) of this section, except that the total amount that may be paid as compensation under paragraphs (3) and (4) of subsection (a) of this section and included as attorneys' fees and other costs under subsection (e) of this section may not exceed $30,000."

Subsec. (e)(1). Pub. L. 101-239, Sec. 6601(l)(2)(A), substituted "In awarding compensation on a petition filed under section 300aa-11 of this title the special master or court shall also award as part of such compensation an amount to cover" for "The judgment of the United States Claims Court on a petition filed under section 300aa-11 of this title awarding compensation shall include an amount to cover".

Pub. L. 101-239, Sec. 6601(l)(2)(B), (C), substituted "the special master or court may award an amount of compensation to cover" for "the court may include in the judgment an amount to cover" and "the special master or court determines that the petition was brought in good faith and there was a reasonable basis for the claim for which the petition" for "the court determines that the civil action was brought in good faith and there was a reasonable basis for the claim for which the civil action".

Subsec. (e)(2). Pub. L. 101-239, Sec. 6601(l)(2)(D), which directed amendment of par. (2) by substituting "the special master or court may also award an amount of compensation" for "the judgment of the court on such petition may include an amount", could not be executed because of the prior amendment by Pub. L. 101-239, Sec. 6601(c)(8)(B), see Amendment note below.

Pub. L. 101-239, Sec. 6601(c)(8), substituted "and petitioned under section 300aa-11(a)(5) of this title to have such action dismissed" for "and elected under section 300aa-11(a)(4) of this title to withdraw such action" and "in awarding compensation on such petition the special master or court may include" for "the judgment of the court on such petition may include".

Subsec. (e)(3). Pub. L. 101-239, Sec. 6601(1)(2) (B), substituted "awarded as compensation by the special master or court under paragraph (1)" for "included under paragraph (1) in a judgment on such petition".

Subsec. (f)(3). Pub. L. 101-239, Sec. 6601(1)(3)(A), inserted "under the Program and the costs of carrying out the Program" after "Payments of compensation".

Subsec. (f)(4)(A). Pub. L. 101-239, Sec. 6601(1)(3)(B), struck out "made in a lump sum" after "the Program shall be" and inserted "and shall be paid from the trust fund in a lump sum of which all or a portion of the proceeds may be used as ordered by the special master to purchase an annuity or otherwise be used, with the consent of the petitioner, in a manner determined by the special master to be in the best interests of the petitioner" after "elements of the compensation".

Subsec. (f)(4)(B). Pub. L. 101-239, Sec. 6601(1)(3)(C), substituted "determined on the basis of the net present value of the elements of compensation and paid in 4 equal annual installments of which all or a portion of the proceeds may be used as ordered by the special master to purchase an annuity or otherwise be used, with the consent of the petitioner, in a manner determined by the special master to be in the best interests of the petitioner. Any reasonable attorneys' fees and costs shall be paid in a lump sum" for "paid in 4 equal annual installments".

Subsec. (g). Pub. L. 101-239, Sec. 6601(1)(4)(A), inserted "(other than under title XIX of the Social Security Act)" after "State health benefits program".

Subsec. (h). Pub. L. 101-239, Sec. 6601(1)(4)(B), inserted before period at end ", except that this subsection shall not apply to the provision of services or benefits under title XIX of the Social Security Act".

Subsec. (i)(1). Pub. L. 101-239, Sec. 6601(1)(5), which directed amendment of par. (1) by substituting "(j)" for "(i)", could not be executed because "(i)" did not appear.

Subsec. (j). Pub. L. 101-239, Sec. 6601(1)(6), struck out "and" after "fiscal year 1991," and inserted ", $80,000,000 for fiscal year 1993" after "fiscal year 1992".

1988 - Subsec. (i)(1). Pub. L. 100-360, Sec. 411(o)(1)(A), substituted "by the Secretary from appropriations under subsection (j)" for "from appropriations under subsection (i)".

Subsec. (j). Pub. L. 100-360, Sec. 411(o)(1)(B), inserted "to the Department of Health and Human Services".

1987 - Subsec. (a). Pub. L. 100-203, Sec. 4302(b)(1), substituted "effective date of this subpart" for "effective date of this part".

Pub. L. 100-203, Sec. 4303(d)(1)(A), struck out last two sentences which read as follows: "Payments for projected expenses shall be paid on a periodic basis (but no payment may be made for a period in excess of 1 year). Payments for pain and suffering and emotional distress and incurred expenses may be paid in a lump sum."

Subsec. (a)(1). Pub. L. 100-203, Sec. 4303(c), struck out last sentence of subpars. (A) and (B) each of which read as follows: "The amount of unreimbursable expenses which may be recovered under this subparagraph shall be limited to the amount in excess of the amount set forth in section 300aa-11(c)(1)(D)(ii) of this title."

Subsec. (b). Pub. L. 100-203, Sec. 4303(e), substituted "may not include the compensation described in paragraph (1)(B) of subsection (a) of this section and may include attorneys' fees and other costs included in a judgment under subsection (e) of this section, except that the total amount that may be paid as compensation under paragraphs (3) and (4) of subsection (a) of this section and included as attorneys' fees and other costs under subsection (e) of this section may not exceed $30,000" for "shall only include the compensation described in paragraphs (1)(A) and (2) of subsection (a) of this section".

Pub. L. 100-203, Sec. 4302(b)(1), substituted "effective date of this subpart" for "effective date of this part".

Subsec. (e)(1). Pub. L. 100-203, Sec. 4307(5), substituted "of the United States Claims Court" for "of a court" in two places.

Subsec. (e)(2). Pub. L. 100-203, Sec. 4302(b), substituted "effective date of this subpart, filed a" for "effective date of this subchapter, filed a" and "effective date of this subpart in preparing" for "effective date of this part in preparing".

Subsec. (f). Pub. L. 100-203, Sec. 4303(d)(1)(B), (g), added par. (4) and redesignated a second subsec. (f), relating to the Program not being primarily liable, as subsec. (g).

Subsec. (f)(2). Pub. L. 100-203, Sec. 4307(6), substituted "United States Claims Court" for "district court of the United States".

Subsecs. (g), (h). Pub. L. 100-203, Sec. 4303(g), redesignated a second subsec. (f), relating to the Program not being liable, as (g) and redesignated former subsec. (g) as (h).

Subsecs. (i), (j). Pub. L. 100-203, Sec. 4303(a), (b), added subsecs. (i) and (j).

EFFECTIVE DATE OF 1992 AMENDMENT

Amendment by Pub. L. 102-572 effective Oct. 29, 1992, see section 911 of Pub. L. 102-572, set out as a note under section 171 of Title 28, Judiciary and Judicial Procedure.

EFFECTIVE DATE OF 1991 AMENDMENT

Amendment by section 201(f) of Pub. L. 102-168 effective as if in effect on and after Oct. 1, 1988, see section 201(i)(2) of Pub. L. 102-168, set out as a note under section 300aa-11 of this title.

EFFECTIVE DATE OF 1990 AMENDMENT

Amendment by Pub. L. 101-502 effective Sept. 30, 1990, see section 5(h) of Pub. L. 101-502, set out as a note under section 300aa-11 of this title.

EFFECTIVE DATE OF 1989 AMENDMENT

Amendment by Pub. L. 101-239 applicable to all pending and

subsequently filed petitions, see section 6601(s)(2) of Pub. L. 101-239, set out as a note under section 300aa-10 of this title.

EFFECTIVE DATE OF 1988 AMENDMENT

Except as specifically provided in section 411 of Pub. L. 100-360, amendment by Pub. L. 100-360, as it relates to a provision in the Omnibus Budget Reconciliation Act of 1987, Pub. L. 100-203, effective as if included in the enactment of that provision in Pub. L. 100-203, see section 411(a) of Pub. L. 100-360, set out as a Reference to OBRA; Effective Date note under section 106 of Title 1, General Provisions.

FOOTNOTE-

(!1) So in original. Probably should be preceded by a closing parenthesis.

-End-

-CITE-
    42 USC Sec. 300aa-16
01/08/2008

-EXPCITE-
    TITLE 42 - THE PUBLIC HEALTH AND WELFARE
    CHAPTER 6A - PUBLIC HEALTH SERVICE
    SUBCHAPTER XIX - VACCINES
    Part 2 - National Vaccine Injury Compensation Program
    subpart a - program requirements

-HEAD-
    Sec. 300aa-16. Limitations of actions

-STATUTE-
    (a) General rule
    In the case of -
        (1) a vaccine set forth in the Vaccine Injury Table which is administered before October 1, 1988, if a vaccine-related injury or death occurred as a result of the administration of such vaccine, no petition may be filed for compensation under the Program for such injury or death after the expiration of 28 months after October 1, 1988, and no such petition may be filed if the first symptom or manifestation of onset or of the significant aggravation of such injury occurred more than 36 months after the date of administration of the vaccine,
        (2) a vaccine set forth in the Vaccine Injury Table which is administered after October 1, 1988, if a vaccine-related injury occurred as a result of the administration of such vaccine, no petition may be filed for compensation under the Program for such injury after the expiration of 36 months after the date of the occurrence of the first symptom or manifestation of onset or of the significant aggravation of such injury, and
        (3) a vaccine set forth in the Vaccine Injury Table which is

administered after October 1, 1988, if a death occurred as a
result of the administration of such vaccine, no petition may be
filed for compensation under the Program for such death after the
expiration of 24 months from the date of the death and no such
petition may be filed more than 48 months after the date of the
occurrence of the first symptom or manifestation of onset or of
the significant aggravation of the injury from which the death
resulted.
(b) Effect of revised table
   If at any time the Vaccine Injury Table is revised and the effect
of such revision is to permit an individual who was not, before
such revision, eligible to seek compensation under the Program, or
to significantly increase the likelihood of obtaining compensation,
such person may, notwithstanding section 300aa-11(b)(2) of this
title, file a petition for such compensation not later than 2 years
after the effective date of the revision, except that no
compensation may be provided under the Program with respect to a
vaccine-related injury or death covered under the revision of the
table if -
   (1) the vaccine-related death occurred more than 8 years before
   the date of the revision of the table, or
   (2) the vaccine-related injury occurred more than 8 years
   before the date of the revision of the table.
(c) State limitations of actions
   If a petition is filed under section 300aa-11 of this title for a
vaccine-related injury or death, limitations of actions under State
law shall be stayed with respect to a civil action brought for such
injury or death for the period beginning on the date the petition
is filed and ending on the date (1) an election is made under
section 300aa-21(a) of this title to file the civil action or (2)
an election is made under section 300aa-21(b) of this title to
withdraw the petition.

-SOURCE-
(July 1, 1944, ch. 373, title XXI, Sec. 2116, as added Pub. L. 99-
660, title III, Sec. 311(a), Nov. 14, 1986, 100 Stat. 3769;
amended Pub. L. 100-203, title IV, Sec. 4302(b)(2), Dec. 22, 1987,
101 Stat. 1330-221; Pub. L. 101-239, title VI, Sec. 6601(m)(1),
Dec. 19, 1989, 103 Stat. 2291; Pub. L. 101-502, Sec. 5(e), Nov. 3,
1990, 104 Stat. 1287; Pub. L. 102-168, title II, Sec. 201(d)(2),
Nov. 26, 1991, 105 Stat. 1103; Pub. L. 103-66, title XIII, Sec.
13632(a)(1), Aug. 10, 1993, 107 Stat. 645.)

-COD-
                         CODIFICATION
   In subsec. (a)(1) to (3), "October 1, 1988" and "October 1,
1988," substituted for "the effective date of this subpart" on
authority of section 323 of Pub. L. 99-660, as amended, set out as
an Effective Date note under section 300aa-1 of this title.

-MISC1-
                       PRIOR PROVISIONS
   A prior section 2116 of act July 1, 1944, was successively
renumbered by subsequent acts and transferred, see section 238m of
this title.

AMENDMENTS

1993 - Subsec. (b). Pub. L. 103-66 substituted "or to significantly increase the likelihood of obtaining compensation, such person may, notwithstanding section 300aa-11(b)(2) of this title, file" for "such person may file".

1991 - Subsec. (c). Pub. L. 102-168 substituted "or (2)" for ", (2)" and struck out ", or (3) the petition is considered withdrawn under section 300aa-21(b) of this title."

1990 - Subsec. (a)(1). Pub. L. 101-502, Sec. 5(e)(1), substituted "28 months" for "24 months" and inserted before comma at end "and no such petition may be filed if the final symptom or manifestation of onset or of the significant aggravation of such injury occurred more than 36 months after the date of administration of the vaccine".

Subsec. (c). Pub. L. 101-502, Sec. 5(e)(2), substituted "and ending on the date (1) an election is made under section 300aa-21(a) of this title to file the civil action, (2) an election is made under section 300aa-21(b) of this title to withdraw the petition, or (3) the petition is considered withdrawn under section 300aa-21(b) of this title" for "and ending on the date a final judgment is entered on the petition".

1989 - Subsec. (c). Pub. L. 101-239 substituted "300aa-11 of this title" for "300aa-11(b) of this title".

1987 - Subsec. (a). Pub. L. 100-203 substituted "effective date of this subpart" for "effective date of this subchapter" in pars. (1) to (3).

EFFECTIVE DATE OF 1991 AMENDMENT

Amendment by Pub. L. 102-168 effective as if in effect on and after Oct. 1, 1988, see section 201(i)(2) of Pub. L. 102-168, set out as a note under section 300aa-11 of this title.

EFFECTIVE DATE OF 1990 AMENDMENT

Amendment by Pub. L. 101-502 effective Sept. 30, 1990, see section 5(h) of Pub. L. 101-502, set out as a note under section 300aa-11 of this title.

EFFECTIVE DATE OF 1989 AMENDMENT

For applicability of amendments by Pub. L. 101-239 to petitions filed after Dec. 19, 1989, petitions currently pending in which the evidentiary record is closed, and petitions currently pending in which the evidentiary record is not closed, with provision for an immediate suspension for 30 days of all pending cases, see section 6601(s)(1) of Pub. L. 101-239, set out as a note under section 300aa-10 of this title.

-End-

-CITE-
    42 USC Sec. 300aa-17
01/08/2008

-EXPCITE-
    TITLE 42 - THE PUBLIC HEALTH AND WELFARE
    CHAPTER 6A - PUBLIC HEALTH SERVICE

```
    SUBCHAPTER XIX - VACCINES
    Part 2 - National Vaccine Injury Compensation Program
    subpart a - program requirements
```

-HEAD-
    Sec. 300aa-17. Subrogation

-STATUTE-
    (a) General rule
    Upon payment of compensation to any petitioner under the Program,
    the trust fund which has been established to provide such
    compensation shall be subrograted (!1) to all rights of the
    petitioner with respect to the vaccine-related injury or death for
    which compensation was paid, except that the trust fund may not
    recover under such rights an amount greater than the amount of
    compensation paid to the petitioner.

    (b) Disposition of amounts recovered
    Amounts recovered under subsection (a) of this section shall be
    collected on behalf of, and deposited in, the Vaccine Injury
    Compensation Trust Fund established under section 9510 of title 26.

-SOURCE-
    (July 1, 1944, ch. 373, title XXI, Sec. 2117, as added Pub. L. 99-
    660, title III, Sec. 311(a), Nov. 14, 1986, 100 Stat. 3770;
    amended Pub. L. 100-203, title IV, Sec. 4307(7), Dec. 22, 1987, 101
    Stat. 1330-225; Pub. L. 101-239, title VI, Sec. 6601(m)(2), Dec.
    19, 1989, 103 Stat. 2291.)

-MISC1-
                            AMENDMENTS
    1989 - Subsec. (b). Pub. L. 101-239 substituted "the Vaccine
    Injury Compensation Trust Fund established under section 9510 of
    title 26" for "the trust fund which has been established to provide
    compensation under the Program".
    1987 - Subsec. (a). Pub. L. 100-203 struck out par. (1)
    designation before "Upon" and struck out par. (2) which read as
    follows: "In any case in which it deems such action appropriate, a
    district court of the United States may, after entry of a final
    judgment providing for compensation to be paid under section 300aa-
    15 of this title for a vaccine-related injury or death, refer the
    record of such proceeding to the Secretary and the Attorney General
    with such recommendation as the court deems appropriate with
    respect to the investigation or commencement of a civil action by
    the Secretary under paragraph (1)."

                 EFFECTIVE DATE OF 1989 AMENDMENT
    For applicability of amendments by Pub. L. 101-239 to petitions
    filed after Dec. 19, 1989, petitions currently pending in which the
    evidentiary record is closed, and petitions currently pending in
    which the evidentiary record is not closed, with provision for an
    immediate suspension for 30 days of all pending cases, see section
    6601(s)(1) of Pub. L. 101-239, set out as a note under section
    300aa-10 of this title.
```
```

-FOOTNOTE-

(!1) So in original. Probably should be "subrogated".

-End-

-CITE-
    42 USC Sec. 300aa-18
01/08/2008

-EXPCITE-
    TITLE 42   THE PUBLIC HEALTH AND WELFARE
    CHAPTER 6A - PUBLIC HEALTH SERVICE
    SUBCHAPTER XIX - VACCINES
    Part 2 - National Vaccine Injury Compensation Program
    subpart a - program requirements

-HEAD-
    Sec. 300aa-18. Repealed.

-MISC1-
    Sec. 300aa-18. Repealed. Pub. L. 100-203, title IV, Sec.
    4303(d)(2)(B), Dec. 22, 1987, 101 Stat. 1330-222.
      Section, act July 1, 1944, ch. 373, title XXI, Sec. 2118, as
    added Nov. 14, 1986, Pub. L. 99-660, title III, Sec. 311(a), 100
    Stat. 3771, provided for annual increases for inflation of
    compensation under subsections (a)(2) and (a)(4) of section 300aa-
    15 of this title and civil penalty under section 300aa-27(b) of
    this title.

-End-

-CITE-
    42 USC Sec. 300aa-19
01/08/2008

-EXPCITE-
    TITLE 42 - THE PUBLIC HEALTH AND WELFARE
    CHAPTER 6A - PUBLIC HEALTH SERVICE
    SUBCHAPTER XIX - VACCINES
    Part 2 - National Vaccine Injury Compensation Program
    subpart a - program requirements

-HEAD-
    Sec. 300aa-19. Advisory Commission on Childhood Vaccines

-STATUTE-
    (a) Establishment
      There is established the Advisory Commission on Childhood
    Vaccines. The Commission shall be composed of:
        (1) Nine members appointed by the Secretary as follows:
          (A) Three members who are health professionals, who are not
        employees of the United States, and who have expertise in the
        health care of children, the epidemiology, etiology, and

prevention of childhood diseases, and the adverse reactions associated with vaccines, of whom at least two shall be pediatricians.

(B) Three members from the general public, of whom at least two shall be legal representatives of children who have suffered a vaccine-related injury or death.

(C) Three members who are attorneys, of whom at least one shall be an attorney whose specialty includes representation of persons who have suffered a vaccine-related injury or death and of whom one shall be an attorney whose specialty includes representation of vaccine manufacturers.

(2) The Director of the National Institutes of Health, the Assistant Secretary for Health, the Director of the Centers for Disease Control and Prevention, and the Commissioner of Food and Drugs (or the designees of such officials), each of whom shall be a nonvoting ex officio member.

The Secretary shall select members of the Commission within 90 days of October 1, 1988. The members of the Commission shall select a Chair from among the members.

(b) Term of office

Appointed members of the Commission shall be appointed for a term of office of 3 years, except that of the members first appointed, 3 shall be appointed for a term of 1 year, 3 shall be appointed for a term of 2 years, and 3 shall be appointed for a term of 3 years, as determined by the Secretary.

(c) Meetings

The Commission shall first meet within 60 days after all members of the Commission are appointed, and thereafter shall meet not less often than four times per year and at the call of the chair. A quorum for purposes of a meeting is 5. A decision at a meeting is to be made by a ballot of a majority of the voting members of the Commission present at the meeting.

(d) Compensation

Members of the Commission who are officers or employees of the Federal Government shall serve as members of the Commission without compensation in addition to that received in their regular public employment. Members of the Commission who are not officers or employees of the Federal Government shall be compensated at a rate not to exceed the daily equivalent of the rate in effect for grade GS-18 of the General Schedule for each day (including traveltime) they are engaged in the performance of their duties as members of the Commission. All members, while so serving away from their homes or regular places of business, may be allowed travel expenses, including per diem in lieu of subsistence, in the same manner as such expenses are authorized by section 5703 of title 5 for employees serving intermittently.

(e) Staff

The Secretary shall provide the Commission with such professional and clerical staff, such information, and the services of such consultants as may be necessary to assist the Commission in carrying out effectively its functions under this section.

(f) Functions

The Commission shall -

(1) advise the Secretary on the implementation of the Program,

(2) on its own initiative or as the result of the filing of a

petition, recommend changes in the Vaccine Injury Table,

(3) advise the Secretary in implementing the Secretary's responsibilities under section 300aa-27 of this title regarding the need for childhood vaccination products that result in fewer or no significant adverse reactions,

(4) survey Federal, State, and local programs and activities relating to the gathering of information on injuries associated with the administration of childhood vaccines, including the adverse reaction reporting requirements of section 300aa-25(b) of this title, and advise the Secretary on means to obtain, compile, publish, and use credible data related to the frequency and severity of adverse reactions associated with childhood vaccines, and

(5) recommend to the Director of the National Vaccine Program research related to vaccine injuries which should be conducted to carry out this part.

-SOURCE-

(July 1, 1944, ch. 373, title XXI, Sec. 2119, as added Pub. L. 99-660, title III, Sec. 311(a), Nov. 14, 1986, 100 Stat. 3771; amended Pub. L. 100-203, title IV, Sec. 4302(b)(1), Dec. 22, 1987, 101 Stat. 1330-221; Pub. L. 102-168, title II, Sec. 201(g), Nov. 26, 1991, 105 Stat. 1104; Pub. L. 102-531, title III, Sec. 312(d)(14), Oct. 27, 1992, 106 Stat. 3505.)

-COD-

CODIFICATION

In subsec. (a), "October 1, 1988" substituted for "the effective date of this subpart" on authority of section 323 of Pub. L. 99-660, as amended, set out as an Effective Date note under section 300aa-1 of this title.

-MISC1

AMENDMENTS

1992 - Subsec. (a)(2). Pub. L. 102-531 substituted "Centers for Disease Control and Prevention" for "Centers for Disease Control".

1991 - Subsec. (c). Pub. L. 102-168 inserted "present at the meeting" before period at end.

1987 - Subsec. (a). Pub. L. 100-203 substituted "effective date of this subpart" for "effective date of this part" in last sentence.

TERMINATION OF ADVISORY COMMISSIONS

Advisory commissions established after Jan. 5, 1973, to terminate not later than the expiration of the 2-year period beginning on the date of their establishment, unless, in the case of a commission established by the President or an officer of the Federal Government, such commission is renewed by appropriate action prior to the expiration of such 2-year period, or in the case of a commission established by the Congress, its duration is otherwise provided by law. See sections 3(2) and 14 of Pub. L. 92-463, Oct. 6, 1972, 86 Stat. 776, set out in the Appendix to Title 5, Government Organization and Employees.

Pub. L. 93-641, Sec. 6, Jan. 4, 1975, 88 Stat. 2275, set out as a note under section 217a of this title, provided that an advisory committee established pursuant to the Public Health Service Act shall terminate at such time as may be specifically prescribed by an Act of Congress enacted after Jan. 4, 1975.

REFERENCES IN OTHER LAWS TO GS-16, 17, OR 18 PAY RATES
 References in laws to the rates of pay for GS-16, 17, or 18, or to maximum rates of pay under the General Schedule, to be considered references to rates payable under specified sections of Title 5, Government Organization and Employees, see section 529 [title I, Sec. 101(c)(1)] of Pub. L. 101-509, set out in a note under section 5376 of Title 5.

-End-

-CITE-
 42 USC subpart b - additional remedies
01/08/2008

-EXPCITE-
 TITLE 42 - THE PUBLIC HEALTH AND WELFARE
 CHAPTER 6A - PUBLIC HEALTH SERVICE
 SUBCHAPTER XIX - VACCINES
 Part 2 - National Vaccine Injury Compensation Program
 subpart b - additional remedies

-HEAD-
                    SUBPART B - ADDITIONAL REMEDIES

-End-

-CITE-
 42 USC Sec. 300aa-21
01/08/2008

-EXPCITE-
 TITLE 42 - THE PUBLIC HEALTH AND WELFARE
 CHAPTER 6A - PUBLIC HEALTH SERVICE
 SUBCHAPTER XIX - VACCINES
 Part 2 - National Vaccine Injury Compensation Program
 subpart b - additional remedies

-HEAD-
 Sec. 300aa-21. Authority to bring actions

-STATUTE-
 (a) Election
   After judgment has been entered by the United States Court of Federal Claims or, if an appeal is taken under section 300aa-12(f) of this title, after the appellate court's mandate is issued, the petitioner who filed the petition under section 300aa-11 of this title shall file with the clerk of the United States Court of Federal Claims -
     (1) if the judgment awarded compensation, an election in writing to receive the compensation or to file a civil action for damages for such injury or death, or

(2) if the judgment did not award compensation, an election in writing to accept the judgment or to file a civil action for damages for such injury or death.

An election shall be filed under this subsection not later than 90 days after the date of the court's final judgment with respect to which the election is to be made. If a person required to file an election with the court under this subsection does not file the election within the time prescribed for filing the election, such person shall be deemed to have filed an election to accept the judgment of the court. If a person elects to receive compensation under a judgment of the court in an action for a vaccine-related injury or death associated with the administration of a vaccine before October 1, 1988, or is deemed to have accepted the judgment of the court in such an action, such person may not bring or maintain a civil action for damages against a vaccine administrator or manufacturer for the vaccine-related injury or death for which the judgment was entered. For limitations on the bringing of civil actions for vaccine-related injuries or deaths associated with the administration of a vaccine after October 1, 1988, see section 300aa-11(a)(2) of this title.
(b) Continuance or withdrawal of petition
A petitioner under a petition filed under section 300aa-11 of this title may submit to the United States Court of Federal Claims a notice in writing choosing to continue or to withdraw the petition if -
(1) a special master fails to make a decision on such petition within the 240 days prescribed by section 300aa-12(d)(3)(A)(ii) of this title (excluding (i) any period of suspension under section 300aa-12(d)(3)(C) or 300aa-12(d)(3)(D) of this title, and (ii) any days the petition is before a special master as a result of a remand under section 300aa-12(e)(2)(C) of this title), or
(2) the court fails to enter a judgment under section 300aa-12 of this title on the petition within 420 days (excluding (i) any period of suspension under section 300aa-12(d)(3)(C) or 300aa-12(d)(3)(D) of this title, and (ii) any days the petition is before a special master as a result of a remand under section 300aa-12(e)(2)(C) of this title) after the date on which the petition was filed.

Such a notice shall be filed within 30 days of the provision of the notice required by section 300aa-12(q) of this title.
(c) Limitations of actions
A civil action for damages arising from a vaccine-related injury or death for which a petition was filed under section 300aa-11 of this title shall, except as provided in section 300aa-16(c) of this title, be brought within the period prescribed by limitations of actions under State law applicable to such civil action.

-SOURCE-
(July 1, 1944, ch. 373, title XXI, Sec. 2121, as added Pub. L. 99-660, title III, Sec. 311(a), Nov. 14, 1986, 100 Stat. 3772; amended Pub. L. 100-203, title IV, Secs. 4304(c), 4307(8), 4308(c), Dec. 22, 1987, 101 Stat. 1330-224, 1330-225; Pub. L. 100-360, title IV, Sec. 411(o)(3)(A), July 1, 1988, 102 Stat. 808; Pub. L. 101-239, title VI, Sec. 6601(n), Dec. 19, 1989, 103 Stat. 2291; Pub. L. 101-502, Sec. 5(f), Nov. 3, 1990, 104 Stat. 1287; Pub. L. 102-

168, title II, Sec. 201(d)(3), Nov. 26, 1991, 105 Stat. 1103; Pub. L. 102-572, title IX, Sec. 902(b)(1), Oct. 29, 1992, 106 Stat. 4516.)

-COD-

CODIFICATION

In subsec. (a), "October 1, 1988," and "October 1, 1988" substituted for "the effective date of this part".

-MISC1-

AMENDMENTS

1992 - Subsecs. (a), (b). Pub. L. 102-572 substituted "United States Court of Federal Claims" for "United States Claims Court" wherever appearing.

1991 - Subsec. (b). Pub. L. 102-168 substituted "Continuance or withdrawal of petition" for "Withdrawal of petition" in heading, redesignated introductory provisions of par. (1) as introductory provisions of subsec. (b) and substituted "a notice in writing choosing to continue or to withdraw the petition" for "a notice in writing withdrawing the petition", redesignated subpars. (A) and (B) of former par. (1) as pars. (1) and (2), respectively, and realigned margins, struck out at end of former par. (1) "If such a notice is not filed before the expiration of such 30 days, the petition with respect to which the notice was to be filed shall be considered withdrawn under this paragraph.", and struck out par. (2) which read as follows: "If a special master or the court does not enter a decision or make a judgment on a petition filed under section 300aa-11 of this title within 30 days of the provision of the notice in accordance with section 300aa-12(g) of this title, the special master or court shall no longer have jurisdiction over such petition and such petition shall be considered as withdrawn under paragraph (1)."

1990 - Subsec. (a). Pub. L. 101-502, Sec. 5(f)(1), in closing provisions, inserted after second sentence "If a person elects to receive compensation under a judgment of the court in an action for a vaccine-related injury or death associated with the administration of a vaccine before October 1, 1988, or is deemed to have accepted the judgment of the court in such an action, such person may not bring or maintain a civil action for damages against a vaccine administrator or manufacturer for the vaccine-related injury or death for which the judgment was entered." and inserted "for vaccine-related injuries or deaths associated with the administration of a vaccine after October 1, 1988" after "actions" in last sentence.

Subsec. (b). Pub. L. 101-502, Sec. 5(f)(2), amended subsec. (b) generally. Prior to amendment, subsec. (b) read as follows: "If the United States Claims Court fails to enter a judgment under section 300aa-12 of this title on a petition filed under section 300aa-11 of this title within 420 days (excluding any period of suspension under section 300aa-12(d) of this title and excluding any days the petition is before a special master as a result of a remand under section 300aa-12(e)(2)(C) of this title) after the date on which the petition was filed, the petitioner may submit to the court a notice in writing withdrawing the petition. An election shall be filed under this subsection not later than 90 days after the date of the entry of the Claims Court's judgment or the appellate court's mandate with respect to which the election is to be made. A person who has submitted a notice under this subsection may, notwithstanding section 300aa-11(a)(2) of this title, thereafter maintain a civil action for damages in a State or Federal court without regard to this subpart and consistent with otherwise applicable law."

1989 - Subsec. (a). Pub. L. 101-239, Sec. 6601(n)(1)(A), amended introductory provisions generally. Prior to amendment, introductory provisions read as follows: "After the judgment of the United States Claims Court under section 300aa-11 of this title on a petition filed for compensation under the Program for a vaccine-related injury or death has become final, the person who filed the petition shall file with the court - ".

Pub. L. 101-239, Sec. 6601(n)(1)(B), amended last sentence generally. Prior to amendment, last sentence read as follows: "If a person elects to receive compensation under a judgment of the court or is deemed to have accepted the judgment of the court, such person may not bring or maintain a civil action for damages against a vaccine manufacturer for the vaccine-related injury or death for which the judgment was entered."

Subsec. (b). Pub. L. 101-239, Sec. 6601(n)(2), substituted "within 420 days (excluding any period of suspension under section 300aa-12(d) of this title and excluding any days the petition is before a special master as a result of a remand under section 300aa-12(e)(2)(C) of this title)" for "within 365 days" in first sentence and amended second sentence generally. Prior to amendment, second sentence read as follows: "Such a notice shall be filed not later than 90 days after the expiration of such 365-day period."

1988 - Subsec. (a). Pub. L. 100-360 added Pub. L. 100-203, Sec. 4308(c), see 1987 Amendment note below.

1987 - Subsec. (a). Pub. L. 100-203, Sec. 4308(c), as added by Pub. L. 100-360, substituted "the court's final judgment" for "the entry of the court's judgment" in concluding provisions.

Pub. L. 100-203, Sec. 4307(8), substituted "the United States Claims Court" for "a district court of the United States" and "the court" for "a court" in three places.

Subsecs. (b), (c). Pub. L. 100-203, Sec. 4304(c), added subsec. (b) and redesignated former subsec. (b) as (c).

EFFECTIVE DATE OF 1992 AMENDMENT

Amendment by Pub. L. 102-572 effective Oct. 29, 1992, see section 911 of Pub. L. 102-572, set out as a note under section 171 of Title 28, Judiciary and Judicial Procedure.

EFFECTIVE DATE OF 1991 AMENDMENT

Amendment by Pub. L. 102-168 effective as in effect on and after Oct. 1, 1988, see section 201(i)(2) of Pub. L. 102-168, set out as a note under section 300aa-11 of this title.

EFFECTIVE DATE OF 1990 AMENDMENT

Amendment by section 5(f)(1) of Pub. L. 101-502 effective Nov. 14, 1986, and amendment by section 5(f)(2) of Pub. L. 101-502 effective Sept. 30, 1990, see section 5(h) of Pub. L. 101-502, set out as a note under section 300aa-11 of this title.

EFFECTIVE DATE OF 1989 AMENDMENT

For applicability of amendments by Pub. L. 101-239 to petitions filed after Dec. 19, 1989, petitions currently pending in which the evidentiary record is closed, and petitions currently pending in which the evidentiary record is not closed, with provision for an immediate suspension for 30 days of all pending cases, except that such suspension be excluded in determining the 420-day period prescribed in subsec. (b) of this section, see section 6601(s)(1) of Pub. L. 101-239, set out as a note under section 300aa-10 of this title.

EFFECTIVE DATE OF 1988 AMENDMENT

Except as specifically provided in section 411 of Pub. L. 100-360, amendment by Pub. L. 100-360, as it relates to a provision in the Omnibus Budget Reconciliation Act of 1987, Pub. L. 100-203, effective as if included in the enactment of that provision in Pub. L. 100-203, see section 411(a) of Pub. L. 100-360, set out as a Reference to OBRA; Effective Date note under section 106 of Title 1, General Provisions.

EFFECTIVE DATE

Subpart effective Oct. 1, 1988, see section 323 of Pub. L. 99-660, set out as a note under section 300aa-1 of this title.

-End-

-CITE-
    42 USC Sec. 300aa-22
01/08/2008

-EXPCITE-
    TITLE 42 - THE PUBLIC HEALTH AND WELFARE
    CHAPTER 6A - PUBLIC HEALTH SERVICE
    SUBCHAPTER XIX - VACCINES
    Part 2 - National Vaccine Injury Compensation Program
    subpart b - additional remedies

-HEAD-
    Sec. 300aa-22. Standards of responsibility

-STATUTE-
    (a) General rule
    Except as provided in subsections (b), (c), and (e) of this section State law shall apply to a civil action brought for damages for a vaccine-related injury or death.
    (b) Unavoidable adverse side effects; warnings
    (1) No vaccine manufacturer shall be liable in a civil action for damages arising from a vaccine-related injury or death associated with the administration of a vaccine after October 1, 1988, if the injury or death resulted from side effects that were unavoidable even though the vaccine was properly prepared and was accompanied by proper directions and warnings.
    (2) For purposes of paragraph (1), a vaccine shall be presumed to be accompanied by proper directions and warnings if the vaccine manufacturer shows that it complied in all material respects with all requirements under the Federal Food, Drug, and Cosmetic Act [21

U.S.C. 301 et seq.] and section 262 of this title (including
regulations issued under such provisions) applicable to the vaccine
and related to vaccine-related injury or death for which the civil
action was brought unless the plaintiff shows -

    (A) that the manufacturer engaged in the conduct set forth in
subparagraph (A) or (B) of section 300aa-23(d)(2) of this title,
or

    (B) by clear and convincing evidence that the manufacturer
failed to exercise due care notwithstanding its compliance with
such Act and section (and regulations issued under such
provisions).

(c) Direct warnings

  No vaccine manufacturer shall be liable in a civil action for
damages arising from a vaccine-related injury or death associated
with the administration of a vaccine after October 1, 1988, solely
due to the manufacturer's failure to provide direct warnings to the
injured party (or the injured party's legal representative) of the
potential dangers resulting from the administration of the vaccine
manufactured by the manufacturer.

(d) Construction

  The standards of responsibility prescribed by this section are
not to be construed as authorizing a person who brought a civil
action for damages against a vaccine manufacturer for a vaccine-
related injury or death in which damages were denied or which was
dismissed with prejudice to bring a new civil action against such
manufacturer for such injury or death.

(e) Preemption

  No State may establish or enforce a law which prohibits an
individual from bringing a civil action against a vaccine
manufacturer for damages for a vaccine-related injury or death if
such civil action is not barred by this part.

-SOURCE-

(July 1, 1944, ch. 373, title XXI, Sec. 2122, as added Pub. L. 99-
660, title III, Sec. 311(a), Nov. 14, 1986, 100 Stat. 3773;
amended Pub. L. 100-203, title IV, Sec. 4302(b)(1), Dec. 22, 1987,
101 Stat. 1330-221.)

-REFTEXT-

REFERENCES IN TEXT

  The Federal Food, Drug, and Cosmetic Act, referred to in subsec.
(b)(2), is act June 25, 1938, ch. 675, 52 Stat. 1040, as amended,
which is classified generally to chapter 9 (Sec. 301 et seq.) of
Title 21, Food and Drugs. For complete classification of this Act
to the Code, see Tables.

-COD-

CODIFICATION

  In subsecs. (b)(1), (c), "October 1, 1988" was substituted for
"the effective date of this subpart" on authority of section 323 of
Pub. L. 99-660, as amended, set out as an Effective Date note under
section 300aa-1 of this title.

-MISC1-

AMENDMENTS

  1987 - Subsecs. (b)(1), (c). Pub. L. 100-203 substituted

"effective date of this subpart" for "effective date of this part".

-End-

-CITE-
    42 USC Sec. 300aa-23
01/08/2008

-EXPCITE-
    TITLE 42 - THE PUBLIC HEALTH AND WELFARE
    CHAPTER 6A - PUBLIC HEALTH SERVICE
    SUBCHAPTER XIX - VACCINES
    Part 2 - National Vaccine Injury Compensation Program
    subpart b - additional remedies

-HEAD-
    Sec. 300aa-23. Trial

-STATUTE-
    (a) General rule
    A civil action against a vaccine manufacturer for damages for a
vaccine-related injury or death associated with the administration
of a vaccine after October 1, 1988, which is not barred by section
300aa-11(a)(2) of this title shall be tried in three stages.
    (b) Liability
    The first stage of such a civil action shall be held to determine
if a vaccine manufacturer is liable under section 300aa-22 of this
title.
    (c) General damages
    The second stage of such a civil action shall be held to
determine the amount of damages (other than punitive damages) a
vaccine manufacturer found to be liable under section 300aa-22 of
this title shall be required to pay.
    (d) Punitive damages
    (1) If sought by the plaintiff, the third stage of such an action
shall be held to determine the amount of punitive damages a vaccine
manufacturer found to be liable under section 300aa-22 of this
title shall be required to pay.
    (2) If in such an action the manufacturer shows that it complied,
in all material respects, with all requirements under the Federal
Food, Drug, and Cosmetic Act [21 U.S.C. 301 et seq.] and this
chapter applicable to the vaccine and related to the vaccine injury
or death with respect to which the action was brought, the
manufacturer shall not be held liable for punitive damages unless
the manufacturer engaged in -
        (A) fraud or intentional and wrongful withholding of
    information from the Secretary during any phase of a proceeding
    for approval of the vaccine under section 262 of this title,
        (B) intentional and wrongful withholding of information
    relating to the safety or efficacy of the vaccine after its
    approval, or
        (C) other criminal or illegal activity relating to the safety
    and effectiveness of vaccines,

which activity related to the vaccine-related injury or death for

which the civil action was brought.
(e) Evidence
   In any stage of a civil action, the Vaccine Injury Table, any
finding of fact or conclusion of law of the United States Court of
Federal Claims or a special master in a proceeding on a petition
filed under section 300aa-11 of this title and the final judgment
of the United States Court of Federal Claims and subsequent
appellate review on such a petition shall not be admissible.

-SOURCE-

   (July 1, 1944, ch. 373, title XXI, Sec. 2114, as added Pub. L. 99-
660, title III, Sec. 311(a), Nov. 14, 1986, 100 Stat. 3774;
amended Pub. L. 100-203, title IV, Secs. 4302(b)(1), 4307(9), Dec.
22, 1987, 101 Stat. 1330-221, 1330-225; Pub. L. 101-239, title VI,
Sec. 6601(o), Dec. 19, 1989, 103 Stat. 2292; Pub. L. 102-572, title
IX, Sec. 902(b)(1), Oct. 29, 1992, 106 Stat. 4516.)

-REFTEXT-

REFERENCES IN TEXT
   The Federal Food, Drug, and Cosmetic Act, referred to in subsec.
(d)(2), is act June 25, 1938, ch. 675, 52 Stat. 1040, as amended,
which is classified generally to chapter 9 (Sec. 301 et seq.) of
Title 21, Food and Drugs. For complete classification of this Act
to the Code, see Tables.

-COD-

CODIFICATION
   In subsec. (a), "October 1, 1988" substituted for "the effective
date of this subpart" on authority of section 323 of Pub. L. 99-
660, as amended, set out as an Effective Date note under section
300aa-1 of this title.

-MISC1-

AMENDMENTS
   1992 - Subsec. (e). Pub. L. 102-572 substituted "United States
Court of Federal Claims" for "United States Claims Court" in two
places.
   1989 - Subsec. (e). Pub. L. 101-239 substituted "finding of fact
or conclusion of law" for "finding", "special master" for "master
appointed by such court", and directed substitution of "the United
States Claims Court and subsequent appellate review" for "a
district court of the United States" which was executed by
inserting "and subsequent appellate review" after "the United
States Claims Court" the second place it appeared to reflect the
probable intent of Congress and the amendment by Pub. L. 100-203,
Sec. 4307(d), see 1987 Amendment note below.
   1987 - Subsec. (a). Pub. L. 100-203, Sec. 4302(b)(1), substituted
"effective date of this subpart" for "effective date of this part".
   Subsec. (e). Pub. L. 100-203, Sec. 4307(9), substituted "the
United States Claims Court" for "a district court of the United
States" in two places.

EFFECTIVE DATE OF 1992 AMENDMENT
   Amendment by Pub. L. 102-572 effective Oct. 29, 1992, see section
911 of Pub. L. 102-572, set out as a note under section 171 of
Title 28, Judiciary and Judicial Procedure.

EFFECTIVE DATE OF 1989 AMENDMENT
For applicability of amendments by Pub. L. 101-239 to petitions
filed after Dec. 19, 1989, petitions currently pending in which the
evidentiary record is closed, and petitions currently pending in
which the evidentiary record is not closed, with provision for an
immediate suspension for 30 days of all pending cases, see section
6601(s)(1) of Pub. L. 101-239, set out as a note under section
300aa-10 of this title.

-End-

-CITE-
    42 USC subpart c - assuring a safer childhood vaccination
        program in united states   01/08/2008

-EXPCITE-
    TITLE 42 - THE PUBLIC HEALTH AND WELFARE
    CHAPTER 6A - PUBLIC HEALTH SERVICE
    SUBCHAPTER XIX - VACCINES
    Part 2 - National Vaccine Injury Compensation Program
    subpart c - assuring a safer childhood vaccination program in
united states

-HEAD-
     SUBPART C - ASSURING A SAFER CHILDHOOD VACCINATION PROGRAM IN
                         UNITED STATES

-End-

-CITE-
    42 USC Sec. 300aa-25
01/08/2008

-EXPCITE-
    TITLE 42 - THE PUBLIC HEALTH AND WELFARE
    CHAPTER 6A - PUBLIC HEALTH SERVICE
    SUBCHAPTER XIX - VACCINES
    Part 2 - National Vaccine Injury Compensation Program
    subpart c - assuring a safer childhood vaccination program in
united states

-HEAD-
    Sec. 300aa-25. Recording and reporting of information

-STATUTE-
    (a) General rule
    Each health care provider who administers a vaccine set forth in
the Vaccine Injury Table to any person shall record, or ensure that
there is recorded, in such person's permanent medical record (or in
a permanent office log or file to which a legal representative
shall have access upon request) with respect to each such vaccine -

(1) the date of administration of the vaccine,

(2) the vaccine manufacturer and lot number of the vaccine,

(3) the name and address and, if appropriate, the title of the health care provider administering the vaccine, and

(4) any other identifying information on the vaccine required pursuant to regulations promulgated by the Secretary.

(b) Reporting

(1) Each health care provider and vaccine manufacturer shall report to the Secretary -

(A) the occurrence of any event set forth in the Vaccine Injury Table, including the events set forth in section 300aa-14(b) of this title which occur within 7 days of the administration of any vaccine set forth in the Table or within such longer period as is specified in the Table or section,

(B) the occurrence of any contraindicating reaction to a vaccine which is specified in the manufacturer's package insert, and

(C) such other matters as the Secretary may by regulation require.

Reports of the matters referred to in subparagraphs (A) and (B) shall be made beginning 90 days after December 22, 1987. The Secretary shall publish in the Federal Register as soon as practicable after such date a notice of the reporting requirement.

(2) A report under paragraph (1) respecting a vaccine shall include the time periods after the administration of such vaccine within which vaccine-related illnesses, disabilities, injuries, or conditions, the symptoms and manifestations of such illnesses, disabilities, injuries, or conditions, or deaths occur, and the manufacturer and lot number of the vaccine.

(3) The Secretary shall issue the regulations referred to in paragraph (1)(C) within 100 days of December 22, 1987.

(c) Release of information

(1) Information which is in the possession of the Federal Government and State and local governments under this section and which may identify an individual shall not be made available under section 552 of title 5, or otherwise, to any person except -

(A) the person who received the vaccine, or

(B) the legal representative of such person.

(2) For purposes of paragraph (1), the term "information which may identify an individual" shall be limited to the name, street address, and telephone number of the person who received the vaccine and of that person's legal representative and the medical records of such person relating to the administration of the vaccine, and shall not include the locality and State of vaccine administration, the name of the health care provider who administered the vaccine, the date of the vaccination, or information concerning any reported illness, disability, injury, or condition resulting from the administration of the vaccine, any symptom or manifestation of such illness, disability, injury, or condition, or death resulting from the administration of the vaccine.

(3) Except as provided in paragraph (1), all information reported under this section shall be available to the public.

-SOURCE-
    (July 1, 1944, ch. 373, title XXI, Sec. 2125, as added Pub. L. 99-
    660, title III, Sec. 311(a), Nov. 14, 1986, 100 Stat. 3774;
    amended Pub. L. 100-203, title IV, Sec. 4302(b)(1), Dec. 22, 1987,
    101 Stat. 1330-221.)

-COD-
                        CODIFICATION
    In subsec. (b)(1), (3), "December 22, 1987" was substituted for
"the effective date of this subpart" on authority of section 323 of
Pub. L. 99-660, as amended, set out as an Effective Date note under
section 300aa-1 of this title.

-MISC1-
                        AMENDMENTS
    1987 - Subsec. (b)(1), (3). Pub. L. 100-203 substituted
"effective date of this subpart" for "effective date of this part".

                        EFFECTIVE DATE
    Subpart effective Dec. 22, 1987, see section 323 of Pub. L. 99-
660, set out as a note under section 300aa-1 of this title.

-End-

-CITE-
    42 USC Sec. 300aa-26
01/08/2008

-EXPCITE-
    TITLE 42 - THE PUBLIC HEALTH AND WELFARE
    CHAPTER 6A - PUBLIC HEALTH SERVICE
    SUBCHAPTER XIX - VACCINES
    Part 2 - National Vaccine Injury Compensation Program
    subpart c - assuring a safer childhood vaccination program in
united states

-HEAD-
    Sec. 300aa-26. Vaccine information

-STATUTE-
    (a) General rule
    Not later than 1 year after December 22, 1987, the Secretary
shall develop and disseminate vaccine information materials for
distribution by health care providers to the legal representatives
of any child or to any other individual receiving a vaccine set
forth in the Vaccine Injury Table. Such materials shall be
published in the Federal Register and may be revised.
    (b) Development and revision of materials
    Such materials shall be developed or revised -
        (1) after notice to the public and 60 days of comment thereon,
    and
        (2) in consultation with the Advisory Commission on Childhood
    Vaccines, appropriate health care providers and parent

organizations, the Centers for Disease Control and Prevention, and the Food and Drug Administration.

(c) Information requirements

The information in such materials shall be based on available data and information, shall be presented in understandable terms and shall include -

(1) a concise description of the benefits of the vaccine,

(2) a concise description of the risks associated with the vaccine,

(3) a statement of the availability of the National Vaccine Injury Compensation Program, and

(4) such other relevant information as may be determined by the Secretary.

(d) Health care provider duties

On and after a date determined by the Secretary which is -

(1) after the Secretary develops the information materials required by subsection (a) of this section, and

(2) not later than 6 months after the date such materials are published in the Federal Register,

each health care provider who administers a vaccine set forth in the Vaccine Injury Table shall provide to the legal representatives of any child or to any other individual to whom such provider intends to administer such vaccine a copy of the information materials developed pursuant to subsection (a) of this section, supplemented with visual presentations or oral explanations, in appropriate cases. Such materials shall be provided prior to the administration of such vaccine.

-SOURCE-

(July 1, 1944, ch. 373, title XXI, Sec. 2126, as added Pub. L. 99-660, title III, Sec. 311(a), Nov. 14, 1986, 100 Stat. 3775; amended Pub. L. 100-203, title IV, Sec. 4302(b)(1), Dec. 22, 1987, 101 Stat. 1330-221; Pub. L. 101-239, title VI, Sec. 6601(p), Dec. 19, 1989, 103 Stat. 2292; Pub. L. 102-531, title III, Sec. 312(d)(15), Oct. 27, 1992, 106 Stat. 3505; Pub. L. 103-183, title VII, Sec. 700, Dec. 14, 1993, 107 Stat. 2242.)

-COD-

CODIFICATION

In subsec. (a), "December 22, 1987" substituted for "the effective date of this subpart" on authority of section 323 of Pub. L. 99-660, as amended, set out as an Effective Date note under section 300aa-1 of this title.

-MISC1-

AMENDMENTS

1993 - Subsec. (a). Pub. L. 103-183, Sec. 708(c), inserted "or to any other individual" after "to the legal representatives of any child".

Subsec. (b). Pub. L. 103-183, Sec. 708(a), struck out "by rule" after "revised" in introductory provisions and substituted "and 60" for ", opportunity for a public hearing, and 90" in par. (1).

Subsec. (c). Pub. L. 103-183, Sec. 708(b), inserted in introductory provisions "shall be based on available data and information," after "such materials", added pars. (1) to (4), and struck out former pars. (1) to (10) which read as follows:

"(1) the frequency, severity, and potential long-term effects of the disease to be prevented by the vaccine,

"(2) the symptoms or reactions to the vaccine which, if they occur, should be brought to the immediate attention of the health care provider,

"(3) precautionary measures legal representatives should take to reduce the risk of any major adverse reactions to the vaccine that may occur,

"(4) early warning signs or symptoms to which legal representatives should be alert as possible precursors to such major adverse reactions,

"(5) a description of the manner in which legal representatives should monitor such major adverse reactions, including a form on which reactions can be recorded to assist legal representatives in reporting information to appropriate authorities,

"(6) a specification of when, how, and to whom legal representatives should report any major adverse reaction,

"(7) the contraindications to (and bases for delay of) the administration of the vaccine,

"(8) an identification of the groups, categories, or characteristics of potential recipients of the vaccine who may be at significantly higher risk of major adverse reaction to the vaccine than the general population,

"(9) a summary of -

"(A) relevant Federal recommendations concerning a complete schedule of childhood immunizations, and

"(B) the availability of the Program, and

"(10) such other relevant information as may be determined by the Secretary."

Subsec. (d). Pub. L. 103-183, Sec. 708(c), (d), in concluding provisions, inserted "or to any other individual" after "to the legal representatives of any child", substituted "supplemented with visual presentations or oral explanations, in appropriate cases" for "or other written information which meets the requirements of this section", and struck out "or other information" after "Such materials".

1992 - Subsec. (b)(2). Pub. L. 102-531 substituted "Centers for Disease Control and Prevention" for "Centers for Disease Control".

1989 - Subsec. (c)(9). Pub. L. 101-239 amended par. (9) generally. Prior to amendment, par. (9) read as follows: "a summary of relevant State and Federal laws concerning the vaccine, including information on -

"(A) the number of vaccinations required for school attendance and the schedule recommended for such vaccinations, and

"(B) the availability of the Program, and".

1987 - Subsec. (a). Pub. L. 100-203 substituted "effective date of this subpart" for "effective date of this part".

EFFECTIVE DATE OF 1989 AMENDMENT

For applicability of amendments by Pub. L. 101-239 to petitions filed after Dec. 19, 1989, petitions currently pending in which the evidentiary record is closed, and petitions currently pending in which the evidentiary record is not closed, with provision for an immediate suspension for 30 days of all pending cases, see section 6601(s)(1) of Pub. L. 101-239, set out as a note under section 300aa-10 of this title.

-End-

-CITE-
    42 USC Sec. 300aa-27
01/08/2008

-EXPCITE-
    TITLE 42 - THE PUBLIC HEALTH AND WELFARE
    CHAPTER 6A - PUBLIC HEALTH SERVICE
    SUBCHAPTER XIX - VACCINES
    Part 2 - National Vaccine Injury Compensation Program
    subpart c - assuring a safer childhood vaccination program in
general

-HEAD-
    Sec. 300aa-27. Mandate for safer childhood vaccines

-STATUTE-
    (a) General rule
    In the administration of this part and other pertinent laws under
the jurisdiction of the Secretary, the Secretary shall -
        (1) promote the development of childhood vaccines that result
    in fewer and less serious adverse reactions than those vaccines
    on the market on December 22, 1987, and promote the refinement of
    such vaccines, and
        (2) make or assure improvements in, and otherwise use the
    authorities of the Secretary with respect to, the licensing,
    manufacturing, processing, testing, labeling, warning, use
    instructions, distribution, storage, administration, field
    surveillance, adverse reaction reporting, and recall of
    reactogenic lots or batches, of vaccines, and research on
    vaccines, in order to reduce the risks of adverse reactions to
    vaccines.
    (b) Task force
        (1) The Secretary shall establish a task force on safer childhood
    vaccines which shall consist of the Director of the National
    Institutes of Health, the Commissioner of the Food and Drug
    Administration, and the Director of the Centers for Disease
    Control.
        (2) The Director of the National Institutes of Health shall serve
    as chairman of the task force.
        (3) In consultation with the Advisory Commission on Childhood
    Vaccines, the task force shall prepare recommendations to the
    Secretary concerning implementation of the requirements of
    subsection (a) of this section.
    (c) Report
    Within 2 years after December 22, 1987, and periodically
thereafter, the Secretary shall prepare and transmit to the
Committee on Energy and Commerce of the House of Representatives
and the Committee on Labor and Human Resources of the Senate a
report describing the actions taken pursuant to subsection (a) of
this section during the preceding 2-year period.

-SOURCE-
   (July 1, 1944, ch. 373, title XXI, Sec. 2127, as added Pub. L. 99-
   660, title III, Sec. 311(a), Nov. 14, 1986, 100 Stat. 3777;
   amended Pub. L. 100-203, title IV, Sec. 4302(b)(1), Dec. 22, 1987,
   101 Stat. 1330-221; Pub. L. 101-239, title VI, Sec. 6601(q), Dec.
   19, 1989, 103 Stat. 2292.)

-COD-
                    CODIFICATION
   In subsecs. (a)(1), (c), "December 22, 1987" substituted for "the
effective date of this subpart" on authority of section 323 of Pub.
L. 99-660, as amended, set out as an Effective Date note under
section 300aa-1 of this title.

-MISC1-
                     AMENDMENTS
   1989 - Subsecs. (b), (c). Pub. L. 101-239 added subsec. (b) and
redesignated former subsec. (b) as (c).
   1987 - Subsecs. (a)(1), (b). Pub. L. 100-203 substituted
"effective date of this subpart" for "effective date of this part".

-CHANGE-
                   CHANGE OF NAME
   Committee on Labor and Human Resources of Senate changed to
Committee on Health, Education, Labor, and Pensions of Senate by
Senate Resolution No. 20, One Hundred Sixth Congress, Jan. 19,
1999.
   Committee on Energy and Commerce of House of Representatives
treated as referring to Committee on Commerce of House of
Representatives by section 1(a) of Pub. L. 104-14, set out as a
note preceding section 21 of Title 2, The Congress. Committee on
Commerce of House of Representatives changed to Committee on Energy
and Commerce of House of Representatives, and jurisdiction over
matters relating to securities and exchanges and insurance
generally transferred to Committee on Financial Services of House
of Representatives by House Resolution No. 5, One Hundred Seventh
Congress, Jan. 3, 2001.
   Centers for Disease Control changed to Centers for Disease
Control and Prevention by Pub. L. 102-531, title III, Sec. 312,
Oct. 27, 1992, 106 Stat. 3504.

-MISC2-
            EFFECTIVE DATE OF 1989 AMENDMENT
   For applicability of amendments by Pub. L. 101-239 to petitions
filed after Dec. 19, 1989, petitions currently pending in which the
evidentiary record is closed, and petitions currently pending in
which the evidentiary record is not closed, with provision for an
immediate suspension for 30 days of all pending cases, see section
6601(s)(1) of Pub. L. 101-239, set out as a note under section
300aa-10 of this title.

-End-

-CITE-
    42 USC Sec. 300aa-28
01/08/2008

-EXPCITE-
    TITLE 42 - THE PUBLIC HEALTH AND WELFARE
    CHAPTER 6A - PUBLIC HEALTH SERVICE
    SUBCHAPTER XIX - VACCINES
    Part 2 - National Vaccine Injury Compensation Program
    subpart c - assuring a safer childhood vaccination program in
united states

-HEAD-
    Sec. 300aa-28. Manufacturer recordkeeping and reporting

-STATUTE-
    (a) General rule
    Each vaccine manufacturer of a vaccine set forth in the Vaccine
Injury Table or any other vaccine the administration of which is
mandated by the law or regulations of any State, shall, with
respect to each batch, lot, or other quantity manufactured or
licensed after December 22, 1987 -
        (1) prepare and maintain records documenting the history of the
    manufacturing, processing, testing, repooling, and reworking of
    each batch, lot, or other quantity of such vaccine, including the
    identification of any significant problems encountered in the
    production, testing, or handling of such batch, lot, or other
    quantity,
        (2) if a safety test on such batch, lot, or other quantity
    indicates a potential imminent or substantial public health
    hazard is presented, report to the Secretary within 24 hours of
    such safety test which the manufacturer (or manufacturer's
    representative) conducted, including the date of the test, the
    type of vaccine tested, the identity of the batch, lot, or other
    quantity tested, whether the batch, lot, or other quantity tested
    is the product of repooling or reworking of previous batches,
    lots, or other quantities (and, if so, the identity of the
    previous batches, lots, or other quantities which were repooled
    or reworked), the complete test results, and the name and address
    of the person responsible for conducting the test,
        (3) include with each such report a certification signed by a
    responsible corporate official that such report is true and
    complete, and
        (4) prepare, maintain, and upon request submit to the Secretary
    product distribution records for each such vaccine by batch, lot,
    or other quantity number.
    (b) Sanction
    Any vaccine manufacturer who intentionally destroys, alters,
falsifies, or conceals any record or report required under
paragraph (1) or (2) of subsection (a) of this section shall -
        (1) be subject to a civil penalty of up to $100,000 per
    occurrence, or
        (2) be fined $50,000 or imprisoned for not more than 1 year, or
    both.

    Such penalty shall apply to the person who intentionally destroyed,

altered, falsified, or concealed such record or report, to the
person who directed that such record or report be destroyed,
altered, falsified, or concealed, and to the vaccine manufacturer
for which such person is an agent, employee, or representative.
Each act of destruction, alteration, falsification, or concealment
shall be treated as a separate occurrence.

-SOURCE-
   (July 1, 1944, ch. 373, title XXI, Sec. 2128, as added Pub. L. 99-
   660, title III, Sec. 311(a), Nov. 14, 1986, 100 Stat. 3777;
   amended Pub. L. 100-203, title IV, Sec. 4302(b)(1), Dec. 22, 1987,
   101 Stat. 1330-221.)

-COD-
                         CODIFICATION
      In subsec. (a), "December 22, 1987" substituted for "the
   effective date of this subpart" on authority of section 323 of Pub.
   L. 99-660, as amended, set out as an Effective Date note under
   section 300aa-1 of this title.

-MISC1-
                         AMENDMENTS
      1987 - Subsec. (a). Pub. L. 100-203 substituted "effective date
   of this subpart" for "effective date of this part".

-End-

-CITE-
   42 USC subpart d - general provisions
01/08/2008

-EXPCITE-
   TITLE 42 - THE PUBLIC HEALTH AND WELFARE
   CHAPTER 6A - PUBLIC HEALTH SERVICE
   SUBCHAPTER XIX - VACCINES
   Part 2 - National Vaccine Injury Compensation Program
   subpart d - general provisions

-HEAD-
                   SUBPART D - GENERAL PROVISIONS

-End-

-CITE-
   42 USC Sec. 300aa-31
01/08/2008

-EXPCITE-
   TITLE 42 - THE PUBLIC HEALTH AND WELFARE
   CHAPTER 6A - PUBLIC HEALTH SERVICE
   SUBCHAPTER XIX - VACCINES
   Part 2 - National Vaccine Injury Compensation Program
   subpart d - general provisions

-HEAD-
    Sec. 300aa-31. Citizen's actions

-STATUTE-
    (a) General rule
    Except as provided in subsection (b) of this section, any person
    may commence in a district court of the United States a civil
    action on such person's own behalf against the Secretary where
    there is alleged a failure of the Secretary to perform any act or
    duty under this part.
    (b) Notice
    No action may be commenced under subsection (a) of this section
    before the date which is 60 days after the person bringing the
    action has given written notice of intent to commence such action
    to the Secretary.
    (c) Costs of litigation
    The court, in issuing any final order in any action under this
    section, may award costs of litigation (including reasonable
    attorney and expert witness fees) to any plaintiff who
    substantially prevails on one or more significant issues in the
    action.

-SOURCE-
    (July 1, 1944, ch. 373, title XXI, Sec. 2131, as added Pub. L. 99-
    660, title III, Sec. 311(a), Nov. 14, 1986, 100 Stat. 3778;
    amended Pub. L. 100-203, title IV, Sec. 4305, Dec. 22, 1987, 101
    Stat. 1330-224.)

-MISC1-
                              AMENDMENTS
    1987 - Subsec. (c). Pub. L. 100-203, which directed that subsec.
    (c) be amended by substituting "to any plaintiff who substantially
    prevails on one or more significant issues in the action" for "to
    any party, whenever the court determines that such award is
    appropriate", was executed by making the substitution for "to any
    party, whenever the court determines such award is appropriate", to
    reflect the probable intent of Congress.

                            EFFECTIVE DATE
    Subpart effective Dec. 22, 1987, see section 323 of Pub. L. 99-
    660, set out as a note under section 300aa-1 of this title.

-End-

-CITE-
    42 USC Sec. 300aa-32
01/08/2008

-EXPCITE-
    TITLE 42 - THE PUBLIC HEALTH AND WELFARE
    CHAPTER 6A - PUBLIC HEALTH SERVICE
    SUBCHAPTER XIX - VACCINES
    Part 2 - National Vaccine Injury Compensation Program

subpart d - general provisions

-HEAD-
    Sec. 300aa-32. Judicial review

-STATUTE-
    A petition for review of a regulation under this part may be
filed in a court of appeals of the United States within 60 days
from the date of the promulgation of the regulation or after such
date if such petition is based solely on grounds arising after such
60th day.

-SOURCE-
    (July 1, 1944, ch. 373, title XXI, Sec. 2132, as added Pub. L. 99-
660, title III, Sec. 311(a), Nov. 14, 1986, 100 Stat. 3778.)

-End-

-CITE-
    42 USC Sec. 300aa-33
01/08/2008

-EXPCITE-
    TITLE 42 - THE PUBLIC HEALTH AND WELFARE
    CHAPTER 6A - PUBLIC HEALTH SERVICE
    SUBCHAPTER XIX - VACCINES
    Part 2 - National Vaccine Injury Compensation Program
    subpart d - general provisions

-HEAD-
    Sec. 300aa-33. Definitions

-STATUTE-
    For purposes of this part:
      (1) The term "health care provider" means any licensed health
    care professional, organization, or institution, whether public
    or private (including Federal, State, and local departments,
    agencies, and instrumentalities) under whose authority a vaccine
    set forth in the Vaccine Injury Table is administered.
      (2) The term "legal representative" means a parent or an
    individual who qualifies as a legal guardian under State law.
      (3) The term "manufacturer" means any corporation,
    organization, or institution, whether public or private
    (including Federal, State, and local departments, agencies, and
    instrumentalities), which manufactures, imports, processes, or
    distributes under its label any vaccine set forth in the Vaccine
    Injury Table, except that, for purposes of section 300aa-28 of
    this title, such term shall include the manufacturer of any other
    vaccine covered by that section. The term "manufacture" means to
    manufacture, import, process, or distribute a vaccine.
      (4) The term "significant aggravation" means any change for the
    worse in a preexisting condition which results in markedly
    greater disability, pain, or illness accompanied by substantial
    deterioration of health.
      (5) The term "vaccine-related injury or death" means an

illness, injury, condition, or death associated with one or more
of the vaccines set forth in the Vaccine Injury Table, except
that the term does not include an illness, injury, condition, or
death associated with an adulterant or contaminant intentionally
added to such a vaccine.

(6)(A) The term "Advisory Commission on Childhood Vaccines"
means the Commission established under section 300aa-19 of this
title.

(B) The term "Vaccine Injury Table" means the table set out in
section 300aa-14 of this title.

-SOURCE-

(July 1, 1944, ch. 373, title XXI, §2133, as added Pub. L. 99-
660, title III, Sec. 311(a), Nov. 14, 1986, 100 Stat. 2778;
amended Pub. L. 107-296, title XVII, Secs. 1714-1716, Nov. 25,
2002, 116 Stat. 2320, 2321; Pub. L. 108-7, div. L, Sec. 102(a),
Feb. 20, 2003, 117 Stat. 528.)

-MISC1-

AMENDMENTS

2003 - Pars. (3), (5), (7). Pub. L. 108-7 repealed Pub. L. 107-
296, Secs. 1714-1717, and provided that this chapter shall be
applied as if the sections repealed had never been enacted. See
2002 Amendment notes below.

2002 - Par. (3). Pub. L. 107-296, Sec. 1714, which directed
amendment of first sentence by substituting "any vaccine set forth
in the Vaccine Injury table, including any component or ingredient
of any such vaccine" for "under its label any vaccine set forth in
the Vaccine Injury Table" and of second sentence by inserting
"including any component or ingredient of any such vaccine" before
period at end, was repealed by Pub. L. 108-7.

Par. (5). Pub. L. 107-296, Sec. 1715, which directed insertion of
"For purposes of the preceding sentence, an adulterant or
contaminant shall not include any component or ingredient listed in
a vaccine's product license application or product label." at end,
was repealed by Pub. L. 108-7.

Par. (7). Pub. L. 107-296, Sec. 1716, which directed addition of
par. (7), was repealed by Pub. L. 108-7, Sec. 102(a). Par. (7) read
as follows: "The term 'vaccine' means any preparation or
suspension, including but not limited to a preparation or
suspension containing an attenuated or inactive microorganism or
subunit thereof or toxin, developed or administered to produce or
enhance the body's immune response to a disease or diseases and
includes all components and ingredients listed in the vaccines's
product license application and product label."

EFFECTIVE DATE OF 2002 AMENDMENT

Pub. L. 107-296, title XVII, Sec. 1717, Nov. 25, 2002, 116 Stat.
2321, which provided that the amendments made by sections 1714,
1715, and 1716 (amending this section) shall apply to all actions
or proceedings pending on or after Nov. 25, 2002, unless a court of
competent jurisdiction has entered judgment (regardless of whether
the time for appeal has expired) in such action or proceeding
disposing of the entire action or proceeding, was repealed by Pub.
L. 108-7, div. L, Sec. 102(a), Feb. 20, 2003, 117 Stat. 528.

CONSTRUCTION OF AMENDMENTS

Pub. L. 108-7, div. L, Sec. 102(b), (c), Feb. 20, 2003, 117 Stat.
528, provided that:

"(b) Application of the Public Health Service Act. - The Public
Health Service Act (42 U.S.C. 201 et seq.) shall be applied and
administered as if the sections repealed by subsection (a)
[repealing sections 1714 to 1717 of Pub. L. 107-296, which amended
this section and enacted provisions set out as a note under this
section] had never been enacted.

"(c) Rule of Construction. - No inference shall be drawn from the
enactment of sections 1714 through 1717 of the Homeland Security
Act of 2002 (Public Law 107-296), or from this repeal [repealing
sections 1714 to 1717 of Pub. L. 107-296], regarding the law prior
to enactment of sections 1714 through 1717 of the Homeland Security
Act of 2002 (Public Law 107-296) [Nov. 25, 2002]. Further, no
inference shall be drawn that subsection (a) or (b) affects any
change in that prior law, or that Leroy v. Secretary of Health and
Human Services, Office of Special Master, No. 02-392V (October 11,
2002), was incorrectly decided."

-End-

-CITE-
    42 USC Sec. 300aa-34
01/08/2008

-EXPCITE-
    TITLE 42 - THE PUBLIC HEALTH AND WELFARE
    CHAPTER 6A - PUBLIC HEALTH SERVICE
    SUBCHAPTER XIX - VACCINES
    Part 2 - National Vaccine Injury Compensation Program
    subpart d - general provisions

-HEAD-
    Sec. 300aa-34. Termination of program

-STATUTE-
    (a) Reviews
    The Secretary shall review the number of awards of compensation
made under the program to petitioners under section 300aa-11 of
this title for vaccine-related injuries and deaths associated with
the administration of vaccines on or after December 22, 1987, as
follows:
        (1) The Secretary shall review the number of such awards made
    in the 12-month period beginning on December 22, 1987.
        (2) At the end of each 3-month period beginning after the
    expiration of the 12-month period referred to in paragraph (1)
    the Secretary shall review the number of such awards made in the
    3-month period.
    (b) Report
        (1) If in conducting a review under subsection (a) of this
    section the Secretary determines that at the end of the period
    reviewed the total number of awards made by the end of that period
    and accepted under section 300aa-21(a) of this title exceeds the
    number of awards listed next to the period reviewed in the table in

paragraph (2) -
    (A) the Secretary shall notify the Congress of such determination, and
    (B) beginning 180 days after the receipt by Congress of a notification under paragraph (1), no petition for a vaccine-related injury or death associated with the administration of a vaccine on or after December 22, 1987, may be filed under section 300aa-11 of this title.

Section 300aa-11(a) of this title and subpart B of this part shall not apply to civil actions for damages for a vaccine-related injury or death for which a petition may not be filed because of subparagraph (B).
    (2) The table referred to in paragraph (1) is as follows:

Period reviewed:	Total number of awards by the end of the period reviewed
12 months after December 22, 1987	150
13th through the 15th month after December 22, 1987	188
16th through the 18th month after December 22, 1987	225
19th through the 21st month after December 22, 1987	263
22nd through the 24th month after December 22, 1987	300
25th through the 27th month after December 22, 1987	330
28th through the 30th month after December 22, 1987	375
31st through the 33rd month after December 22, 1987	413
34th through the 36th month after December 22, 1987	450
37th through the 39th month after December 22, 1987	488
40th through the 42nd month after December 22, 1987	525
43rd through the 45th month after December 22, 1987	563
46th through the 48th month after December 22, 1987	600.

-SOURCE-
    (July 1, 1944, ch. 373, title XXI, Sec. 2134, as added Pub. L. 100-203, title IV, Sec. 4303(f), Dec. 22, 1987, 101 Stat. 1330-222.)

-COD-

CODIFICATION

    In subsecs. (a) and (b), "December 22, 1987" substituted for "the effective date of this subpart" on authority of section 323 of Pub. L. 99-660, as amended, set out as an Effective Date note under section 300aa-1 of this title.

-End-

Source: http://uscode.house.gov/download/pls/42C6A.txt, extracted
12/08/2009

NOTES

Chapter 1. How to Use This Book

1. *Health Resources and Services Administration (HRSA) Statistics Report on the National Vaccine Injury Compensation Program,* Department of Health and Human Services (HHS), March 5, 2014.
2. Johns Hopkins Bloomberg School of Public Health, Institute for Vaccine Safety, *Vaccine Adverse Event Reporting System (VAERS)—Usefulness and Limitations*, Miles Braun, MD MPH, February 12, 2014.
3. United States Court of Federal Claims, *Vaccine Claims/Office of Special Masters, Vaccine Attorneys—Complete List*, June 1, 2014

Chapter 2. A Brief History of Vaccination

1. Roger G. Kennedy, *Hidden Cities: The Discovery and Loss of Ancient North American Civilization;* Toronto, Free Press, 1994, p 12.
2. Harvard University Library, *Contagion: Historical Views of Disease and Epidemics*, June 2014.
3. Howard Markel, M.D., "Life, Liberty and the Pursuit of Vaccines," *New York Times*, February 28, 2011
4. Byrd S. Leavell, M.D., "Thomas Jefferson and Smallpox Vaccination," *Transactions of the American Clinical and Climatological Association*, 1977, 119 – 127.
5. J.T. BIGGS J.P., *LEICESTER: SANITATION versus VACCINATION*, 1912, WHALE 2006/7, Book supplied by John Wantling.
6. Ibid.
7. Ibid.
8. Ibid.

Chapter 3. *Jacobson v. Massachusetts*

1. U.S. Supreme Court, *Jacobson v. Massachusetts*, 197 U.S. 11 (1905), No. 70, Argued December 6, 1904, Decided February 20, 1905.
2. "Toward a Twenty-First-Century *Jacobson v. Massachusetts*." *Harvard Law Review* (The Harvard Law Review Association) 121 (7): 1822. May 2008. Retrieved March 13, 2014

Chapter 4. Contaminated "Biologics" and a Horse Named Jim

1. US Food and Drug Administration, *Science and the Regulation of Biological Products: The St. Louis Tragedy and Enactment of the 1902 Biologics Control Act,* April 4, 2009.
2. Ibid.
3. Suzanne Humphries, M.D., and Roman Bystriank, Dissolving Illusions: *Disease, Vaccines, and The Forgotten History*, Create Space Independent Publishing Platform, July 27, 2013.

Chapter 5. The Cutter Crisis

1. Centers for Disease Control and Prevention *Vaccines and Immunizations: Poliomyelitis Epidemiology and Prevention of Vaccine-Preventable Diseases,* May 7, 2012.
2. Edward Shorter, Ph.D., *The Health Century*, New York, Doubleday, 1987, 67–70.
3. Ibid.
4. Arthur Allen, *Vaccine—The Controversial Story of Medicine's Greatest Lifesaver*, Norton, 2007, 209–212.
5. Ibid.

Chapter 6. The Rise of "Vaccinology"

1. Mary Holland, Louis Conte, Robert Krakow, and Lisa Colin, "Unanswered Questions from the Vaccine Injury Compensation Program: A Review of Compensated Cases of Vaccine-Induced Brain Injury," 28 *Pace Envtl. L. Rev.* 480 (2011). Available at: http://digitalcommons.pace.edu/pelr/vol28/iss2/6
2. *Conflicts of Interest in Vaccine Policy Making*, Majority Staff Report, Committee on Government Reform, US House of Representatives, June 15, 2000.

Chapter 7. DPT: Seizures and Encephalopathy

1. Harris S. Coulter and Barbara Loe Fisher, *A Shot in the Dark: Why the P in the DPT Vaccination May be Hazardous to Your Child's Health*, Harcourt Brace Jovanovich, 1985.

Chapter 8. The National Vaccine Injury Compensation Program—Reflection of Reality or Betrayal of a Promise?

1. Slide courtesy of Rebecca Estepp.
2. Arthur Allen, "Shots in the Dark," *The Washington Post Magazine*, Sunday, August 30, 1998.
3. Ibid.
4. Ibid.
5. Ibid.

Chapter 9. The Omnibus Autism Proceedings

1. Amy Pisani, Executive Director of Every Child By Two, November 12, 2013. Letter to Members of the Committee on Government Oversight and Reform, www.ecbt. org

2. J. B. Handley, "Every Child By Two: A Front Group for Wyeth," *Age of Autism*, August 1, 2008, http://www.ageofautism.com/2008/08/every-child-by.html

3. Mary Holland, Louis Conte, Robert Krakow, and Lisa Colin, *Unanswered Questions from the Vaccine Injury Compensation Program: A Review of Compensated Cases of Vaccine-Induced Brain Injury*, 28 Pace Envtl. L. Rev. 480 (2011). Available at: http:// digitalcommons.pacc.edu/pelr/vol28/iss2/6